The Role of Health Literacy in Major Healthcare Crises

Vassilios Papalois
Royal Berkshire Hospital NHS Foundation Trust, UK

Kyriaki Papalois
Royal Berkshire Hospital NHS Foundation Trust, UK

A volume in the Advances in Human Services and Public Health (AHSPH) Book Series

IGI Global
PUBLISHER of TIMELY KNOWLEDGE

Published in the United States of America by
IGI Global
Information Science Reference (an imprint of IGI Global)
701 E. Chocolate Avenue
Hershey PA, USA 17033
Tel: 717-533-8845
Fax: 717-533-8661
E-mail: cust@igi-global.com
Web site: http://www.igi-global.com

Library of Congress Cataloging-in-Publication Data

Names: Papalois, Vassilios E., editor. | Papalois, Kyriaki, editor.
Title: The role of health literacy in major healthcare crises / Vassilios Papalois, Kyriaki Papalois, editors.
Description: Hershey, PA : Medical Information Science Reference, [2024] | Includes bibliographical references and index. | Summary: "This book examines the role of health literacy not only in informing the public but also on building a culture of cooperation between the healthcare systems and their users, helping readers navigate through the health-related information, accessing accurate and reliable information and acting upon it "-- Provided by publisher.
Identifiers: LCCN 2022001651 (print) | LCCN 2022001652 (ebook) | ISBN 9781799896524 (hardcover) | ISBN 9781799896531 (paperback) | ISBN 9781799896548 (ebook)
Subjects: MESH: Health Literacy | Health Promotion | Public-Private Sector Partnerships | Social Media
Classification: LCC RA425 (print) | LCC RA425 (ebook) | NLM WA 590 | DDC 362.1--dc23/eng/20220120
LC record available at https://lccn.loc.gov/2022001651
LC ebook record available at https://lccn.loc.gov/2022001652

This book is published in the IGI Global book series Advances in Human Services and Public Health (AHSPH) (ISSN: 2475-6571; eISSN: 2475-658X)

British Cataloguing in Publication Data
A Cataloguing in Publication record for this book is available from the British Library.
All work contributed to this book is new, previously-unpublished material.

For electronic access to this publication, please contact: eresources@igi-global.com.

Advances in Human Services and Public Health (AHSPH) Book Series

ISSN:2475-6571
EISSN:2475-658X

Editor-in-Chief: Jennifer Martin, RMIT University, Australia

MISSION

The well-being of the general public should be a primary concern for any modern civilization. Ongoing research in the field of human services and public healthcare is necessary to evaluate, manage, and respond to the health and social needs of the global population.

The **Advances in Human Services and Public Health (AHSPH)** book series aims to publish high-quality reference publications focused on the latest methodologies, tools, issues, and strategies for managing the health and social welfare of the public. The AHSPH book series will be especially relevant for healthcare professionals, policy makers, government officials, and students seeking the latest research in this field.

COVERAGE

- Healthcare Reform
- Social Welfare Policy
- Youth Development
- Access to Healthcare Services
- Public Welfare
- Poverty
- Public Funding
- Health Policy
- Assistance Programs
- Social Work

IGI Global is currently accepting manuscripts for publication within this series. To submit a proposal for a volume in this series, please contact our Acquisition Editors at Acquisitions@igi-global.com or visit: http://www.igi-global.com/publish/.

The Advances in Human Services and Public Health (AHSPH) Book Series (ISSN 2475-6571) is published by IGI Global, 701 E. Chocolate Avenue, Hershey, PA 17033-1240, USA, www.igi-global.com. This series is composed of titles available for purchase individually; each title is edited to be contextually exclusive from any other title within the series. For pricing and ordering information please visit http://www.igi-global.com/book-series/advances-human-services-public-health/102256. Postmaster: Send all address changes to above address.

Titles in this Series

For a list of additional titles in this series, please visit:
http://www.igi-global.com/book-series/advances-human-services-public-health/102256

Dealing With Regional Conflicts of Global mportance
Piotr Pietrzak (Sofia University, Bulgaria)
Information Science Reference • © 2024 • 320pp • H/C (ISBN: 9781668494677) • US $215.00

Analyzing Global Responses to Contemporary Regional Conflicts
Piotr Pietrzak (Sofia University, Bulgaria)
Information Science Reference • © 2024 • 350pp • H/C (ISBN: 9798369328378) • US $245.00

Ecological and Evolutionary Perspectives on Infections and Morbidity
P.A. Azeez (Salim Ali Centre for Ornithology and Natural History, Coimbatore, India) P.P. Nikhil Raj (Amrita School of Engineering, Amrita Vishwa Vidyapeetham, India) and R. Mohanraj (Bharathidasan University, India)
Medical Information Science Reference • © 2023 • 331pp • H/C (ISBN: 9781799894148) • US $325.00

Transformation and Efficiency Enhancement of Public Utilities Systems Multidimensional Aspects and Perspectives
Jordan Gjorchev (International Slavic University, North Macedonia) Samoil Malcheski (International Slavic University, North Macedonia) Tamara Rađenović (University of Niš, Serbia) Dejan Vasović (University of Niš, Serbia) and Snežana Živković (University of Niš, Serbia)
Information Science Reference • © 2023 • 457pp • H/C (ISBN: 9781668477304) • US $215.00

For an entire list of titles in this series, please visit:
http://www.igi-global.com/book-series/advances-human-services-public-health/102256

IGI Global
PUBLISHER of TIMELY KNOWLEDGE

701 East Chocolate Avenue, Hershey, PA 17033, USA
Tel: 717-533-8845 x100 • Fax: 717-533-8661
E-Mail: cust@igi-global.com • www.igi-global.com

Table of Contents

Detailed Table of Contents

of comprehending and effectively utilizing health information has emerged as a pressing and critical concern. This study investigates the paramount importance of health information comprehension in India's response to the COVID-19 pandemic.

The chapter explores the critical role of health information communication in rural settings during pandemics. It looks into rural populations' unique challenges in accessing health information, information dissemination, and improving health outcomes. The chapter discusses the current health information communication in rural settings, the need for tailoring health information, the barriers, and the potential of technology and innovations in improving access to rural information. It also highlights the importance of cultural sensitivity and policy considerations in effectively addressing health information disparities in rural areas.

The aim of this chapter is to determine the areas of using digital technology to cope with the COVID 19 pandemic. PubMed and Google Scholar article content analysis was conducted, the governments' good practices were examined and Turkish filiation implementation studies were combined to obtain digital technologies to deal with COVID-19. The areas have been determined as planning and monitoring, contact tracing, infection screening, quarantine and self-isolation, clinical management, and medical procurement. As a result of the investigation, efforts coordinated by governments around the world have focused on successfully isolating and mitigating COVID-19 to varying degrees. Countries that maintain low COVID-19 mortality rates per person are implementing strategies that include early surveillance, testing, contact tracing, and strict quarantine. The low mortality rate in Turkey has been concluded due to Turkey's Filiation application. Turkey quickly locates and isolates the contacts at the rate, of 99.9%, and filiation success is based on the detection of cases through 10 hours.

The 21st Century has experienced a global pandemic caused by a highly infectious viral disease called COVID-19. It spread globally and put a wide impact on human

immunity products. This study attempts to analyse the factors influencing immunity literacy among people and to determine predictor variables for people's immunity consciousness. A sample of 391 respondents was collected and analyzed using descriptive and determinant analysis. The findings of the study highlight important factors behind consumers' literacy and their buying behaviour towards immunity products. In conclusion, a high variance is observed on the basis of the length of time, use of products and money spent in buying immunity products. A function mapping based on their buying intention towards immunity products categorized people as immunity aware or immunity ignorant.

This study delves into personal narratives of mental health crises and psychiatric treatment, comparing them with an extended Caplan's Crisis Theory. The objective is to unravel identifiable phases and turning points in these narratives, challenging traditional diagnostic categories and advocating for a paradigm shift in crisis intervention strategies. Through meticulous analysis, distinct phases of mental health crises emerged, showcasing the impact of interventions on recovery trajectories. Proposed alternative crisis categories highlighted the universal quest for safety and professional care, countered by social barriers. The study calls for a paradigm shift in mental health services, emphasizing psychosocial factors and community support. Through empathetic understanding and strategic interventions, mental health services can be restructured to be more responsive, fostering recovery and resilience among individuals facing mental health crises.

Health management and sustained mental comfort requires a multidisciplinary approach, with a holistic strategy for maintenance of overall wellbeing. Therapeutic interventions for maternal health need to be designed in such a way that it permits mitigation and prevention of the adverse influences on the health of mother and child both. Good gut health has a significant impact on motivation, and higher cognitive functions involving the neuro-immuno-endocrine mediators. The study aimed to understand the knowledge, attitude and practices of expectant mothers during their pregnancy towards the use of probiotics from different cities of Rajasthan, India.

Results of the survey study suggested that a considerable number of mothers were unaware about the health benefits of probiotics consumption during and post-pregnancy and due to partial and ambiguous knowledge towards probiotics, maternal subjects also showed characteristics of disbelief on probiotics consumption during and post-pregnancy, which further contributed towards the decreased consumption of probiotics during and post-pregnancy.

To understand the causes and consequences of the rising rates of teenage pregnancy, we utilized the National Family Health Survey (NFHS-5) dataset to explore various factors, including contraception methods employed across India. Employing Python programming, we conducted a cluster analysis to examine data patterns and similarities. Our investigation aimed to establish a potential causal link between adolescent pregnancy and variables such as age, educational attainment, and internet usage. The findings suggest that higher literacy levels are associated with a reduction in teenage pregnancies. Additionally, teenage pregnancies contribute to an increased risk of anemia among pregnant women aged 15-19. Over the past two decades, the prevalence of anemia among Indian women of reproductive age has been 20% higher than the global average. In India, one in every two women is anemic, exceeding the global ratio of one in every three women. Among pregnant women, the incidence of anemia varies from 33% to 89%, with adolescent girls experiencing a rate exceeding 60%.

Since the 1990s, more than 500,000 deaths have been recorded in the U.S. due to opioids, and the opioid crisis has become a leading cause of death. This risk is higher for individuals with cancer as they are prone to becoming addicted but need these drugs to manage chronic pain. In fact, about 75% of cancer patients use opioids but at least 19% of them show signs of misuse. The crisis has cost the U.S. billions of dollars in federal funding. Although the U.S. has increased the accessibility of substance abuse treatments and patient education programs, the stigma of seeking treatment for substance abuse and the necessity of opioids as an analgesic for cancer patients remain. To solve the American opioid crisis's impact on individuals with

Preface

In the midst of unprecedented global challenges, the pivotal role of health literacy has come to the forefront, shaping the narrative of healthcare crises. The COVID-19 pandemic has underscored the undeniable need for accurate, reliable information to safeguard public health. In this edited reference book, titled *The Role of Health Literacy in Major Healthcare Crises*, we delve into the multifaceted dimensions of health literacy and its profound impact on navigating and mitigating crises within healthcare systems.

Allow editors Professor Vassilios Papalois and Dr. Kyriaki-Barbara Papalois to guide you through an exploration of health literacy that extends beyond the immediate concerns of patients. It encompasses the broader needs of the general population, highlighting the imperative for not just compliance with health advice but a genuine understanding of the severity of health crises and the subsequent informed response.

Healthcare systems are confronted with an array of crises, from pandemics and natural catastrophes to terrorist attacks and outbreaks of illnesses. Yet, there are also internal challenges within healthcare structures, such as resource shortages and workforce constraints, which, if not efficiently managed, can lead to inefficiencies and inequalities in health provision.

This book probes into the intricate interplay between health literacy, communication strategies, and educational activities at local, national, and global levels. We examine ethical considerations associated with healthcare crises and how they are negotiated within the realm of health campaigns. The goal is not only to inform the public but also to foster a culture of cooperation between healthcare systems and their users.

Health campaigns play a pivotal role in raising awareness, motivating individuals to seek information and services, and catalyzing attitudinal and behavioral change. While an abundance of health-related information is available through diverse media channels, the process of navigating, accessing accurate information, and translating it into action is far from straightforward.

The chapters in this book cover a spectrum of crucial topics, including health literacy crises, the nexus between health literacy and vaccination, the impact of health literacy on healthcare organizations, the significance of e-health literacy, ethical challenges in healthcare communication, and the role of health literacy in blood and organ donation.

We invite contributions from a diverse array of stakeholders—healthcare professionals, academics, researchers, charities, patients' associations, and the general population. The collective perspectives and experiences shared within these pages will not only facilitate the exchange of best practices but also offer insights that may guide future actions.

As we navigate the complex landscape of healthcare crises, this book stands as a testament to the vital role that health literacy plays in shaping the trajectory of informed decision-making, cooperation, and resilience in the face of challenges.

ORGANIZATION OF THE BOOK

Chapter 1: Navigating Healthcare in a Crisis: Understanding Health Literacy and Medical Tourism

Sunil Kumar, Nishi patel, Paturi Reddy

This chapter examines the emerging trend of medical tourism in India, focusing on two specific cases: cardiovascular surgery in Kozhikode, Kerala, and a total hip replacement in New Delhi. Through a thematic analysis, the research elucidates the significant role of health literacy in guiding patients' decisions to seek medical interventions abroad. This chapter highlights several themes. One is balancing concerns about healthcare costs with the care quality in India. Another is how online research and patient stories affect decisions. Planning before the trip is detailed. After-treatment care is vital. The chapter also looks at how cultural experiences in medical trips can help patients. It emphasizes the need to understand and use health information, especially in medical tourism. The study examines how health knowledge influences patient choices.

Chapter 2: Beyond the Virus: Health Literacy's Crucial Role in India's Pandemic Story

Soumya Sankar Ghosh

The accessibility and efficacy of healthcare services rely on a fundamental element that is often underestimated: the capacity to understand and engage with health information. It's universally acknowledged that access to healthcare is a basic right for all individuals. In the Indian context, a country marked by significant socio-economic disparities and a rich mosaic of cultural and linguistic diversity, the matter of comprehending and effectively utilizing health information has emerged as a pressing and critical concern. This study investigates the paramount importance of health information comprehension in India's response to the COVID-19 pandemic.

Chapter 3: Health Information Communication in Rural Settings During Crises

Hilda Mwangakala

This chapter explores the critical role of health information communication in rural settings during pandemics. It looks into rural populations' unique challenges in accessing health information, information dissemination, and improving health outcomes. The chapter discusses the current health information communication in rural settings, the need for tailoring health information, the barriers, and the potential of technology and innovations in improving access to rural information. It also highlights the importance of cultural sensitivity and policy considerations in effectively addressing health information disparities in rural areas.

Chapter 4: Use of Digital Technology to Deal with Covid-19

Alaattin Parlakkılıç

The aim of this chapter is to determine the areas of using digital technology to cope with the pandemic. PubMed and Google Scholar article content analysis was conducted, the governments' good practices were examined and Turkish filiation implementation studies were combined to obtain digital technologies to deal with Covid-19. The areas have been determined as planning and monitoring, contact tracing, infection screening, quarantine and self-isolation, clinical management, and medical procurement. As a result of the investigation, efforts coordinated by governments around the world have focused on successfully isolating and mitigating COVID-19 to varying degrees. Countries that maintain low COVID-19 mortality rates per person are implementing strategies that include early surveillance, testing, contact tracing, and strict quarantine. The low mortality rate in Turkey has been concluded due to Turkey's Filiation application. Turkey quickly locates and isolates the contacts at the rate, of 99.9%, and filiation success is based on the detection of cases through 10 hours.

Chapter 5: An Analytical Review of the Roles of Digital Media and the Health in India during the Pandemic of COVID-19

Subir Sinha

The 21st Century has experienced a global pandemic caused by a highly infectious viral disease called COVID-19. It spread globally and had a wide impact on human civilization. In India, the scenario of the pandemic was not different. The Indian government took several serious steps to resist the COVID-19 and several other health issues during the pandemic. India initially focuses on the health literacy, information dissemination and awareness program to resist the spread of infection. Digital media played some significant roles in it. The article entitled "An Analytical Review of the Roles of Digital Media and the Health in India during the Pandemic of COVID-19" analyzed five case studies and justify significances. The article reflected how digital media disseminates information on Corona virus and the diseases called COVID-19, creates awareness among the public and helps to resist the spread of infection. During the pandemic, digital media also acts as a platform which provided comfort to mental stress and support in the vaccination process.

Chapter 6: Inductive Ontology for Specifying the Contexture of Web Health Information System

Minaxi Parmar

Inductive ontology helps to describe the algorithm of process, application, architecture, plan, design, etc. It is easily pertinent for elaborating the concept. An ontology creator shows all connectivity of the core concept to another concept, procedures, and application with the five fundamentals i.e., properties, matter, energy, space, and time; hence, it made broader the idea plan of its users/reader enables to find out various connected elements relevant to the query on the direct and indirect way. The services sector has two main property-level functions first to develop/produce the service and second to provide the service. Both the property has specific phases of multiple processes i.e., creating services, owner/authority functions, user functions, identity, process, etc. phase can be easily described in a graphical way. Here, a researcher describes the ontology for web-based health information systems by explaining two websites namely Web MD, and drugs.com. Both the WHISs are rich in information and data relevant to mankind's health and lifestyle.

Chapter 7: Predictive Analysis of Consumers' Immunity Literacy towards Immunity Products - A Statistical Study using Discriminant Method

Poonam Arora, Nidhi Arora

The outbreak of COVID-19 pandemic and the subsequent recurrences have profound effect on psychological, social and physical health of people. The fear of Corona virus has posed unexampled stress on all the population segments of country. The perceived threat has made people more conscious about their health and immunity. This has triggered a significant change in consumer buying behaviour towards immunity products. This study attempts to analyse the factors influencing immunity literacy among people and to determine predictor variables for people's immunity consciousness. A sample of 391 respondents was collected and analyzed using descriptive and determinant analysis. The findings of the study highlight important factors behind consumers' literacy and their buying behaviour towards immunity products. In conclusion, a high variance is observed on the basis of the length of time, use of products and money spent in buying immunity products. A function mapping based on their buying intention towards immunity products categorized people as immunity aware or immunity ignorant.

Chapter 8: Navigating Mental Health Crises: Understanding Pivotal Phases, Health Campaigns, and Community Resilience for Recovery and Reform

Rita Komalasari

This study delves into personal narratives of mental health crises and psychiatric treatment, comparing them with an extended Caplan's Crisis Theory. The objective is to unravel identifiable phases and turning points in these narratives, challenging traditional diagnostic categories and advocating for a paradigm shift in crisis intervention strategies. Through meticulous analysis, distinct phases of mental health crises emerged, showcasing the impact of interventions on recovery trajectories. Proposed alternative crisis categories highlighted the universal quest for safety and professional care, countered by social barriers. The study calls for a paradigm shift in mental health services, emphasizing psychosocial factors and community support. Through empathetic understanding and strategic interventions, mental health services can be restructured to be more responsive, fostering recovery and resilience among individuals facing mental health crises.

Chapter 9: Knowledge, Attitude and Practices Towards the use of Psychobiotics for Maternal Health and Well-Being

Suyesha Singh, Geeta Khanwani, Manali Datta

Health management and sustained mental comfort requires a multidisciplinary approach, with a holistic strategy for maintenance of overall wellbeing. Therapeutic interventions for maternal health need to be designed in such a way that it permits mitigation and prevention of the adverse influences on the health of mother and child both. Good gut health has a significant impact on motivation, and higher cognitive functions involving the neuro-immuno-endocrine mediators. The study aimed to understand the knowledge, attitude and practices of expectant mothers during their pregnancy towards the use of probiotics from different cities of Rajasthan, India.

Results of the survey study suggested that a considerable number of mothers were unaware about the health benefits of probiotics consumption during and post-pregnancy and due to partial and ambiguous knowledge towards probiotics, maternal subjects also showed characteristics of disbelief on probiotics consumption during and post-pregnancy, which further contributed towards the decreased consumption of probiotics during and post-pregnancy.

Chapter 10: Analysis of Teenage Pregnancy and Contraception Methods on National Family Health Survey (NFHS5) Data

Lakshmi D, Shreya Shetye, Karishni Mehta, Vaishnavi Patil

To understand the causes and consequences of the rising rates of teenage pregnancy, we utilized the National Family Health Survey (NFHS-5) dataset to explore various factors, including contraception methods employed across India. Employing Python programming, we conducted a cluster analysis to examine data patterns and similarities. Our investigation aimed to establish a potential causal link between adolescent pregnancy and variables such as age, educational attainment, and internet usage. The findings suggest that higher literacy levels are associated with a reduction in teenage pregnancies. Additionally, teenage pregnancies contribute to an increased risk of anemia among pregnant women aged 15-19. Over the past two decades, the prevalence of anemia among Indian women of reproductive age has been 20% higher than the global average. In India, one in every two women is anemic, exceeding the global ratio of one in every three women. Among pregnant women, the incidence of anemia varies from 33% to 89%, with adolescent girls experiencing a rate exceeding 60%.

Chapter 11: The Intersectionality of the Opioid Crisis and Cancer Treatment

Siddhi Surawkar

Since the 1990s, more than 500,000 deaths have been recorded in the U.S. due to opioids, and the opioid crisis has become a leading cause of death. This risk is higher for individuals with cancer as they are prone to becoming addicted but need these drugs to manage chronic pain. In fact, about 75% of cancer patients use opioids but at least 19% of them show signs of misuse (3). The crisis has cost the U.S. billions of dollars in federal funding. Although the U.S. has increased the accessibility of substance abuse treatments and patient education programs, the stigma of seeking treatment for substance abuse and the necessity of opioids as an analgesic for cancer patients remain. To solve the American opioid crisis's impact on individuals with cancer, an awareness campaign is proposed, allowing for a decrease in stigmatization.

Chapter 12: Health Literacy for Disabled Students: A Case Study of Curriculum Development in Japanese Special Schools

Taku Murayama

Health literacy and related practical issues have been the subject of discussion in recent research. In with-COVID 19 times, the discussion and practice on the health literacy are also critical in the schooling, for the safe schooling and classroom activities. The purpose of this chapter is to discuss the chief issues on health literacy for the children with the special educational needs, especially focused on the intellectually and developmentally disabled students. In this chapter, the case for the curriculum development and lesson studies in the special educational schools for the intellectually and developmentally disabled are studied. The author of chapter plays a role as a supervisor for the school and have been in the participant observation in lesson study for the practice on the theme of the difference between COVID-19 virus and influenza virus.

Chapter 13: Health Literacy Initiatives in the Donation Landscape: Educating for Impact

Susmita Chakrabarty, Monali Mishra

Health literacy plays a pivotal role in the landscape of organ and blood donation, influencing individuals' understanding of the process, its benefits, and the critical need for donations. This abstract provides an overview of a comprehensive study that examines health literacy initiatives and their impact on the donation landscape. The research delves into the various strategies employed to enhance health literacy, including educational campaigns, digital platforms, and community engagement. The study aims to shed light on the effectiveness of these initiatives in increasing awareness, dispelling myths, improving comprehension of the donation process, and ultimately driving higher participation in life-saving donations. Additionally, the research explores the challenges faced in promoting health literacy and suggests recommendations to further optimize educational approaches in the context of organ and blood donation.

IN SUMMARY

As we draw the curtains on this comprehensive exploration into *The Role of Health Literacy in Major Healthcare Crises*, the collective wisdom shared by our esteemed contributors has illuminated the intricate tapestry of challenges and opportunities in the realm of health literacy. Vassilios Papalois and Sundy Papalois have guided us through a nuanced journey, unraveling the layers that underscore the indispensability of health literacy in the face of healthcare crises.

From the impactful lessons of the COVID-19 pandemic to the perennial challenges within healthcare systems, this book has ventured into the core of health literacy, dissecting its role not only in informing but in cultivating a symbiotic relationship between healthcare providers and the public. Our exploration into communication strategies, educational initiatives, and ethical considerations associated with healthcare crises has provided a roadmap for a more resilient and informed future.

Health campaigns, as discussed in these pages, serve as crucial catalysts for attitudinal and behavioral change. Navigating the complexities of language, cultural backgrounds, and individual attitudes, the book underscores the imperative of clear and accessible health information. The symbiosis between health-related information, intermediary campaigns, and public response emerges as a critical juncture that demands ongoing attention.

The diverse perspectives presented by healthcare professionals, academics, researchers, charities, patients' associations, and the broader public have woven a rich tapestry of insights. This collective wisdom not only reflects the current landscape but also offers a foundation for future actions and interventions.

In the ever-evolving landscape of healthcare, where crises manifest in myriad forms, health literacy emerges as a powerful tool for empowerment. This book stands as a testament to the profound impact that health literacy can have in shaping a resilient, informed, and cooperative response to the challenges that define our times.

As editors, we extend our sincere gratitude to all contributors who have shared their expertise and experiences within these pages. It is our hope that this reference book serves as a valuable resource for those navigating the complexities of healthcare crises and inspires continued collaboration and innovation in the pursuit of a healthier, more informed society.

Acknowledgment

We would like to extend our grateful thanks to:

Dr Maria Theodosopoulou, PhD,BA (Hons)

Dr Zoe-Athena Papalois, BSc (Hons),MBBS

Dr Charlotte Phillips Clarke, MBio, MBBS

Dr Maria Roma, MD

Chapter 1
Navigating Healthcare in a Crisis:
Understanding Health Literacy and Medical Tourism

Sunil Kumar
https://orcid.org/0000-0002-2362-1972
Shoolini University, India

Nishi Patel
Lovely Professional University, India

Paturi Jagadeeswar Reddy
Lovely Professional University, India

ABSTRACT

This chapter examines the emerging trend of medical tourism in India, focusing on two specific cases: cardiovascular surgery in Kozhikode, Kerala, and a total hip replacement in New Delhi. Through a thematic analysis, the research elucidates the significant role of health literacy in guiding patients' decisions to seek medical interventions abroad. This chapter highlights several themes. One is balancing concerns about healthcare costs with the care quality in India. Another is how online research and patient stories affect decisions. Planning before the trip is detailed. After-treatment care is vital. The chapter also looks at how cultural experiences in medical trips can help patients. It emphasizes the need to understand and use health information, especially in medical tourism, examining how health knowledge influences patient choices.

DOI: 10.4018/978-1-7998-9652-4.ch001

1. INTRODUCTION

Health literacy is one's capability to understand and utilize health information, facilitating informed decision-making. It aids in effective communication with healthcare professionals and helps navigate complex healthcare systems (Berkman *et al.,* 2011; Rudd & Anderson, 2006). Factors such as education, culture, and language proficiency influence health literacy. Misunderstandings related to health issues and treatments due to low health literacy can lead to adverse health outcomes and increased healthcare costs (Nutbeam, 2008). Several tools, like the Test of Functional Health Literacy in Adults (TOFHLA) and the Health Literacy Universal Precautions Toolkit, assess health literacy. Efforts to boost health literacy include patient education, transparent communication, and the development of accessible health resources (Lunt & Carrera, 2010).

On the other hand, medical tourism is travelling abroad for medical procedures. It is driven by factors such as the availability of quality healthcare services in other countries, cost disparities, reduced wait times, and the quest for specific treatments unavailable or restricted in one's home nation. This industry encompasses various medical services and involves healthcare professionals and agencies assisting patients in medical travel logistics. When combining health literacy and medical tourism, challenges arise. It becomes essential to bridge health literacy gaps in the global healthcare setting to ensure patient safety and optimal outcomes.

1.1 Health Literacy

Health literacy, emerging in the 1970s, denotes an individual's ability to navigate today's health demands and has gained importance due to the rising prevalence of non-communicable diseases and healthcare costs (Liu *et al.,* 2020). This literacy influences healthcare access, quality, and fairness, with Santana *et al.* (2021) expanding it to include understanding and using health information and services for decision-making. Liu et al., (2020) identifies three key elements of health literacy: knowledge of health, healthcare, and health systems; processing and using information in various formats related to health and healthcare; and the ability to maintain health through self-management and working with health providers. The study emphasizes the diverse needs of individuals and the importance of interaction between consumers, healthcare providers, and systems in understanding and improving health literacy.

Hayran & Özer (2018) highlighted that effective communication of health information by healthcare organizations in Istanbul positively influences patient contentment. Such literacy is essential for preventive healthcare, enhancing patient-provider communication, and reducing healthcare disparities. Digital health literacy has emerged with the advent of digital healthcare, emphasizing the importance of evaluating online health information and leveraging telehealth services. This literacy is crucial for individual empowerment and refining the overall quality and equity of healthcare (Levy & Janke, 2016).

In diverse regions like India, health literacy is particularly significant due to linguistic and cultural variations. The digital rise in the healthcare system highlighted the need for health information tailored to cultural and linguistic nuances, especially for marginalized populations like women (Sørensen *et al.,* 2015). Community-based interventions have been proposed to address these challenges (Grimmer-Somers, et al., 2010), emphasizing community empowerment and addressing the nuances of rural contexts (Choudhury *et al.,* 2016; Perry, 2014). Furthermore, the relationship between socioeconomic disparities and health literacy underscores the need for specialized interventions for vulnerable communities (Agarahari et al., 2023).

1.2 Health Literacy Tools

Various tools and evaluation methods exist to gauge an individual's capacity to comprehend and apply health-related data. Below are some frequently referenced health literacy instruments, accompanied by their respective authors:

- Test of Functional Health Literacy in Adults (TOFHLA) - Developed by Parker et al. (1995).
- Rapid Estimate of Adult Literacy in Medicine (REALM) - Created by Murphy et al. (1993).
- Newest Vital Sign (NVS) - Developed by Weiss et al. (2005) and sponsored by Pfizer.
- Short Test of Functional Health Literacy in Adults (S-TOFHLA) - An abbreviated version of TOFHLA by Baker et al. (1999).
- Health Literacy Questionnaire (HLQ) - Developed by Osborne et al. (2013).
- European Health Literacy Survey Questionnaire (HLS-EU-Q) - Created as part of the European Health Literacy Project by Sørensen et al. (2013).
- Health Literacy Skills Instrument (HLSI) - Developed by McCormack et al. (2010).
- All Aspects of Health Literacy Scale (AAHLS) - Created by Chinn and McCarthy (2013).
- Functional Communicative and Critical Health Literacy Scale (FCCHL) - Developed by Ishikawa et al. (2008).
- Health Activities Literacy Scale (HALS) - A product of the National Center for Education Statistics in the U.S.

1.3 Medical Tourism

Medical tourism involves individuals venturing outside their native countries to seek medical or dental care. Often, they might pursue treatments unavailable in their home countries (Ormond & Sulianti, 2017). Several drivers, including escalating healthcare costs, gaps in insurance coverage, availability of specialty treatments, and advanced facilities, fuel this trend. Moreover, the enticing opportunity to merge medical procedures with vacationing plays a role.

Globally, numerous destinations have established their prominence in medical tourism, catering to various medical needs, from elective to complex procedures. As defined by Pollard (2012), this phenomenon is an expedition of individuals outside their domiciles for surgeries or elective treatments. These can range from elective aesthetic endeavors to intricate surgeries and holistic wellness services.

One of the substantial catalysts behind the medical tourism sector's impressive growth trajectory is the allure of considerable economic savings. Patients can now access similar high-quality procedures overseas, often at a fraction of what they would expend domestically. Additionally, reduced wait times, combined with specialized care often unavailable in their native territories, are enticing (Wang, 2012). Taking India as an illustrative case, cities like Kozhikode and New Delhi are emerging as potentates in medical tourism. These cities offer superior healthcare in globally accredited institutions, amalgamating medical treatment with recuperative and wellness experiences (Malhotra & Dave, 2022).

The experience, however, transcends mere treatment. It fuses healthcare with the joy of travelling, underpinning a more holistic paradigm (Pollard, 2012). However, this burgeoning sector is not devoid of challenges. Navigating language barriers, deciphering cultural nuances, ensuring the sanctity of patient safety, and upholding ethical standards remain persistent concerns (Turner, 2012).

In essence, while the mushrooming medical tourism arena promises hope, quality, and affordability, it concurrently surfaces multifaceted challenges warranting continual introspection and redressal. The industry encapsulates not merely medical care but an amalgamation of treatment, travel, cultural immersion, and comprehensive well-being.

1.4 Market Size of Medical Tourism

The medical tourism market in India was valued at US$ 7,417 million in 2022. It is projected to experience significant growth, reaching an estimated value of US$ 42,237.47 Million by 2032. This growth trajectory suggests an impressive Compound Annual Growth Rate (CAGR) of 19% over the decade from 2022 to 2032 ("India Medical Tourism Market," 2022). The medical tourism market in the Asia-Pacific region is experiencing significant growth. It is projected to expand at an annual rate of 16.8%. Over the span from 2023 to 2032, it is anticipated that this market will grow to a size of US$ 774,464.3 million ("Research and Markets," 2023). The global medical tourism market reached US$ 10.4 billion in 2021 and is anticipated to experience significant growth over the next decade. Projections indicate that the market will advance at a CAGR of 13.0% from 2022 to 2031. By the end of 2031, it is expected to expand to an estimated value of US$ 72.8 billion. This robust growth reflects the increasing trend of individuals seeking healthcare services abroad, driven by cost savings, high-quality medical care, and access to specialized treatments ("Medical Tourism Market," 2022). In term of medical procedure, the market share of medical tourism is dominated by cosmetic surgery (25%), dental procedures (15%), fertility treatment (12%), ophthalmic procedures (10%), orthopedic surgeries (10%), and 8 percent of cardiac treatments (Statista, 2023).

1.5 Health Literacy and Medical Tourism

Medical tourism refers to individuals travelling for medical treatments, often searching for procedures unavailable in their home countries. Health literacy, the ability to understand and use health information for decision-making, is paramount for medical travelers (Berkman *et al.,* 2011; Nutbeam, 2000; Rudd et al., 2004). Access to clear health information empowers these individuals to grasp details about their condition, treatment options, risks, and post-care instructions. Digital platforms like websites and social media play a significant role in influencing destination choices for these travelers.

Culture also plays a crucial role in medical tourism. Healthcare professionals with cultural competence can better cater to patients from diverse backgrounds, leading to better patient experiences (Betancourt *et al.,* 2005). Such competence is vital, especially when treating international patients. Connell (2013) investigated into the modern perspective of medical tourism, its cultural implications, and its commodification. The notion of "health diplomacy" is introduced as a collaboration between nations to enhance healthcare experiences for medical tourists.

Additionally, given India's rich history of traditional medicine, there is potential to merge these treatments into medical tourism offerings, providing a unique experience for international patients (Patwardhan & Mashelkar, 2009). This integration not only respects cultural competencies but also differentiates the healthcare experience for foreign patients.

The repercussions of the recent COVID-19 pandemic on the sector are inescapable. As COVID-19 spread, individuals well-informed about health issues were better positioned to evaluate the dangers of medical travel, considering potential exposures and the challenges posed by quarantine measures, which caused many to defer non-critical treatments. These knowledgeable individuals often sought guidance from trusted organizations like the WHO to make travel decisions, helping them avoid areas heavily affected by COVID-19. The limitations on movement and the inherent risks of face-to-face medical interactions led to a surge in the use of telemedicine, with these informed individuals at the forefront of this transition. Furthermore, when countries renowned for medical tourism implemented new safety protocols for international patients, those with a strong understanding of health matters were more proficient in adapting to and adhering to such updated guidelines, including enforced quarantines and testing requirements.

Paakkari & Okan (2020) examines health literacy challenges during the COVID-19 pandemic, emphasizing its importance in managing health information and responses. There was a widespread difficulty in understanding health information, with many Europeans struggling. The pandemic highlighted the need for both individual and systemic preparedness, underscoring health literacy's role in handling communicable diseases. The study also stresses the importance of social responsibility and collective action in public health. The more effective public information campaigns and education to enhance health literacy and help people make informed health decisions during the pandemic (Okan et al., 2020).

2. CASE STUDY: CARDIOVASCULAR SURGERY MEDICAL TOURISM IN KOZHIKODE, KERALA, INDIA

A 60-year-old man from Chicago was dealing with a heart problem called coronary artery disease (CAD). CAD gave him chest pain and breathing trouble, especially when he was active or stressed. Also, treating it in the U.S. was very expensive. After five years of dealing with CAD and many tests in Chicago, doctors found blockages in his heart's arteries. His doctor said he urgently needed a heart surgery called CABG to prevent possible heart attacks. Because of the high medical bills in the US, the man and his wife thought about getting the surgery in another country. They researched and talked to doctors online and chose Kozhikode in Kerala, India. They heard good things about the hospitals there, the skills of the doctors, the lower cost, and the good experiences of others.

When they reached Kozhikode, they were welcomed warmly. A person from the medical travel company helped them reach their hotel near the hospital. The next day, the man met the heart doctor at the Kozhikode Cardiac Care Center. They talked about his health history, did some tests, and discussed the upcoming surgery. The surgery was done on April 15, 2023, and took about 4 hours. It was a kind of surgery where they used three new paths to improve blood flow to the heart. He stayed in the hospital for seven days to prepare for the surgery and recover after.

The total cost of everything was about INR 17,05,000. Cost included the surgery, doctor's charges, hospital stay, medicines, tests, other doctor visits, and other costs. After the surgery, the man was taken care of in a special part of the hospital for heart patients. At the same time, the hospital staff made sure his wife knew everything and felt okay.

As the man felt better, they travelled around Kerala. They enjoyed boat rides and visited beautiful places. Before returning to Chicago, the main heart surgeon gave the man a detailed health report and told him what to do next and how to continue his treatment back home. Ultimately, their trip to Kozhikode in Kerala for medical care was successful. They got good treatment without spending too much. With his health now better and with happy memories from Kerala, the man and his wife went back to Chicago. Their story shows how medical travel to India is becoming more popular and helpful.

2.1 Case Thematic Analysis

- *Healthcare Cost Concerns:* The story sheds light on the growing practice of medical tourism to combat the exorbitant healthcare expenditures in the USA. The patient and his family's worries about the cost and availability of high-quality healthcare led him and her to investigate options abroad. This subject highlights a larger trend of people travelling overseas for medical treatment to save costs.
- *Quality of care and expertise:* A few considerations, including the medical personnel's qualifications and the hospital's reputation, played a role in the choice to visit Kozhikode, Kerala. The choice of destination demonstrates how important it is for patients to receive top-notch medical treatment, even if they want to travel for medical purposes.
- *Patient empowerment and informed decision-making:* Before choosing the venue and facility, the patient and his family conducted a thorough investigation, had virtual consultations with a heart surgeon, and carefully considered a few criteria. Their proactive stance in healthcare illustrates patient empowerment and well-informed decision-making.
- *Pre-Trip planning:* The story emphasizes how crucial it is to organize a medical trip well in advance, considering things like getting medical visas, booking airfare, and finding lodging close to the hospital. The theme illustrates the administrative and logistical challenges that people have while travelling for medical care.
- *Cost breakdown:* An understanding of the financial elements of medical tourism may be gained from the comprehensive analysis of the Coronary Artery Bypass Grafting (CABG) surgical expenses, which include the

surgeon's fees, inpatient charges, and prescription prices. This subject reflects the cost and transparency that might influence patients' choices.

- *Post-Treatment Care:* William's post-surgery treatment, which included specialized cardiac recovery, 24-hour monitoring, and wife's support, highlights the significance of all-encompassing recovery and aftercare services in medical tourism.
- *Cultural exploration and tourism:* The Patient's example illustrates how medical tourism enables patients to experience the local natural and cultural attractions while their health stabilizes. This subject illustrates the possibility of a comprehensive therapeutic encounter.
- *Follow-up care:* The instance highlights how crucial it is for the patient to have a seamless return to their country, complete with a thorough medical report, follow-up appointments with the local healthcare practitioner, and a final examination. This subject emphasizes the value of seamless integration with the patient's healthcare journey and continuity of care.
- *Patient feedback and contentment:* The gratitude William and Mary expressed for the excellent medical treatment and kind hospitality they enjoyed in Kozhikode highlights the benefits and happy endings that may come from medical tourism. Patient testimonials are a great way to promote medical tourism locations and institutions.

3. CASE STUDY: TOTAL HIP REPLACEMENT IN NEW DELHI, INDIA

A 58-year-old retired male from Seattle, Washington, experienced significant mobility challenges and pain stemming from osteoarthritis in his right hip. Osteoarthritis, a condition characterized by the deterioration of joint cartilage over time, had been impinging on his day-to-day life and retirement activities for half a decade. Several years prior to the current events, he was diagnosed with osteoarthritis in his right hip. As the protective tissue at the ends of his bones eroded, he began to face increased pain, stiffness, and mobility restrictions. While living in Seattle, he initially explored treatments such as physical therapy, medications, and walking aids. These interventions offered transient relief, but they failed to provide a lasting solution.

The ongoing discomfort prompted him to consult multiple hip specialists in Seattle. After thorough assessments, including X-rays and MRI scans, the experts highlighted extensive damage to his hip joint. Medical examinations led to a unanimous recommendation: a Total Hip Replacement (THR) surgery, where the damaged hip is substituted with an artificial counterpart to alleviate pain and restore movement. Aware of the potentially prohibitive costs of the procedure in the U.S., he began considering international healthcare alternatives. India, especially New Delhi, emerged as a prominent option due to its reputation for quality healthcare at a fraction of U.S. prices. His research indicated that many hospitals in New Delhi are known for their orthopedic excellence. In addition, patient testimonials and reviews further solidified his confidence in choosing this route.

After extensive online consultations with healthcare facilities in New Delhi, he decided on the National Orthopedic Institute, where Dr. Sharma, a reputed orthopedic surgeon, would oversee his THR surgery. The decision was not only driven by cost considerations but also by the potential for a unique cultural experience in the heart of India. On reaching New Delhi in early June, he underwent further diagnostic tests to confirm the severity of his osteoarthritis. Dr. Sharma and his team reviewed these findings to finalize their surgical plan. The surgery was scheduled for July 15, 2023. The medical team employed a minimally invasive anterior approach, ensuring a reduced recovery time.

Regarding expenses, the surgery and associated medical costs amounted to 555,000 INR. Accommodations, local travel, sightseeing, food, return flights, and travel insurance led to additional expenses, bringing the total to approximately 760,000 INR. During Post-surgery, his time at the hospital was marked by a regimented rehabilitation program. This involved pain management, infection prevention, and a structured physical therapy regimen to ensure optimal recovery. As days progressed, his mobility improved, enabling him to explore the vibrant city of New Delhi and its myriad cultural offerings.

In conclusion, this case underscores the potential advantages of medical tourism. The patient not only received top-tier medical care at a fraction of the cost he would have faced in the United States, but he also enriched his life with a unique cultural experience. Upon his return to Seattle, he did so with significantly improved hip functionality, showcasing the effectiveness of his medical journey in India.

3.1 Case Thematic Analysis

- *Healthcare costs and access:* The patient's situation highlights the expanding trend of medical tourism as a workable solution to the U.S.'s exorbitant healthcare expenses and protracted waiting lists for elective surgery. Getting timely and reasonably priced medical care overseas has become a viable option for many people with life-threatening illnesses.
- *Quality of life:* The instance highlights the severe effects that degenerative joint conditions, such as osteoarthritis, may have on a person's quality of life. Patient experience serves as a reminder of the necessity for efficient procedures like total hip replacements (THR) to reduce discomfort, increase range of motion, and improve general health.

- *Multifaceted decision-making process:* The decision the patient made to go after medical tourism was the result of several factors. Cost concerns, medical knowledge, reputation, treatment quality, wait times, and cultural experiences were among the aspects that were considered. This theme reflects the thorough assessment that patients do when they make such a big healthcare choice.
- *Surgical planning:* It emphasized how crucial comprehensive diagnostic testing is to precise diagnosis and surgical planning. In addition to confirming the necessity of THR, the testing gave the surgical team crucial information to be ready for the treatment.
- *Cost breakdown:* A thorough description of the surgical process, including the surgical method and cost breakdown, is given in the case. Patients can better comprehend the financial implications of their therapy when medical charges are transparently disclosed.
- *Rehabilitation and post-surgery care:* The patient's post-operative rehabilitation and care underscore the critical importance that pain management, physical therapy, and a progressive recuperation strategy play in ensuring favourable results after orthopedic procedures.
- *Personal and cultural aspects of medical tourism:* The cultural and personal elements of medical tourism are reflected in the patient's wish to make the most of his medical trip and immerse himself in New Delhi society. Patients frequently want to combine receiving medical care with learning about a new location's cultural history.
- *Patient testimonials*: The patient made several decisions based partly on recommendations from friends and relatives who had good experiences receiving medical care in India. Testimonials emphasize how important word-of-mouth recommendations and patient testimonies are in medical tourism decisions.
- *Affordability and quality of care in medical tourism:* The patient's story demonstrates the accessibility of high-quality healthcare and the low cost of medical operations in nations like India. Medical tourism is mostly driven by the allure of receiving excellent treatment at a lower cost.
- *Healthcare infrastructure and specialist surgeons:* New Delhi's specialized surgeons and robust healthcare system made it a popular destination for medical tourism. Travellers frequently look for places with a robust medical community and professionals in their area.

4. FINDINGS OF CASE STUDIES

Both highlighted cases emphasize the challenges Americans face due to high healthcare costs, prompting many to consider medical tourism, given the significant price disparities between treatments in the U.S. and countries like India. Despite the lower costs, patients do not compromise on quality, as evidenced by their choice of renowned medical institutions in Kozhikode and New Delhi, known for their international reputation and expertise. These patients were empowered, taking charge of their healthcare journey from diagnosis to researching overseas treatment options. Their experiences underscore the importance of thorough pre-trip planning, including consultations and logistical preparations. Transparent cost breakdowns in both cases reveal clear financial benefits of overseas treatment, even when factoring in travel and accommodation expenses. Furthermore, the emphasis on comprehensive post-operative care, encompassing physical therapy, pain management, and consistent follow-ups, highlights its integral role in the medical tourism experience. Beyond medical care, both patients embraced cultural exploration, turning their medical trips into enriching, holistic experiences.

4.1 Health Literacy and medical tourism themes

Health literacy encompasses the ability to access, interpret, understand, and utilize medical information for making informed healthcare choices and adhering to therapeutic instructions. In the context of the two medical tourism cases in India, certain themes highlight elements of health literacy:

- *Patient decision-making:* This theme emphasizes a patient's proficiency in researching, interpreting, and determining based on health data. Leveraging online resources and analyzing patient testimonials demonstrates their adeptness at sifting through and making sense of healthcare information, particularly when looking at international healthcare options.
- *Pre-Trip Planning:* Effectively managing tasks like obtaining visas, selecting appropriate lodgings, and coordinating travel logistics indicates a patient's competence in understanding and acting on multifaceted details and procedures.
- *Treatment planning:* The capacity to comprehend medical diagnoses, evaluate treatment alternatives, and be aware of associated risks and benefits reflects a patient's health literacy. Their readiness to engage in conversations about the treatment, its preparation, and potential outcomes signals their understanding of their health condition.

- *Post-Treatment care:* A patient's grasp of health literacy is evident when they understand and comply with post-operative or treatment guidelines. Their ability to follow medical directives, be aware of possible aftereffects, and discern when to seek medical assistance is closely linked to their health literacy.
- *Follow-up care:* Transitioning medical supervision to their native country and consistently adhering to prescribed healthcare practices demonstrates the cognizance of their health condition and the essentials of continuous care.

These themes underscore the various facets where patients can effectively engage with, decipher, and act upon health-related details, encapsulating the essence of health literacy. Figure 1 presents the factors of medical tourism and healthcare literacy that affects patients care and satisfaction.

Figure 1.

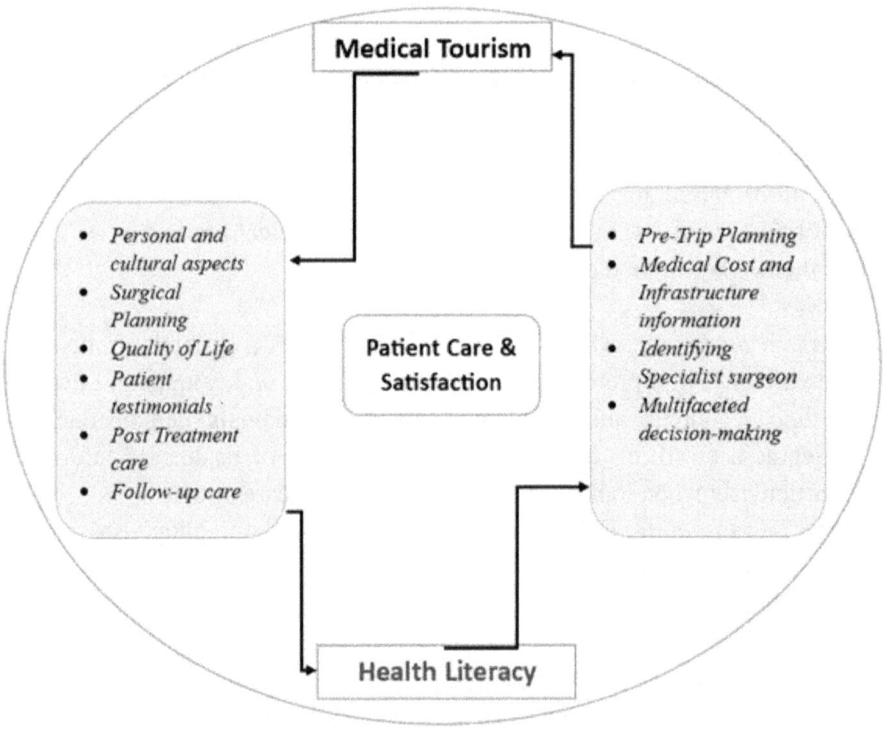

Medical tourism, as depicted by the two cases, offers an efficient and effective alternative to high healthcare costs without compromising quality. Countries like

India are becoming favourable destinations because of their blend of medical expertise, affordability, and rich cultural experiences. The success stories of these patients emphasize the need for thorough research, informed decision-making, and the potential benefits of combining healthcare with cultural exploration. They highlight a growing trend where individuals are empowered to make choices based on health literacy that best suits their medical and personal needs.

4.2 Legal issues in Medical Tourism

In medical tourism cases like the cardiovascular surgery in Kerala and hip replacement in New Delhi, legal issues in India may include:

- *Patient Rights:* Ensuring international patients' rights are protected, similar to local patients, particularly in cases of malpractice or disputes.
- *Medical Malpractice Laws:* Understanding the legal recourse available to international patients in cases of medical negligence or complications.
- *Insurance and Liability:* Issues related to insurance coverage, especially how it applies to international patients and what liabilities the hospitals assume.
- *Regulatory Standards:* Ensuring medical facilities and procedures meet both Indian and international healthcare standards.
- *Ethical Concerns:* Navigating ethical issues, like prioritization of medical tourists over local patients, and ensuring ethical standards in treatment and care.

These legal considerations are crucial for protecting both the patients and the healthcare providers involved in medical tourism.

Case Based Questions

Q.1 How did health literacy play a role in the patients' decision-making processes, from researching potential medical destinations to understanding the complexity of their diagnoses and treatments?

Q.2 How did the comparative cost advantages of seeking treatment in India, combined with the perceived quality of care, influence the patients' decisions? And, what were the health outcomes post-treatment compared to the expected outcomes if the treatments were sought in their home country?

Q.3 In what ways did the cultural experiences in Kozhikode and New Delhi contribute to the overall patient experience and satisfaction, and how did these experiences potentially impact their post-treatment recovery and overall well-being?

REFERENCES

Agarahari, P., Jain, A., Pandey, S. M., Agrahari, A. K., Yadav, J., Srivastava, R., & Pandey, S. M. (2023). Exploring the Synergistic Association Between Oral Health Status and Oral Health Literacy Among College Students: A Cross-Sectional Study. *Cureus*, *15*(7), 1–8. doi:10.7759/cureus.41885 PMID:37581155

Baker, D. W., Williams, M. V., Parker, R. M., Gazmararian, J. A., & Nurss, J. (1999). Development of a brief test to measure functional health literacy. *Patient Education and Counseling*, *38*(1), 33–42. doi:10.1016/S0738-3991(98)00116-5 PMID:14528569

Berkman, N. D., Sheridan, S. L., Donahue, K. E., Halpern, D. J., & Crotty, K. (2011). Low health literacy and health outcomes: An updated systematic review. *Annals of Internal Medicine*, *155*(2), 97–107. doi:10.7326/0003-4819-155-2-201107190-00005 PMID:21768583

Betancourt, J. R., Green, A. R., Carrillo, J. E., & Park, E. R. (2005). Cultural competence and health care disparities: Key perspectives and trends. *Health Affairs*, *24*(2), 499–505. doi:10.1377/hlthaff.24.2.499 PMID:15757936

Chinn, D., & McCarthy, C. (2013). All Aspects of Health Literacy Scale (AAHLS): Developing a tool to measure functional, communicative and critical health literacy in primary healthcare settings. *Patient Education and Counseling*, *90*(2), 247–253. doi:10.1016/j.pec.2012.10.019 PMID:23206659

Choudhury, S. M., Arora, T., Alebbi, S., Ahmed, L., Aden, A., Omar, O., & Taheri, S. (2016). How do Qataris source health information? *PLoS One*, *11*(11), e0166250. doi:10.1371/journal.pone.0166250 PMID:27832112

Connell, J. (2013). Contemporary medical tourism: Conceptualisation, culture and commodification. *Tourism Management*, *34*, 1–13. doi:10.1016/j.tourman.2012.05.009

Deloitte. (2014). L. L. P. (2009). Medical tourism: Update and implications. *Retrieved*, (September), 29.

Grimmer-Somers, K., Johnston, K., Somers, E., Luker, J., Alemao, L. A., & Jones, D. (2010). A holistic client-centred program for vulnerable frequent hospital attenders: Cost efficiencies and changed practices. *Australian and New Zealand Journal of Public Health*, *34*(6), 609–612. doi:10.1111/j.1753-6405.2010.00616.x PMID:21134064

Hayran, O., & Özer, O. (2018). Organizational health literacy as a determinant of patient satisfaction. *Public Health, 163*, 20–26. doi:10.1016/j.puhe.2018.06.011 PMID:30041046

India Medical Tourism Market. (2022, October). Retrieved September 20, 2023, from https://www.futuremarketinsights.com/reports/india-medical-tourism-market#:~:text=The%20Indian%20medical%20tourism%20industry%20is%20estimated%20to,a%20healthy%2019%25%20CAGR%20from%202022%20to%202032

Ishikawa, H., Takeuchi, T., & Yano, E. (2008). Measuring functional, communicative, and critical health literacy among diabetic patients. *Diabetes Care, 31*(5), 874–879. doi:10.2337/dc07-1932 PMID:18299446

Levy, H., & Janke, A. (2016). Health literacy and access to care. *Journal of health communication, 21*(sup1), 43-50.

Liu, C., Wang, D., Liu, C., Jiang, J., Wang, X., Chen, H., Ju, X., & Zhang, X. (2020). What is the meaning of health literacy? A systematic review and qualitative synthesis. *Family Medicine and Community Health, 8*(2), e000351. doi:10.1136/fmch-2020-000351 PMID:32414834

Lunt, N., & Carrera, P. (2010). Medical tourism: Assessing the evidence on treatment abroad. *Maturitas, 66*(1), 27–32. doi:10.1016/j.maturitas.2010.01.017 PMID:20185254

Malhotra, N., & Dave, K. (2022). An assessment of competitiveness of medical tourism industry in India: A case of Delhi NCR. *International Journal of Global Business and Competitiveness, 17*(2), 215–228. doi:10.1007/s42943-022-00060-0

McCormack, L., Bann, C., Squiers, L., Berkman, N. D., Squire, C., Schillinger, D., Ohene-Frempong, J., & Hibbard, J. (2010). Measuring health literacy: A pilot study of a new skills-based instrument. *Journal of Health Communication, 15*(sup2, S2), 51–71. doi:10.1080/10810730.2010.499987 PMID:20845193

Medical Tourism market. (2022, October). Retrieved October 15, 2023, from https://www.transparencymarketresearch.com/medical-tourism.html#:~:text=The%20global%20market%20for%20medical%20tourism%20was%20valued,US%24%2072.8%20Bn%20by%20the%20end%20of%202031

Murphy, P. W., Davis, T. C., Long, S. W., Jackson, R. H., & Decker, B. C. (1993). Rapid estimate of adult literacy in medicine (REALM): A quick reading test for patients. *Journal of Reading, 37*(2), 124–130.

Nutbeam, D. (2000). Health literacy as a public health goal: A challenge for contemporary health education and communication strategies into the 21st century. *Health Promotion International, 15*(3), 259–267. doi:10.1093/heapro/15.3.259

Nutbeam, D. (2008). The evolving concept of health literacy. *Social Science & Medicine, 67*(12), 2072–2078. doi:10.1016/j.socscimed.2008.09.050 PMID:18952344

Okan, O., Bollweg, T. M., Berens, E. M., Hurrelmann, K., Bauer, U., & Schaeffer, D. (2020). Coronavirus-related health literacy: A cross-sectional study in adults during the COVID-19 infodemic in Germany. *International Journal of Environmental Research and Public Health, 17*(15), 5503. doi:10.3390/ijerph17155503 PMID:32751484

Ormond, M., & Sulianti, D. (2017). More than medical tourism: Lessons from Indonesia and Malaysia on South–South intra-regional medical travel. *Current Issues in Tourism, 20*(1), 94–110. doi:10.1080/13683500.2014.937324

Osborne, R. H., Batterham, R. W., Elsworth, G. R., Hawkins, M., & Buchbinder, R. (2013). The grounded psychometric development and initial validation of the Health Literacy Questionnaire (HLQ). *BMC Public Health, 13*(1), 1–17. doi:10.1186/1471-2458-13-658 PMID:23855504

Paakkari, L., & Okan, O. (2020). COVID-19: Health literacy is an underestimated problem. *The Lancet. Public Health, 5*(5), e249–e250. doi:10.1016/S2468-2667(20)30086-4 PMID:32302535

Parker, R. M., Baker, D. W., Williams, M. V., & Nurss, J. R. (1995). The test of functional health literacy in adults: A new instrument for measuring patients' literacy skills. *Journal of General Internal Medicine, 10*(10), 537–541. doi:10.1007/BF02640361 PMID:8576769

Patwardhan, B., & Mashelkar, R. A. (2009). Traditional medicine-inspired approaches to drug discovery: Can Ayurveda show the way forward? *Drug Discovery Today, 14*(15-16), 804–811. doi:10.1016/j.drudis.2009.05.009 PMID:19477288

Perry, E. L. (2014). Health literacy in adolescents: An integrative review. *Journal for Specialists in Pediatric Nursing, 19*(3), 210–218. doi:10.1111/jspn.12072 PMID:24612548

Pollard, K. (2012). Medical tourism: Key facts. *Treatment Abroad*. The Foam Company (intuitionconnect.com).

Research and Markets. (2023, May). Asia Pacific Medical Tourism Market 2022-2032 by specialty type (Cosmetic, cardiac, orthopedic, dental, fertility, organ transplant, Bariatric), tourism type, consumer group, tour type, and country: trend forecast and growth opportunity. Retrieved October 10, 2023, from https://www.researchandmarkets.com/reports/5681816/asia-pacific-medical-tourism-market-2022-2032-by#:~:text=Asia%20Pacific%20medical%20tourism%20market%20will%20grow%20by,growing%20lifestyle-related%20disorders%20along%20with%20the%20aging%20population

Rudd, R., Kirsch, I., & Yamamoto, K. (2004). *Literacy and health in America. Policy information report*. Educational Testing Service.

Rudd, R. E., & Anderson, J. E. (2006). *The Health Literacy Environment of Hospitals and Health Centers. Partners for Action: Making Your Healthcare Facility Literacy-Friendly. National Center for the study of adult learning and literacy*. NCSALL.

Santana, S., Brach, C., Harris, L., Ochiai, E., Blakey, C., Bevington, F., Kleinman, D., & Pronk, N. (2021). Practice full report: Updating health literacy for healthy people 2030: Defining its importance for a new decade in public health. *Journal of Public Health Management and Practice*, *27*(6, Supplement 6), S258–S264. doi:10.1097/PHH.0000000000001324 PMID:33729194

Sørensen, K., Pelikan, J. M., Röthlin, F., Ganahl, K., Slonska, Z., Doyle, G., Fullam, J., Kondilis, B., Agrafiotis, D., Uiters, E., Falcon, M., Mensing, M., Tchamov, K., Broucke, S., & Brand, H. (2015). Health literacy in Europe: Comparative results of the European health literacy survey (HLS-EU). *European Journal of Public Health*, *25*(6), 1053–1058. doi:10.1093/eurpub/ckv043 PMID:25843827

Sørensen, K., Van den Broucke, S., Pelikan, J. M., Fullam, J., Doyle, G., Slonska, Z., Kondilis, B., Stoffels, V., Osborne, R. H., & Brand, H. (2013). Measuring health literacy in populations: Illuminating the design and development process of the European Health Literacy Survey Questionnaire (HLS-EU-Q). *BMC Public Health*, *13*(1), 1–10. doi:10.1186/1471-2458-13-948 PMID:24112855

Statista. (2023, September 26). Medical tourism worldwide as of 2023, by procedure. Retrieved from https://www.statista.com/statistics/1414337/share-medical-tourism-worldwide-by-medical-procedure/

Turner, L. (2012). Beyond medical tourism: Canadian companies marketing medical travel. *Globalization and Health*, *8*(1), 1–11. doi:10.1186/1744-8603-8-16 PMID:22703873

Wang, H. Y. (2012). Value as a medical tourism driver. *Managing Service Quality*, *22*(5), 465–491. doi:10.1108/09604521211281387

Weiss, B. D., Mays, M. Z., Martz, W., Castro, K. M., DeWalt, D. A., Pignone, M. P., ... Hale, F. A. (2005). Quick assessment of literacy in primary care: The newest vital sign. *Annals of Family Medicine*, *3*(6), 514–522. doi:10.1370/afm.405 PMID:16338915

Chapter 2
Beyond the Virus:
Health Literacy's Crucial Role in India's Pandemic Story

Soumya Sankar Ghosh
https://orcid.org/0000-0002-4469-4070
VIT Bhopal University, India

ABSTRACT

The accessibility and efficacy of healthcare services rely on a fundamental element that is often underestimated: the capacity to understand and engage with health information. It's universally acknowledged that access to healthcare is a basic right for all individuals. In the Indian context, a country marked by significant socio-economic disparities and a rich mosaic of cultural and linguistic diversity, the matter of comprehending and effectively utilizing health information has emerged as a pressing and critical concern. This study investigates the paramount importance of health information comprehension in India's response to the COVID-19 pandemic.

1. INTRODUCTION

The experience of India during the epidemic serves as a compelling example of the critical significance of knowledge related to well-being in the realm of public health crises. The limited understanding of the population has had a significant impact on their comprehension of and adherence to public health guidelines, vaccine hesitancy, access to healthcare, and the overall effectiveness of the response to the pandemic. According to a recent publication by Saluja (2023) in the Times of India, the COVID-19 pandemic has starkly revealed substantial disparities in this field.

DOI: 10.4018/978-1-7998-9652-4.ch002

Individuals with restricted knowledge in this domain face obstacles in grasping essential health-related information. This lack of awareness leads to a state of ignorance regarding preventive measures, making individuals more vulnerable to infection. Several factors contribute to the reduced comprehension of health matters among individuals, including a heavy reliance on traditional healing practices, high levels of illiteracy, limited access to healthcare, inadequate dissemination of health awareness initiatives in rural areas, and a widespread lack of knowledge. It is crucial to emphasise that the global pandemic has exacerbated these challenges, and the spread of misinformation and conspiracy theories has further complicated matters.

This study is motivated by the pressing recognition of the intricate interplay between health knowledge and the COVID-19 pandemic in the Indian context. Competence in health has been established as a well-documented determinant of health outcomes, and its significance has been especially highlighted during the pandemic, particularly in a diverse and dynamic nation like India. The significant disparities across various regions have exposed the vulnerabilities of specific populations and underscored the importance of targeted interventions during public health crises. Furthermore, this study aims to integrate contemporary knowledge and incorporate a range of case studies to provide a nuanced and comprehensive understanding of the complex challenges posed by limited health awareness in India during the COVID-19 pandemic. The objectives of this study are as follows:

- To Illuminate the Role of Health Knowledge: This study seeks to elucidate the consequences of deficiencies in health-related knowledge on public health understanding, vaccine acceptance, healthcare accessibility, and the overall effectiveness of the pandemic response.
- To Investigate Regional Disparities: It aims to delineate how health illiteracy manifests in urban areas, rural regions, and tribal populations by examining case studies from diverse contexts. This investigation will enhance understanding of the intersection between health-related knowledge and geographical disparities within the context of the pandemic.
- To Propose Practical Insights and Solutions: This involves not only the current pandemic situation but also the strengthening of public health preparedness. The objective of this study is to analyze experiences from diverse locations and offer evidence-based techniques and solutions that can empower individuals to make informed health decisions by providing them with essential information and skills.
- To Contribute to Public Health Resilience: The objective is to advocate for a fair and informed approach to the diverse health challenges that India may face in the future, addressing gaps in knowledge. This aligns with the

overarching goal of improving public health outcomes and preparedness in the face of increasing health crises.

To achieve these objectives, this paper is structured into four distinct sections. Section 2 conducts a comprehensive review of the existing body of research on health-related knowledge and its relevance in the field of public health. This section emphasizes the importance of health awareness in the context of the ongoing pandemic. In Section 3, the article outlines the research methodology, highlighting the use of case studies to gain in-depth insights into the impact of health awareness in various regions of India. It further elaborates on the reasons for choosing this research approach. Section 4 serves as a platform within the study to conduct a comparative analysis of the case surveys. This investigation aims to identify commonalities and recurring trends in the consequences of limited health awareness.

2. LITERATURE REVIEW

The concept of health consciousness is complex and diverse, extending beyond an individual's basic understanding of health information. It encompasses an individual's capacity to grasp, evaluate, and employ health-related knowledge to make well-informed choices regarding their overall state of welfare. The study conducted by Kumar in 2019 brought to light a significant worry regarding the level of health knowledge in India. It was observed that a substantial proportion, around 90%, of the country's population had weaknesses in this crucial area. It is imperative to underscore the fact that India has substantial issues with pervasive illiteracy and profound poverty, both of which exert a deleterious influence on health literacy. Indeed, a considerable segment of the populace may face financial limitations when it comes to obtaining crucial healthcare services and prescriptions, despite possessing the necessary financial resources to cover expenses related to transportation. The insufficiency of health insurance coverage in India can be attributed to a lack of comprehensive understanding, as indicated by Neelima et al. (2018). Despite an observable rise in the prevalence of insurance coverage among the populace over the previous five-year period, a significant discrepancy in the distribution of said coverage continues to exist throughout the country, with rural regions shouldering an inequitable share of this burden. The findings of the fifth phase of the National Family Health Survey (NFHS) highlight that, except in Andhra Pradesh, Telangana, Assam, and Kerala, a significant proportion of citizens in most states and Union Territories have limited access to a comprehensive health safety net, with coverage rates falling below 50% (Nankani, 2022). As a result, the healthcare system in India is confronted with substantial dangers that hurt the health and overall welfare of the population.

It is imperative to acknowledge that there is a significant dearth of comprehensive countrywide research within the Indian context about the thorough assessment of health consciousness. However, several independent research regularly demonstrates deficiencies in health literacy and understanding among persons of Indian descent, hence impacting their capacity to make educated decisions. In a recent study done by Nankani (2022), a notable proportion of patients diagnosed with ovarian cancer had limited pre-existing knowledge and comprehension of the disease. More than two-thirds of the participants had a significant lack of knowledge of ovarian cancer. Moreover, as indicated in the research, a survey conducted in 2016 among adult persons seeking oral health treatments at a private clinic in Bengaluru revealed that over 65% of patients exhibited poor knowledge regarding preventative oral care and dental hygiene services. Nankani (2022) cites research conducted in 2015 that examines disease-specific literacy among the Saharia tribe dwelling in Central India. The findings indicate that around 50% of the participants possessed little understanding of the incidence of TB. The results highlight the extensive consequences of inadequate health awareness in India, surpassing factors such as gender, socioeconomic position, and geographical location. Although there may be disparities across different demographic groups, a considerable portion of the population exhibits a limited grasp of their health status and the essential steps required for its enhancement.

The significance of understanding and utilizing health-related knowledge has been prominently highlighted within the context of the COVID-19 pandemic, an era characterized by the emergence of a global health crisis (Abel & Mcqueen, 2020; Sentell et al., 2020). The worldwide spread of the COVID-19 virus has not only exposed the lack of readiness of governments, healthcare systems, and social support networks to effectively respond to the evolving health needs of the population but has also introduced substantial challenges for governments, organizations, and individuals alike (Duan et al., 2020; Nguyen et al., 2020; Rosenbaum, 2020). To address this, the World Health Organization (WHO) and many countries have established communication platforms to disseminate information to educate the public about COVID-19 symptoms, preventative measures, and authoritative sources for the latest guidance. Unfortunately, the proliferation of false information, deliberate spread of misinformation, and harmful content through social media and mainstream media have worsened the impact of the COVID-19 pandemic on the general population (Naeem et al., 2020). These circumstances have not only created fear among the broader population but have also posed unprecedented challenges for health education and healthcare systems (Nguyen et al., 2020).

Recognizing the importance of being well-informed about health is crucial for improving healthcare quality, promoting healthy behaviours, enhancing overall well-being, instilling health-protective actions, and reducing health disparities. A healthy environment not only facilitates the achievement of health-related goals but also improves healthcare outcomes, reduces financial burdens, and eases the strain on healthcare infrastructure. Existing research indicates that individuals with limited health knowledge are more likely to experience suboptimal health outcomes. These individuals have a reduced inclination to engage in preventative measures, make increased use of healthcare services, and may unintentionally take inappropriate medications, leading to hospitalization and morbidity. Furthermore, a direct connection between limited health knowledge and increased hospitalization costs, elevated mortality rates, and a decreased quality of life is evident.

Seng et al. (2020) conducted a comprehensive investigation of the phenomenon of health consciousness in the context of pandemics, which is considered a key research in the field. The results of their study indicated suboptimal levels of health consciousness among both healthcare professionals and the general population. The primary objective of this study was to gather data about symptoms, mechanisms of viral transmission, concerns connected to infection, and preventative measures, including the use of masks and strict adherence to hand hygiene practices. In the Indian environment, particularly in rural regions, the response to the COVID-19 pandemic is significantly influenced by insufficient health knowledge, which is further exacerbated by challenges in adhering to preventative measures. Individuals with restricted comprehension may struggle to grasp the subtleties associated with behaviours such as the utilisation of masks, adherence to hand hygiene practises, and the maintenance of physical separation. Rural regions, which are defined by their limited resources and infrastructure, encounter increased challenges in achieving compliance as a result of many variables such as high population density, inadequate access to clean water, and substandard sanitation facilities. As a result, these regions exhibit increased susceptibility to the occurrence of outbreaks and the spread of viral infections. Moreover, individuals residing in rural areas consistently have difficulties associated with the inadequate availability of healthcare facilities, and their low awareness might further intensify their difficulties in acknowledging the significance of accessing healthcare services. Community health workers, with specialised knowledge of local languages and cultural intricacies, assume a crucial function in the efficient dissemination of comprehensible information and enhancement of healthcare service accessibility, whenever they are present.

Bazua et al. (2021) conducted an investigation and found that a considerable proportion of persons residing in rural Odisha had little understanding of COVID-19 symptoms, high-risk demographic categories, and the aetiology of the illness. This highlights the necessity for accurate and focused educational outreach initiatives, specifically aimed at demographic cohorts with less awareness, such as women and young persons who assume caregiving responsibilities. These initiatives may encompass tactics for engaging with these groups through door-to-door interactions, which are considered the most effective method of connection. Individuals who engage with social media, the internet, and conventional media platforms are more inclined to hold a greater understanding of high-risk groups and the underlying causes of diseases. This implies the potential advantages of educational initiatives offered by organisations such as Anganwadi and ASHA workers. The present study is of considerable importance within the contemporary environment, as it offers significant insights into the effects of health awareness initiatives in rural regions of India during the COVID-19 pandemic. This research endeavour effectively fills a preexisting void in the academic literature. Gaining a comprehensive understanding of the impact of health consciousness on individual behaviour, access to healthcare, and disease transmission within rural communities is of utmost importance to devising efficacious treatments and formulating well-informed policy choices. The objective of this research endeavour is to offer evidence-based strategies for improving the implementation of health service and health education initiatives. The overarching objective is to mitigate discrepancies and foster parity in health outcomes. The use of community health practitioners and the construction of health education initiatives that are culturally suitable serve to enhance community engagement, foster trust, and encourage empowerment. This study surpasses the constraints given by the pandemic, providing useful insights that are advantageous for long-term public health strategizing and the enhancement of community resilience in the presence of diverse health hazards.

3. METHODOLOGY

The methodology utilised in this study is carefully crafted to offer a thorough comprehension of the crucial significance of health knowledge in influencing India's approach to the COVID-19 epidemic. As we go further into our research technique, we investigate the complex correlation between health knowledge and the repercussions of the pandemic, with a specific emphasis on rural environments. The research technique employed in our study is specifically designed to comprehensively capture the many subtleties associated with health knowledge issues across a range of varied cultures. The study employs a qualitative research methodology and adopts numerous case study techniques. This approach facilitates a comprehensive exploration of health knowledge concerns in various geographical areas, providing the chance to do cross-case analysis and derive meaningful comparisons. Now, let us proceed to examine the methodological framework, first with the crucial aspect of selecting case studies.

3.1 Research Design: Selection of Case Studies

The research design used in this study is qualitative with a concentration on several case studies. The qualitative methodology is highly appropriate for acquiring a comprehensive understanding of the intricacies of health intelligence and its significance within the framework of the COVID-19 epidemic in rural India. The utilisation of many case studies facilitates a comprehensive examination of the subject matter, enabling the researcher to conduct cross-case analysis to establish significant parallels and find overarching trends. Three different rural districts were chosen as the case study locations to fully investigate the impact of health intelligence in rural India's pandemic response. The selection of these areas was carefully made to encompass a wide range of difficulties and features. The first case study investigates the obstacles encountered in a predominantly agrarian area situated in northern India, specifically focusing on rural Rajasthan. It explores the effects of inadequate awareness on individuals' health-seeking behaviours, the spread of disinformation, and comprehension. The topic of discussion pertains to the COVID-19 pandemic. The choice of Rural Rajasthan is intended to represent areas in which there may be limited availability of health services, hence highlighting the problems related to accessing health. The second case study is based on urban areas of Mumbai slums. Despite their urban classification, some slum districts in Mumbai exhibit resemblances to rural regions, including the presence of low-income residents, language variety, and constrained availability of high-quality health facilities. This particular environment offers significant perspectives on the health literacy encountered by persons residing in metropolitan areas that resemble rural situations. The third case study examines the challenges prevalent among indigenous tribal people residing in the state of Madhya Pradesh. The aforementioned settlements exhibit notable traits such as a wide range of languages spoken, geographical seclusion, and unique cultural customs. It is crucial to comprehend the problems in these distinct contexts to effectively tackle health inequalities.

3.2 Data Collection Methods

The research will involve the use of a standardised survey tool to evaluate the knowledge related to the health of people residing in each respective case study location. The survey included inquiries about the understanding of COVID-19, awareness of vaccinations, and sources of information. It aims to assess the dimensions of functional, interactive, and critical health understanding. In addition to collecting demographic information, the survey aims to ascertain the impact of variables such as educational attainment, age, and socioeconomic standing. The research methodology will further involve the use of in-depth interviews with key informants, encompassing health practitioners, community health workers, and local leaders. The primary objective of these interviews is to offer valuable perspectives on the difficulties encountered and approaches adopted in tackling health education concerns within the designated regions of the case study. Additionally, the authors investigate the significance of community participation and culturally responsive health education programmes in the dissemination of information and the facilitation of health access. The analysis will focus on documents about the COVID-19 pandemic, including instructional materials, booklets, posters, and local public health messages. The objective of this document analysis is to evaluate the level of clarity, ease of comprehension, and cultural appropriateness of the health-related information that is being disseminated to rural communities.

The data obtained through surveys, interviews, document analysis, and observations will be subjected to a thorough and rigorous analytical process. The analysis will utilise a combination of quantitative and qualitative methodologies. The survey results will undergo quantitative analysis to discover and examine trends and patterns in health knowledge levels. The data collected from interviews and observations will undergo thematic coding to uncover significant themes and gain insights into the problems of health literacy and the tactics used to tackle them. It is important to mention here that the investigation was done with rigorous ethical principles. All survey participants and interviewers have provided informed consent, indicating their comprehensive comprehension of the research's objectives and the intended use of their data. Anonymity and confidentiality were upheld for all participants. The research adhered to all pertinent ethical protocols.

4. CASE STUDIES

The impact of health literacy transcended geographic and demographic boundaries, thus delineating distinctive narratives of the COVID-19 pandemic within the Indian context. This research endeavours to delve into the intricate role of health literacy in three distinct locales, namely Rural Rajasthan, Urban Mumbai Slums, and Tribal Communities in Madhya Pradesh, employing a case study-centred analytical approach. This analysis will illuminate the manifold facets of the mentioned in these environments, particularly in the context of the ongoing pandemic. Each of these settings offers a unique vantage point for scrutinizing the repercussions of deficient education on information dissemination, vaccine acceptance, access to health resources, and comprehension of vaccine-related information. A closer examination of select cases from our studies will facilitate a deeper comprehension:

Case Study 1

The rural expanse of Rajasthan, characterized by remote villages and limited health infrastructure, confronted substantial challenges during the COVID-19 pandemic. The absence of robust health facilities and the logistical difficulties of reaching health resources posed formidable barriers to health accessibility.

Challenges in Health Literacy:

- Deciphering COVID-19 Symptoms: A considerable segment of the population in this region grappled with limited health awareness, leading to difficulties in identifying COVID-19 symptoms. Many residents struggled to differentiate between commonplace maladies and potential COVID-19 symptoms. This dearth of symptom awareness resulted in delayed testing and potential viral transmission.
- Accessing Health Information: Owing to constrained digital access and educational resources, residents encountered impediments in acquiring accurate and current pandemic-related information. Misinformation and misconceptions often prevailed, impeding the promotion of effective preventive measures.
- Digital Literacy Obstacle: The introduction of mobile health units brought to light the challenges faced by some residents in utilizing digital applications for appointments and health information. Navigating this technology proved daunting for them, underscoring the digital divide's influence on health understanding.

In response to these challenges, local health workers and non-governmental organizations (NGOs) recognized the issue and initiated community health awareness programs. These initiatives encompassed educating villagers about recognizing COVID-19 symptoms, the importance of early testing, and the establishment of a local support network for emergencies. This resulted in earlier testing, diminished viral transmission, and improved health-seeking behaviour, contributing to a more effective pandemic response. This case study underscores the pivotal role of health literacy in bolstering health access and responsiveness during crises.

Case Study 2

The densely populated slums of Mumbai, characterized by cramped living conditions and limited access to quality health, confronted exacerbated challenges during the COVID-19 pandemic. Many residents encountered difficulties in comprehending and implementing fundamental preventive measures, such as mask usage, hand hygiene, and physical distancing. These challenges substantially elevated their vulnerability to the virus.

Health Literacy Challenges:

- Misuse of Masks: In numerous instances, community health workers observed residents wearing masks incorrectly. Some individuals would wear masks below their noses or leave them hanging from one ear, mistakenly believing this practice to be sufficient. This erroneous usage stemmed from a lack of awareness regarding the correct method of mask-wearing and the pivotal role of masks in preventing viral transmission.
- Misconceptions Regarding Hand Hygiene: General awareness issues surfaced in residents' hand hygiene practices. Some believed that merely rinsing their hands with water sufficed, disregarding the significance of soap and thorough handwashing. Others remained unaware of the recommended frequency for handwashing, a particularly vital aspect in crowded living conditions.
- Challenges in Maintaining Physical Distancing: Upholding physical distancing presented challenges within the tightly-knit slum communities. Many residents did not fully comprehend the concept of physical distancing and its role in curbing transmission. Constrained living spaces and shared facilities further exacerbated adherence to these measures.

Recognizing these issues, local NGOs and community organizations implemented health literacy programs tailored to the specific needs of the slum residents. These programs employed simple, culturally relevant messaging and visual aids to educate residents about COVID-19 preventive measures. This case study exemplifies how local interventions and culturally sensitive health awareness programs effectively addressed the challenges in understanding and implementing COVID-19 preventive measures within urban Mumbai slum communities. These endeavours played a pivotal role in enhancing health literacy and diminishing residents' susceptibility to the virus.

These illustrative case studies laid the groundwork for an exhaustive survey encompassing 135 participants, distributed evenly across these three states. The survey was conceived in response to these real-world challenges, to systematically appraise the state of health knowledge and its ramifications on COVID-19 responses.

By encompassing participants from these diverse regions, the survey sought to capture a comprehensive understanding of the multifaceted impact it has on information dissemination, vaccine acceptance, health access, and the overall response to the pandemic, bridging the chasm between vivid case studies and empirical research.

4.1 Survey Questionnaire

The survey questionnaire used in this research was designed to capture critical insights into this field of health and its impact on responses to the COVID-19 pandemic in diverse regions of India. The questionnaire encompassed a range of questions tailored to the unique challenges faced in the case study settings of Rural Rajasthan, Urban Mumbai Slums, and Tribal Communities in Madhya Pradesh. The key sections of the survey included:

- Demographic Information: Participants were asked to provide basic demographic information, such as age, gender, education level, occupation, and household size.
- Health Awareness Assessment: Questions in this section aimed to evaluate respondents' ability to understand and interpret health-related information, including COVID-19 guidelines, symptoms, and vaccine-related instructions.
- Access to Health Services: This section focused on participants' experiences in accessing health services during the pandemic, with questions addressing factors like distance to health facilities, digital access for telemedicine, and challenges faced in seeking health care.
- COVID-19 Knowledge and Beliefs: Participants were asked about their knowledge of COVID-19, including preventive measures and the importance of vaccination. The questionnaire also explored participants' beliefs and perceptions about the virus and the vaccine.
- Mistrust in the Health System: This section sought to understand the level of trust or mistrust participants had in the health system and health providers, exploring whether past experiences and health literacy played a role in shaping their perceptions.
- Cultural and Linguistic Factors: Given the diverse linguistic and cultural settings of the case studies, the survey included questions about the influence of local culture, traditions, and language on health decisions.
- Impact of Regional Disparities: Questions in this section were designed to assess how regional disparities affected access to health and the overall pandemic response in the case study regions.

The survey was administered to a total of 135 participants, with an equal distribution of respondents in each of the three case study regions. The data collected through this comprehensive questionnaire provided valuable insights into the multifaceted impact of health education on the COVID-19 pandemic, highlighting how it influenced information dissemination, vaccine acceptance, access to health services, and the overall understanding and response to the pandemic in India's diverse settings.

4.2 Survey Summary and Result

The COVID-19 epidemic presented significant obstacles in the context of inadequate knowledge in the dry rural landscapes of Rajasthan. The impact of the lack of understanding and awareness on the progression of the pandemic has been significant in areas where access to high-quality education and health services is limited. The importance of insufficient health literacy became notably evident in the dissemination of information. The proliferation of misconceptions and superstitions among locals resulted in a belief that traditional cures or religious rites may protect against the virus. Consequently, this led to a delay in the implementation of testing and treatment measures. Moreover, the aforementioned geographical area faced significant challenges due to a deep-seated lack of confidence in the health system, hence exacerbating the difficulties in properly disseminating crucial information. The investigation into rural Rajasthan reveals the serious effects of poor health education, emphasising the urgent need for community engagement initiatives and targeted health education interventions in areas with limited access to formal education and health facilities. In the context of our second case study, located among the densely populated and dynamic slums of Mumbai, the impact of health literacy on the COVID-19 outbreak exhibited distinct characteristics. While the urban population enjoyed somewhat improved educational opportunities in comparison to their rural counterparts, the challenges were further exacerbated by the densely populated metropolitan environment. The proliferation of inaccurate information has contributed to the phenomenon of vaccination hesitancy and inconsistent compliance with preventative measures. The issue of digital literacy has presented hurdles for people in enrolling for vaccinations online since many individuals struggle to comprehend complicated health communications. This investigation provides valuable insights into the significant importance of community-oriented health education initiatives, the streamlining of health procedures, and the strategic use of technology to engage with inhabitants efficiently. The urban population has several obstacles that emphasise the necessity of implementing customised solutions to tackle health illiteracy in densely populated areas. As we continue along this similar route and approach our third case study, we see that the tribal people of Madhya Pradesh present distinctive difficulties because of their isolation from the outside world, linguistic diversity, and reliance on traditional treatment modalities. The impact of health literacy on the COVID-19 outbreak in this particular area was especially substantial. The understanding of the virus was hindered by insufficient health knowledge throughout the pandemic, hence posing challenges in differentiating COVID-19 from other illnesses. The impact of traditional beliefs and local dialects on health-seeking behaviour was substantial, as it added to the intricacy of testing and vaccination programmes owing to distrust towards foreign entities and the health system.

The case studies listed above offer a thorough comprehension of the intricate characteristics of health illiteracy, highlighting the necessity for customised and situation-specific approaches to successfully tackle this matter in the field of public health. The subsequent section will now centre on the results of these investigations, which will provide a comprehensive understanding of the consequences of health illiteracy on India's response to the pandemic and offer useful insights on how to mitigate this dilemma. The result is as follows:

1. Health Literacy Assessment:
    - In Urban Mumbai Slums, 45% of respondents demonstrated difficulty in understanding and interpreting COVID-19-related health information. This was notably higher than in Rural Rajasthan (30%) and Tribal Communities in MP (35%).
    - Around 70% of respondents in all three regions struggled with comprehending complex vaccine-related instructions.
2. Access to Health Services:
    - In Rural Rajasthan, 60% of participants reported that they faced challenges in accessing health services due to the distance to health facilities. In Urban Mumbai Slums and Tribal Communities in MP, this figure was lower at 40% and 45%, respectively.
    - Digital access to telemedicine was significantly limited in Rural Rajasthan, where only 20% had access, whereas it was more accessible in Urban Mumbai Slums (45%) and Tribal Communities in MP (30%).
3. COVID-19 Knowledge and Beliefs:
    - In all three regions, a substantial majority (around 80%) of respondents displayed a solid understanding of COVID-19 symptoms and preventive measures.
    - Approximately 70% of participants believed that COVID-19 vaccines were effective and necessary in Rural Rajasthan and Tribal Communities in MP, while this percentage was higher at 85% in Urban Mumbai Slums.
4. Mistrust in the Health System:

  - The mistrust in the health system was pronounced in all regions but highest in Urban Mumbai Slums, with 65% of participants expressing concerns about the health system's integrity.
  - Rural Rajasthan and Tribal Communities in MP showed lower levels of mistrust at 50% and 45%, respectively.
5. Cultural and Linguistic Factors:
  - In Rural Rajasthan, 70% of respondents highlighted the influence of local traditions and culture on health decisions.
  - Cultural and linguistic factors played a significant role in Tribal Communities in MP (75%), while this influence was somewhat lower in Urban Mumbai Slums (60%).
6. Impact of Regional Disparities:
  - The impact of regional disparities was particularly pronounced in Tribal Communities in MP, with 65% of participants citing significant challenges in health access due to their remote geographical location.
  - In Rural Rajasthan, 55% reported experiencing such challenges, whereas Urban Mumbai Slums saw the lowest percentage at 40%.

These results provide valuable insights into the influence of health knowledge on the response to the COVID-19 pandemic in different regions of India. Notably, they illustrate the diverse challenges faced by respondents, including difficulties in understanding health information, limited access to health services, variations in vaccine acceptance and hesitancy, mistrust in the health system, the impact of cultural and linguistic factors, and the pronounced effects of regional disparities. These findings underscore the importance of tailored strategies and interventions to address health illiteracy in each of these regions and offer valuable considerations for policymakers and health providers. The results emphasize the need for a nuanced approach to public health preparedness and promotion, taking into account the unique challenges faced by diverse populations during public health crises like the COVID-19 pandemic.

5. DISCUSSION

The discussion component of this study examines and compares the case studies, focusing on identifying trends and similarities in the effects of health illiteracy across various areas. Additionally, this section offers policy implications and suggestions based on the findings. This highlights the need to implement customised health education and communication tactics to successfully combat health illiteracy in times of public health emergencies like as the COVID-19 epidemic. The findings reported in this research study demonstrate a thorough and nuanced comprehension of the influence of health awareness on the reaction to the COVID-19 epidemic throughout various areas of India. The respondents encountered a range of challenges that highlight the complex connection between health literacy and pandemic response. These challenges include disparities in literacy levels, limited health access, mistrust in the health system, the impact of cultural and linguistic factors, and the pronounced effects of regional disparities. The aforementioned findings offer significant contributions to the field of public health preparedness and emphasise the crucial nature of interventions and methods tailored to specific regions to effectively combat health illiteracy.

5.1 Comparative Analysis of the Case Studies

The comparative study of the case studies reveals important trends and connections between how health illiteracy affects the COVID-19 pandemic response in various Indian regions. Although there are differences in literacy levels related to health across various locations, the results consistently highlight common patterns that surpass regional borders. It is worth noting that respondents from all areas demonstrate a consistent and strong comprehension of COVID-19 symptoms and preventative actions. This indicates the effectiveness of public health initiatives in effectively distributing essential knowledge. Nonetheless, a common issue arises within the domain of vaccine literacy, since almost 70% of respondents in every location face challenges in understanding complex instructions about vaccines. The aforementioned collective obstacle underscores the imperative nature of employing concise, comprehensible, and geographically tailored communication tactics to tackle vaccine hesitancy, considering the pivotal significance of immunisation in managing pandemics. Furthermore, a prevalent and persistent motif across society is the lack of faith in the health system. While the degrees of distrust may vary, it is noteworthy that Urban Mumbai Slums have the highest recorded level at 65%. Nonetheless, it is important to recognise that this issue is pervasive across all areas. Elevated distrust in urban areas may be attributed to the complexity of health services and unpleasant prior experiences. On the other hand, rural and tribal regions, characterised by relatively lower levels of distrust, may possess distinct motivations for apprehensions regarding trust. The process of addressing and resolving this lack of trust necessitates the use of tactics that foster openness, active involvement of the community, and the redressal of past injustices.

Cultural and linguistic characteristics continually have an influence over health decisions throughout all regions. The significance of culturally responsive health education is emphasised in several contexts, such as local customs and culture in Rural Rajasthan, cultural and linguistic elements in Tribal Communities in

MP, and to a somewhat lesser level in Urban Mumbai Slums. These programmes must demonstrate due regard for and integration of local customs and languages, therefore functioning as important instruments for actively involving communities and augmenting health literacy. The discernible influence of geographical variations on health accessibility is likewise evident. Tribal communities in Madhya Pradesh have significant obstacles in terms of accessing resources and services, mostly owing to their distant geographical locations. Similar difficulties are observed in rural Rajasthan, although urban Mumbai slums exhibit the lowest rate. The necessity to address these discrepancies in health accessibility is apparent, underscoring the requirement for focused initiatives, particularly in geographically isolated and disadvantaged regions. The importance of tailoring health awareness approaches to specific regions is emphasised in this comprehensive comparative analysis. It recognises the complex interactions that influence health education and emphasises the need for flexible and nuanced public health policies and interventions. This is crucial to ensure that diverse populations have the necessary skills and knowledge to effectively navigate public health emergencies such as the COVID-19 pandemic.

5.2 Policy Implications and Recommendations

At this point, the integration of health literacy theories plays a crucial role in developing customized solutions and recommendations. The Health Belief Model (HBM), a significant theory proposed by Hochbaum & Rosenstock, (1952), suggests that individuals are more likely to adopt health-related behaviours when they perceive susceptibility to a specific health issue and believe that suggested actions will mitigate the threat. In our study, the HBM guides our understanding of participants' perceptions regarding susceptibility to COVID-19 and the effectiveness of recommended preventive measures. The case study in urban Mumbai slums, where residents faced challenges in understanding and implementing preventive measures, aligns with the HBM. It underscores the need for interventions addressing residents' perceived susceptibility, emphasizing proper mask usage, hand hygiene, and physical distancing to reduce vulnerability to the virus. Solutions influenced by the HBM stress personalized health communication to enhance participants' perceived susceptibility and efficacy. Additionally, Ajzen (1991)'s Theory of Planned Behaviour (TPB) contributes by emphasizing attitudes, subjective norms, and perceived behavioural control in shaping health-related behaviours. In the rural Rajasthan case study with limited healthcare access, the TPB informs discussions on attitudes toward seeking healthcare, societal norm influences on healthcare decisions, and individuals' perceived control over accessing medical services. TPB-derived solutions emphasize community-driven initiatives to reshape societal norms, promote positive attitudes toward healthcare-seeking behaviour, and enhance perceived control over accessing medical care. The survey's focus on culturally sensitive health education programs aligns with the Cultural Competence Model (Bauce 2014), emphasizing tailoring healthcare practices to individuals' cultural backgrounds. The Tribal Communities case study in Madhya Pradesh, where cultural factors influenced healthcare decisions, resonates with this model. The discussion advocates for culturally sensitive interventions, leveraging local influencers, and incorporating traditional beliefs into health education programs. Case study results on how health illiteracy impacted the COVID-19 response in diverse parts of India offer valuable insights for targeted policy actions. Implementing these strategies is vital for effectively addressing the intricate challenges posed by health illiteracy during public health emergencies. Within this realm, we will present a thorough examination of policy implications and suggestions derived from the principal results.

(i) Restoring Trust in the Health System: The observed disparities in levels of distrust across various geographical areas underscore the imperative for implementing targeted interventions aimed at restoring trust in the health system. In areas characterised by a pervasive lack of trust, it is imperative to give precedence to endeavours that aim to reinstate confidence. There is a need to augment transparency to guarantee that communities are adequately informed about health practices, policies, and decision-making processes. The provision of transparent information should encompass the elucidation of the underlying reasoning behind health determinations. Enhancing transparency may be achieved by implementing consistent channels of communication and feedback, which enable individuals to express their apprehensions and obtain justifications for health-related determinations. Moreover, the involvement of the community plays a crucial role in the process of restoring confidence. By engaging community leaders, local legislators, and esteemed individuals, health choices may be reached through collaborative efforts with the community, therefore cultivating a feeling of ownership towards health services. When mistrust arises due to historical grievances or poor past experiences, it is crucial to address these issues, provide compensation, and acknowledge previous injustices to restore confidence.

(ii) Culturally Sensitive Health Education Initiatives: The effect of cultural and linguistic elements on health decisions has been consistently documented across all investigated locations. To adequately respond to this impact, it is imperative to advocate for the promotion of health education efforts that are culturally responsive. These efforts are formulated to recognise, value, and incorporate indigenous customs and rituals within health educational curricula. The inclusion of local languages and dialects is of utmost importance to facilitate the accessibility and comprehensibility of health information within the community. Furthermore, the use of community leaders and local influencers within these places may greatly augment the efficacy of health communication. These individuals are frequently held in high regard and enjoy the trust of the community, rendering them influential conveyors of health-related information. The engagement of community leaders can facilitate the bridging of cultural and linguistic divides, thus enhancing the community's ability to relate to and perceive the information as trustworthy.

(iii) Addressing Inequities in Health Access: The results of the study emphasise that geographical differences have a substantial impact on individuals' access to health services. The issue of access problems is particularly evident in geographically isolated and underdeveloped regions. To mitigate these discrepancies, policymakers must provide priority to efforts that are specifically designed to diminish these gaps and guarantee equal access to health services. One proposed approach entails the expansion of telemedicine services, which facilitate rural and underprivileged populations' access to health consultations through digital means. This method not only addresses geographical limitations but also capitalises on the increasing adoption of digital technology in India. By implementing measures to improve telemedicine services and expanding their availability to remote areas, health consultations and the dissemination of information may be conducted with more efficiency and timeliness. Furthermore, it is imperative to enhance the physical health infrastructure in these places. This involves the establishment and ongoing management of additional health institutions and clinics. The proximity of physical health infrastructure to local populations can effectively mitigate obstacles to health accessibility, hence enhancing the reach and responsiveness of health services.

(iv) Community Engagement: Community participation plays a crucial role in tackling health illiteracy and fostering community resilience in the face of public health emergencies. Promoting active engagement of the community in health decision-making and pandemic response has the potential to augment and cultivate a collective feeling of community ownership over matters of public health. It is imperative for policymakers to actively promote and support community involvement through a range of strategies and mechanisms. The implementation of community health worker programmes has demonstrated significant efficacy. These workers function as community-based spokespeople who effectively communicate health-related information to local populations, hence facilitating the connection between health practitioners and community members. Outreach programmes can also assume a pivotal function in effectively engaging populations who have restricted availability of health services. These projects have the potential to disseminate information, give assistance, and promote the adoption of health-seeking behaviour. Furthermore, the utilisation of local community leaders and influencers has the potential to augment community participation. These individuals have the potential to serve as exemplars, instructors, and champions for health-related endeavours, so fostering greater community engagement and acceptance of public health interventions.

(v) The practice of continuous monitoring and evaluation: To enhance the effectiveness of public health awareness initiatives, it is advisable to incorporate continuous monitoring and evaluation techniques. Decision-makers should establish a systematic framework for appraising the impacts of health education efforts. Regular evaluations can yield valuable insights into the performance of various programs and help pinpoint areas that require enhancements. Policymakers can enrich their strategies with data-informed decision-making, scrutinizing literacy rates, vaccination adoption, and community engagement. Additionally, gathering feedback from communities and participants can contribute to shaping future projects promoting health awareness that better aligns with the evolving needs of the population.

These concepts underscore the ever-evolving nature of promoting awareness in the context of the COVID-19 pandemic and its potential implications. A comprehensive plan for public health should encompass several vital components, such as the digitalization of health information, the engagement of community-based health advocates, the adoption of collaborative strategies involving multiple agencies, the establishment of continuous monitoring and assessment mechanisms, and the dissemination of inclusive information. By incorporating these recommendations, decision-makers can effectively respond to the changing dynamics of public health, fostering robust initiatives that are equitable and accessible to all segments of society.

6. CONCLUSION

This in-depth study presents a comprehensive and multifaceted understanding of how the ability to comprehend and utilize health information plays a crucial role in shaping responses to the COVID-19 pandemic in various regions of India. The findings uncover a complex interplay of factors, both common and unique, contributing to the intricate landscape of preparedness in public health. While there is a reasonably strong understanding of COVID-19 symptoms and preventive measures across regions, the challenge of effectively conveying information about vaccines emerges as a substantial hurdle. It necessitates the development of clear, accessible, and region-specific communication strategies tailored to the informational needs of each community. The prevailing lack of trust in the healthcare system, though varying in intensity, underscores the urgent need for interventions designed to rebuild trust through transparency, community engagement, and addressing region-specific concerns. Cultural and linguistic factors consistently influence health decisions, underscoring the critical importance of culturally sensitive health education initiatives that respect and incorporate local practices and languages. Moreover, the profound impact of regional disparities on health access emphasizes the urgency of targeted interventions to ensure equitable access to health services, especially in remote and underserved areas. These findings offer valuable insights for policymakers, health providers, and public health practitioners, highlighting the importance of customized health education and communication strategies to address the unique and multifaceted challenges faced by diverse populations during public health crises. As we navigate the ongoing complexities of the COVID-19 pandemic and prepare for future public health emergencies, it is crucial to emphasize the role of health information comprehension in promoting better health outcomes and building a more resilient healthcare system.

While it has yielded substantial insights into the relationship between understanding health information and responding to the COVID-19 pandemic in India, it's essential to acknowledge certain limitations. The study primarily focused on three distinct regions: Urban Mumbai Slums, Rural Rajasthan, and Tribal Communities in MP. While these regions were selected for their diverse characteristics, India's vast geographic and demographic diversity suggests that a more extensive representation of regions could yield even more comprehensive findings. Therefore, the conclusions drawn may not universally apply to all of India's varied contexts. Additionally, the cross-sectional approach used in this study provides insights about health information comprehension and related responses within a specific timeframe, but a longitudinal or cohort research approach could offer valuable insights into the development of health information comprehension and its influence on pandemic responses over time. This study examined the topic of health information comprehension and its outcomes but did not comprehensively investigate the socioeconomic factors that may impact an individual's health information comprehension. Future research may delve more deeply into these variables and their interaction with health information comprehension.

The primary focus of this study centred on examining individuals' knowledge and attitudes regarding COVID-19 and health services. To provide a more comprehensive view of the impact of health information comprehension on health outcomes during a pandemic, future studies may employ more comprehensive outcome measures, such as health-seeking behaviour. Nevertheless, this study opens up several avenues for future research and exploration. Expanding the research to encompass a more diverse array of regions and demographic groups would contribute to a more comprehensive understanding of how health information comprehension impacts pandemic responses in India. Different regions and communities may present distinct challenges and opportunities, and a broader perspective would allow for more nuanced insights. Furthermore, future research could delve deeper into the complexities of vaccine hesitancy, examining the underlying reasons and barriers contributing to hesitancy in various regions. This approach would enable the development of more targeted strategies to effectively address vaccine-related concerns. Exploring the role of local leaders and community engagement in promoting health information comprehension and encouraging health-seeking behaviours is another promising area of study. Assessing the influence and effectiveness of local leadership and community-based initiatives can provide valuable insights into successful approaches for enhancing health information comprehension in diverse communities. Finally, the ongoing COVID-19 pandemic has underscored the need for proactive public health preparedness. Future research can expand on this by exploring how interventions to improve health information comprehension can be integrated into public health policies and strategies to enhance overall preparedness for public health crises.

REFERENCES

Abel, T., & Mcqueen, D. (2020). Critical health literacy and the COVID-19 crisis. *Health Promotion International*, *35*(6), 1612–1613. doi:10.1093/heapro/daaa040 PMID:32239213

Ajzen, I. (1991). The theory of planned behavior. *Organizational Behavior and Human Decision Processes*, *50*(2), 179–211. doi:10.1016/0749-5978(91)90020-T

Baker, D. W., Gazmararian, J. A., Williams, M. V., Scott, T., Parker, R. M., Green, D., Ren, J., & Peel, J. (2002). Functional health literacy and the risk of hospital admission among Medicare managed care enrollees. *American Journal of Public Health*, *92*(8), 1278–1283. doi:10.2105/AJPH.92.8.1278 PMID:12144984

Baker, D. W., Wolf, M. S., Feinglass, J., Thompson, J. A., Gazmararian, J. A., & Huang, J. (2007). Health literacy and mortality among elderly persons. *Archives of Internal Medicine*, *167*(14), 1503–1509. doi:10.1001/archinte.167.14.1503 PMID:17646604

Bauce, K. (2014). Cultural competence model. In J. J. Fitzpatrick & G. McCarthy (Eds.), *Theories guiding nursing research and practice* (pp. 159–171). Springer., doi:10.1891/9780826164056.0010

Bauza, V., Sclar, G. D., Bisoyi, A., Owens, A., Ghugey, A., & Clasen, T. (2021). Experience of the COVID-19 Pandemic in Rural Odisha, India: Knowledge, Preventative Actions, and Impacts on Daily Life. International Journal of Environmental Research and Public Health, 18(6), 2863. MDPI AG. Retrieved from doi:10.3390/ijerph18062863

Cho, Y. I., Lee, S. Y. D., Arozullah, A. M., & Crittenden, K. S. (2008). Effects of health literacy on health status and health service utilization amongst the elderly. *Social Science & Medicine*, *66*(8), 1809–1816. doi:10.1016/j.socscimed.2008.01.003 PMID:18295949

Duan, H., Wang, S., & Yang, C. (2020). Coronavirus: Limit short-term economic damage. *Nature*, *578*(7796), 515. doi:10.1038/d41586-020-00522-6 PMID:32099120

Greenhalgh, T. (2015). Health literacy: Towards system level solutions. *British Medical Journal*, *350*(feb24 13), h1026. doi:10.1136/bmj.h1026 PMID:25712067

Hochbaum, G., Rosenstock, I., & Kegels, S. (1952). Health belief model. United States Public Health Service, 1, 78-80.

Howard, D. H., Gazmararian, J., & Parker, R. (2005). The impact of low health literacy on the medical costs of Medicare managed care enrollees. *The American Journal of Medicine*, *118*(4), 371–377. doi:10.1016/j.amjmed.2005.01.010 PMID:15808134

Ishikawa, H., & Yano, E. (2008). Patient health literacy and participation in the healthcare process. *Health Expectations*, *11*(2), 113–122. doi:10.1111/j.1369-7625.2008.00497.x PMID:18494956

Kumar, R. (2019, April). Health literacy a must to empower patients. Retrieved October 2023, from The Tribune: https://www.tribuneindia.com/news/archive/comment/health-literacy-a-must-to-empower-patients-752945

Naeem, S. B., Bhatti, R., & Khan, A. (2020). An exploration of how fake news is taking over social media and putting public health at risk. *Health Information and Libraries Journal*. Advance online publication. doi:10.1111/hir.12320 PMID:32657000

Nankani, M. (2022, January). COVID Has Exposed the Low Health Literacy in India. We Must Up the Communication Game. Retrieved September 2023, from News18: https://www.news18.com/news/opinion/covid-has-exposed-the-low-health-literacy-in-india-we-must-up-the-communication-game-4693484.html

Neelima, M., Chandrashekar, B. R., Thetakala, R. K., Sai, Y., Arzu, F., & Sali, M. N. M. (2018). Rapid estimate of adult literacy in medicine and dentistry-20 and oral health status among adolescents, India: A cross-sectional study. *Journal of Education and Health Promotion*, 7. PMID:30693296

Nguyen, H. C., Nguyen, M. H., Do, B. N., Tran, C. Q., Nguyen, T. T., Pham, K. M., Pham, L. V., Tran, K. V., Duong, T. T., Tran, T. V., Duong, T. H., Nguyen, T. T., Nguyen, Q. H., Hoang, T. M., Nguyen, K. T., Pham, T. T. M., Yang, S.-H., Chao, J. C.-J., & Duong, T. V. (2020). People with suspected COVID-19 symptoms were more likely depressed and had lower health-related quality of life: The potential benefit of health literacy. *Journal of Clinical Medicine*, *9*(4), 965. doi:10.3390/jcm9040965 PMID:32244415

Nguyen, H. T., Do, B. N., Pham, K. M., Kim, G. B., Dam, H. T. B., Nguyen, T. T., Nguyen, T. T. P., Nguyen, Y. H., Sørensen, K., Pleasant, A., & Duong, T. V. (2020). Fear of COVID-19 Scale—Associations of Its Scores with Health Literacy and Health-Related Behaviors among Medical Students. *International Journal of Environmental Research and Public Health*, *17*(11), 4164. doi:10.3390/ijerph17114164 PMID:32545240

Nielsen-Bohlman, L., Panzer, A., & Kindig, D. (2004). *Health literacy: A prescription to end confusion*. National Academy Press. doi:10.17226/10883

Qin, W., Yu, P. S., Chen, J. J., Mehta, G., & Kuo, G. M. (2015). The effect of health literacy on medication knowledge and medication discrepancy in Chinese Americans. *The Journal of Pharmacy Technology*, *31*(6), 262–269. doi:10.1177/8755122515588370 PMID:34860950

Rosenbaum, L. (2020). The untold toll—The pandemic's effects on patients without Covid-19. *The New England Journal of Medicine*, *382*(24), 2368–2371. doi:10.1056/NEJMms2009984 PMID:32302076

Saluja, S. (2023, July). Enhancing health literacy: A call to action in the post-pandemic era. Retrieved October 2023, from The Times of India: https://timesofindia.indiatimes.com/blogs/voices/enhancing-health-literacy-a-call-to-action-in-the-post-pandemic-era/

Schillinger, D., Grumbach, K., Piette, J., Wang, F., Osmond, D., Daher, C., & Bindman, A. B. (2002). Association of health literacy with diabetes outcomes. *Journal of the American Medical Association*, *288*(4), 475–482. doi:10.1001/jama.288.4.475 PMID:12132978

SengJ. J. B.YeamC. T.HuangW. C.TanN. C.LowL. L. (2020). Pandemic related Health literacy-A Systematic Review of literature in COVID-19, SARS and MERS pandemics. medRxiv. doi:10.1101/2020.05.07.20094227

Sentell, T., Vamos, S., & Okan, O. (2020). Interdisciplinary perspectives on health literacy research around the world: More important than ever in a time of COVID-19. *International Journal of Environmental Research and Public Health*, *17*(9), 3010. doi:10.3390/ijerph17093010 PMID:32357457

Watson, R. (2011). Europeans with poor "health literacy" are heavy users of health services. *British Medical Journal*, *343*(nov29 4), d7741. doi:10.1136/bmj.d7741 PMID:22127773

Chapter 3
Health Information Communication in Rural Settings During Crises

Hilda Abraham Mwangakala
The University of Dodoma, Tanzania

ABSTRACT

The chapter explores the critical role of health information communication in rural settings during pandemics. It looks into rural populations' unique challenges in accessing health information, information dissemination, and improving health outcomes. The chapter discusses the current health information communication in rural settings, the need for tailoring health information, the barriers, and the potential of technology and innovations in improving access to rural information. It also highlights the importance of cultural sensitivity and policy considerations in effectively addressing health information disparities in rural areas.

INTRODUCTION

The impact of pandemics on a country's healthcare systems is profound, challenging the very core of governments' capacity to respond to public health emergencies. While pandemics such as COVID-19 have resonated globally, they have also spotlighted the unique challenges rural communities face in accessing timely and accurate health information. Effective health information communication is paramount during pandemics, as it serves as a lifeline for individuals seeking guidance and reassurance and plays a pivotal role in the overall containment and management of the crisis.

DOI: 10.4018/978-1-7998-9652-4.ch003

Generally, access to health information is crucial in empowering individuals to make informed decisions on their health and well-being (Gale et al., 2020; Kelley et al., 2016). However, one of the persisting challenges is ensuring equitable access to health information, particularly in rural areas. Rural communities often face limited healthcare infrastructure, geographical isolation, and a lack of resources (MacLeod et al., 2020). which impede their access to timely and reliable health information (Gale et al., 2020; Kelley et al., 2016; McIlhenny et al., 2011), exacerbating the effect of the pandemic when it arises.

Technological advances have caused a growing recognition of their potential to bridge this gap and improve health information access in rural areas during a pandemic. In particular, digital and mobile health (mHealth) solutions have emerged as promising tools for delivering health information and services to underserved populations. These technologies leverage the widespread adoption of mobile devices and the increasing connectivity of rural areas to overcome traditional barriers to access (Oliver-Williams et al, 2017).

The book chapter explores the status of health information access and the technology's potential to address the challenges of health information access in rural areas. Examination of the role of technology in facilitating equitable access to health information during pandemics looks into the opportunities and implications technology offers for enhancing health outcomes in rural populations. Specifically, it discusses the practices, barriers, and implementation considerations associated with technology-driven solutions in rural healthcare settings.

LITERATURE REVIEW

Health Information Communication in Rural Communities

Community access to health information is pivotal for a healthier population as it helps them take responsibility for their health and make better-informed decisions about their health. The research shows that well-informed individuals are likely to be more responsible for their health, e.g., by doing regular health check-ups, complying with treatment and immunizations, and staying healthy for longer than their uninformed counterparts (Mwangakala et al., 2021). Moreover, better access to and use of health information helps individuals improve their knowledge, increase the use of health services, reduce healthcare costs, adopt healthier behaviors, and promote health (Chen et al., 2018).

Davenport (1997) defined information behavior as "how people approach and handle information," which includes searching for it, modifying it, sharing it, hoarding it, and even ignoring it (p.83-84). He further described 'information sharing' as a voluntary act of making information available to others, 'handling information overload' as filtering and overabundance of available information for usefulness, and 'dealing with multiple meanings as recognizing that information items may have different meanings across different functional groups (Davenport, 1997, p87).

Normally, people seek health information because they feel that it will help them make informed health decisions and eventually improve their health outcomes (Warner & Procaccino, 2004). However, it is not always that a person with information needs to actually access the particular information (Szwajcer et al., 2005). After hospital visits, patients seek additional information from other sources, e.g., relatives, pharmacies, friends, and the Internet, for more detailed explanations of their health problems (Tang et al., 1997). Patients' tendency to seek additional health information besides the information provided by the care providers shows the gap between the community's needs and those provided by care providers (Tang et al., 1997). Usually, care providers use hospital visit encounters to provide patients with health education and health information. However, due to limited time during encounters, the health information usually does not meet the information needs of the patients. Typically, people need more detailed information about their health issues rather than short descriptions and instructions.

The health information needs are different and vary among patients. Patients normally need different types of information at different times and for different purposes; however, they often do not access the health information they need. Scott & Thompson (2003) stated that the major barriers to meeting a patient's health information needs include learning difficulties, language or cultural differences, and the practitioner's failure to listen and respond to the patient's concerns. Health information needs to be communicated with sensitivity, respect, and emotional support.

Patients' lack of adequate health information from care providers causes individuals to search for information from other sources, e.g., the Internet and printed materials.

Before the internet and technological boom in the 1990s, the general public used traditional media to access health information. The most commonly used health information media were magazines, newspapers, televisions, radios), and other printed materials like leaflets, pamphlets, flyers, and books (Kelley et al., 2015; Warner & Procaccino, 2004; Szwajcer et al., 2005).

Electronic media has also been used in many African countries to promote the population's health. For example, radio soap operas were used in Zimbabwe, Gambia, and Ghana to promote family planning (Babalola et al., 1993). Television programs, e.g., 'Ijue Afya yako' and 'Afya ni Uhai,' are used in Tanzania to disseminate health information on public health, e.g., Heart diseases, women's health, and prostate cancers. Siera-Leone used radio programs called 'The Doctor Says' to disseminate health information on various health issues, including sickle cell, diabetes, stroke, abortion, and infertility (M'Jimtsu-Sie, 2003).

However, despite its wide reach, the effect of the disseminated information is found to be very low, which may have been due to the generic nature of the information provided, which fails to meet the specific information needs of the target audience. Also, this may be due to the type of communication channel used, as it is only one-way communication, not allowing recipients to contact senders (care providers) in case of any queries or uncertainties on the received information. Nevertheless, despite its weaknesses, the traditional media still plays an important role in health information dissemination and promotion of health programs.

In rural areas, messages are usually communicated through songs, drama, role-play, and stories. In Nigeria, health workers use songs and dances to disseminate health information on maternal health to pregnant women and nursing mothers during antenatal clinic visits (Anasi, 2012). In other rural populations, information is disseminated through town criers and women leaders (Anasi, 2012).

Nonetheless, the advent of the Internet in the 2000s subsumed the traditional media functions in the developed world and urban areas in developing countries by reaching a much wider population with easier and more cost-effective ubiquitous accessibility. Patients and the general public can now access a wide range of health information at their fingertips anywhere and anytime. Patients are also increasingly searching the Internet for additional health information on their health issues.

However, there is still a language barrier problem where most information is presented in English, limiting access to other ethnic groups. Hence, care providers and health planners must take the lead and become the primary health information sources and disseminators to the general public.

Tailoring Health Communication to Rural Audiences

Effective health information communication in rural communities is critical to public health and healthcare delivery. However, rural areas often face unique challenges when disseminating health information to promote health literacy. Understanding rural populations' specific needs, cultural nuances, and limitations is essential for crafting effective health communication strategies. Most developing countries use print, broadcast, and other mass media to communicate health information to communities (Mwangakala, 2021; Jacobs et al., 2017). Besides normal dialogue, health messages are also conveyed as songs, shows, stories, and talks (Mwangakala, 2021; Anasi, 2012). In some rural towns, town messengers and religious leaders also tend to be used to communicate health information (Sokey et al., 2018).

Nonetheless, studies show that conveying health information to rural areas requires properly introducing communication material so that people are acquainted with it and community members can share it. On most occasions, cultural awareness influences how medical information is successfully imparted in the community

(Sokey et al., 2018). Acknowledging and respecting rural communities' cultural beliefs, traditions, and practices is fundamental. Health messages must align with these cultural values to resonate effectively. For instance, community members can easily utilize traditional medicine over Western medicine because the former is just incorporated into populations' ways of life, and they are more comfortable with it than with modern medicine. The comprehension of the weight given to known information sources is an important part of population culture that should be understood when conveying medical health information (Sokey et al., 2018; Tang et al, 1997).

Some studies have been carried out to identify the best communication channels to reach rural populations and radio remains a powerful tool for reaching rural audiences. Collaborating with local radio stations to broadcast health information and programs can be highly effective. Radio has been the best communication medium because many rural dwellers either own a radio or have access to one (Sokey et al., 2018). Radio broadcasts can reach remote areas where internet access is limited. It was further revealed that information sources such as town criers and market announcements were very popular and more effective than TV, billboards, and newspapers.

Moreover, clear and concise messaging is crucial for enhancing comprehension among individuals with varying levels of education. Thus, using plain language without medical jargon ensures that health information on the pandemic is easily understood. Also, incorporating visuals, infographics, and diagrams can convey complex health information effectively, especially to those with limited literacy. Visual aids transcend language barriers, making information accessible to diverse populations.

Peer education also tends to increase the behavioral change of adults and adolescents due to the similarities that may exist between the educator and the target. When health communication campaigns began decades ago, attempts at showing film clips and using other innovative technology were unsuccessful (Sokey et al., 2018). It was only through the utilization of specially designed puppet shows and performances directed to the specific ethnic groups that the expected conduct and awareness level change happened (Du Sautoy, 1958). However, merely improving a person's understanding of an issue might not necessarily lead to a change in behavior, and improving consciousness alone does not hold people responsible for their health (Mwangakala, 2016; Sokey et al., 2018). Ford et al. (2005) discourse that adopting participation, self-determination, and the inclusion attitude in the information delivery strategy have a fundamental impact on helping people understand why certain health behaviors are wrong. They further explain that it is essential to permit people to deliver input on how health information will help them change by talking over different communication channels. The closer a message is to individuals' culture, expectations, and lifestyle, the more integrated the health campaign is and the more effective health information can be passed on and behavioral change achieved.

Generally, facilitating the population's access to important health information at the grassroots increases the individual's sense of responsibility for their health, resulting in more informed health decisions (Mwangakala, 2021). Well-informed individuals will likely adopt healthy behaviors and stay healthy longer than their less informed counterparts (Mwangakala, 2021; Wathen & Harris, 2007). When the majority of the population adopts healthy behaviors, the number of ill individuals will likely be minimized, as well as a pandemic effect in the society and healthcare system. Thus, adopting healthy behaviors will reduce the effect of the acute health staff shortage in most rural areas, particularly during crises.

METHODS

Study Site

The book chapter utilized a case study design to explore and analyze health information communication in rural settings. The aim was to thoroughly examine health information communication within a specific rural setting. The case study focused on a representative rural community in Dodoma, Tanzania. Selection criteria included geographical location, socio-economic factors, and healthcare infrastructure to ensure relevance and applicability to broader rural contexts. The investigation, spanning six months, was carried out in Chamwino District, an administrative district within the Dodoma Region. The chosen community exhibited characteristics emblematic of the challenges and opportunities in rural settings, making it a pertinent case for in-depth analysis.

Participant Population

The study employed purposive sampling to select participants with a focus on obtaining community members who are information-rich and homogeneous, facilitating the attainment of the saturation point. The study participants included 35 individuals, encompassing 25 community members, five traditional birth attendants (TBAs), and five healthcare providers in the selected communities. A total of 29 community members were approached for participation, with 25 providing consent.

The selection of skilled healthcare providers (SHPs) depended on the number of health staff available in a particular health facility, specifically those dealing with community's health. The selection of TBAs was random and contingent on their availability and willingness to participate. Five TBAs were chosen from the two wards, three from Buigiri ward and two from Msanga ward.

Data Collection Methods

Preliminary data was collected by reviewing existing documents, including community health reports, local media coverage, and relevant publications. The review provided context and background information on the selected community. Also, in-depth, semi-structured interviews and focus groups were conducted with key stakeholders, including community members, healthcare providers, and local leaders. Interviews explored the community's health information access, sources, communication preferences, and perceptions of the effectiveness of existing health communication initiatives. Focused group discussions with community members encouraged open dialogue and uncovered shared experiences and perceptions related to health communication.

Data Analysis

Qualitative data from interviews, and focus group discussions undergo thematic analysis. Identified themes were categorized and organized to comprehensively understand health information communication dynamics within the selected rural community. Further, the findings were compared with broader trends and patterns reported in other rural communities. Cross-case analysis highlighted similarities, differences, and unique features, contributing to the generalizability of the study.

Findings integration provided a comprehensive understanding of health information communication in rural settings. The findings triangulation offered a nuanced portrayal of the challenges and opportunities faced by rural communities.

RESULTS

Barriers to Effective Health Communication in Rural Areas

Sources of Health Information

In developed countries and most urban areas in developing countries, patients usually access health information from healthcare providers during hospital visits through one-on-one counseling or leaflets, brochures, or books, which are usually offered free of charge. Other media used to access maternal health information include TVs, radios, and the Internet (Lagan et al., 2010). However, in rural areas people, women are underprivileged; while TV and the internet were not possible options, with radio accessed only by a few then, healthcare providers remained the main source of reliable health information, as shown in Figure 1.

The predominant reliance on healthcare providers (42%) highlights the central role of formal healthcare services in rural health information dissemination. It underscores the significance of established medical structures as the primary source of trustworthy health information. The prevalence of healthcare providers as a source also suggests a high level of trust in the expertise and guidance offered by trained medical professionals. This trust is crucial for effective health communication, as it can influence community members to seek and follow professional medical advice. Thus, given the influence of healthcare providers, there is an opportunity to design targeted health campaigns that leverage the credibility of medical professionals. Collaborative efforts between healthcare institutions and community organizations can enhance the reach and impact of such campaigns.

Figure 1. Health Information Sources

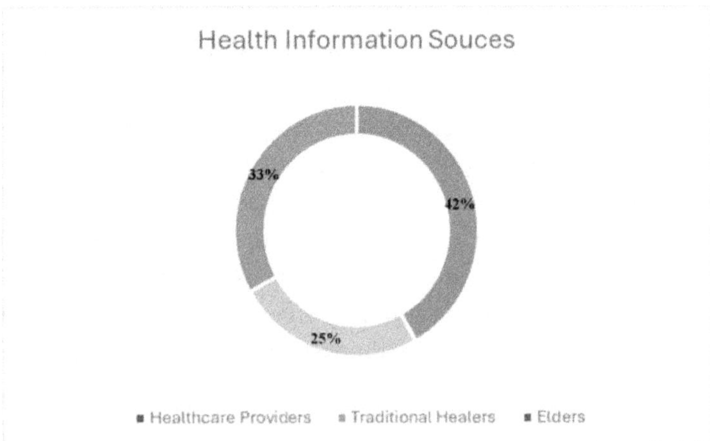

Moreover, the elderly community members were also widely used. The reliance on elders (33%) signifies the esteemed role of older community members as pillars of wisdom and knowledge. Elders serve as influential figures whose guidance shapes community perceptions and practices. Engaging elders in health education initiatives can facilitate intergenerational knowledge transfer. This approach not only disseminates health information but also strengthens community bonds by involving older and younger generations. Therefore, health communication strategies should be designed to deeply respect cultural norms and community structures. Recognizing the influential role of elders ensures that health messages align with established community values.

Nonetheless, Traditional healers were also used as a source of health information. The reliance on traditional birth attendants (25%) underscores the deeply embedded cultural practices in rural health-seeking behavior. The finding suggests a preference for traditional approaches, emphasizing the need for culturally sensitive health communication strategies. Thus, health communication initiatives should be inclusive, recognizing the role of traditional birth attendants. Collaborative programs that integrate traditional practices with modern healthcare approaches can bridge gaps and enhance the overall effectiveness of health messaging.

The findings emphasize the importance of culturally sensitive health communication in rural areas. Tailoring messages to align with cultural beliefs and practices ensures that the community receives and embraces health information. A holistic approach integrating formal healthcare, traditional practices, and community wisdom can result in more comprehensive health communication strategies. Recognizing and respecting the coexistence of these sources can enhance the overall impact on health literacy.

Collaborative efforts between formal healthcare institutions, traditional practitioners, and community leaders are essential for designing and implementing successful health communication initiatives. This collaboration ensures a united and culturally grounded approach to health education.

Limited Access to Health Information Media

The digital age has transformed the way individuals access and utilize health information. However, this transformation has not been uniform, and rural communities worldwide continue to grapple with the "Rural Health Information Divide." The divide represents a significant gap in the accessibility and availability of healthcare information among rural populations, resulting in disparities in health outcomes and healthcare access, which have profound impacts for the community's health (Kelley et al., 2016; Scantlebury et al., 2017).

In many rural populations, particularly in developing countries, access to health information is still a major challenge (Chen et al., 2019: Anasi, 2012; Kelley et al., 2016). It was found that majority community members do not have access to potential media for health information as shown in figure 2. Further, many rural areas lack reliable high-speed internet access, making it difficult for residents to browse health websites, access telehealth services, or engage in online health communities. They lack broadband access, making accessing online health resources and health-related information challenging (Greenberg et al., 2018; Lustria et al., 2011). The adequacy and ease of access to information are important factors when seeking health information. According to Eysenbach et al. (2002), if the information is adequate and can be accessed efficiently and effectively at the first level of the information system, then that information could be accessed by every information seeker at any level (national to international) without a need for further processing.

Figure 2. Health Information Media in Rural Areas

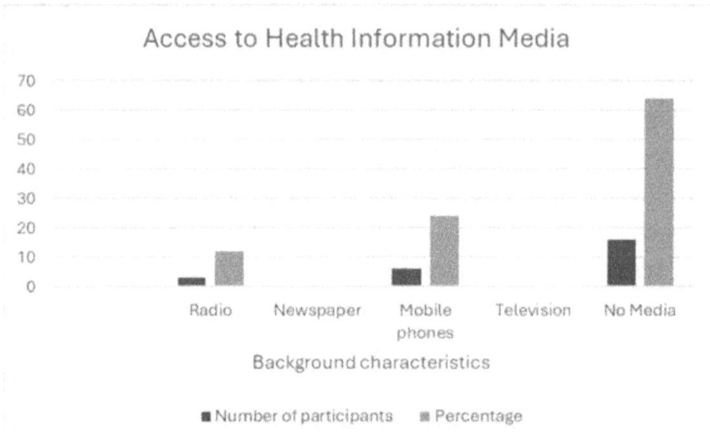

Furthermore, doctors normally assume the power of health professionals and perceive patients as just health illiterates who cannot understand medical terms and do not need to know everything. Further, doctors' perception that patients are just medical conditions rather than a person contributes to their attitudes and non-communication of health information with their patients, as indicated in Figure 3, where the majority reported not being given any health information when visiting the health facility. Thus, addressing the increasing tendency of patients seeking additional health information out of those provided during encounters, care providers must ensure effective health information communication to all patients.

Figure 3. Health Information Provision

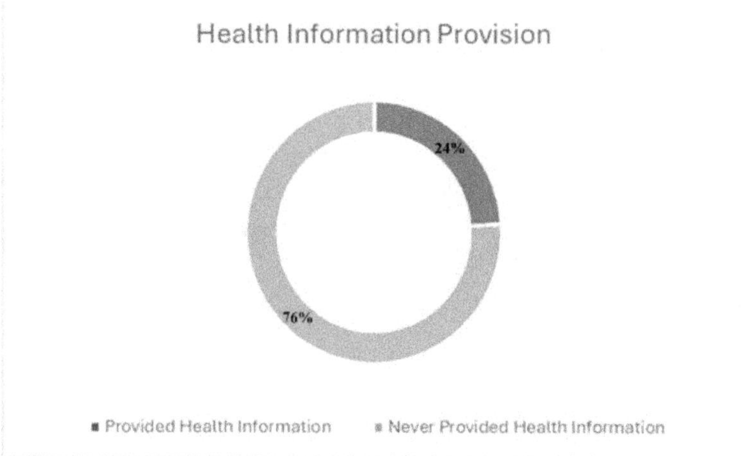

Moreover, other studies found that an individual's self-efficacy and high internal locus of control also significantly influence an individual's actual health information communication. The extent to which an individual believes she has control over his/her health and the ability to access and act on the information determines whether to seek the health information or not (Lambert & Loiselle, 2007). People usually seek information perceived as easily accessible and act upon. A person who has limited access to health information and lacks decision-making power about her health condition is less likely to be an active seeker and user of health information.

Low Health Literacy

Furthermore, rural populations often face lower health literacy levels due to limited access to educational resources and low education levels as shown in figure 4. Health literacy is the degree to which a person can access, process, and understand basic health information and services needed to make proper decisions regarding their health. Lower health literacy leads to difficulties in understanding medical information, managing chronic conditions, and making informed healthcare decisions (Golboni et al., 2018), particularly in crises such as COVID-19. It also hinders their ability to understand and act upon health information, such as pandemic control measures, leading to potentially harmful decisions or delayed medical care.

Figure 4. Participants Education Level

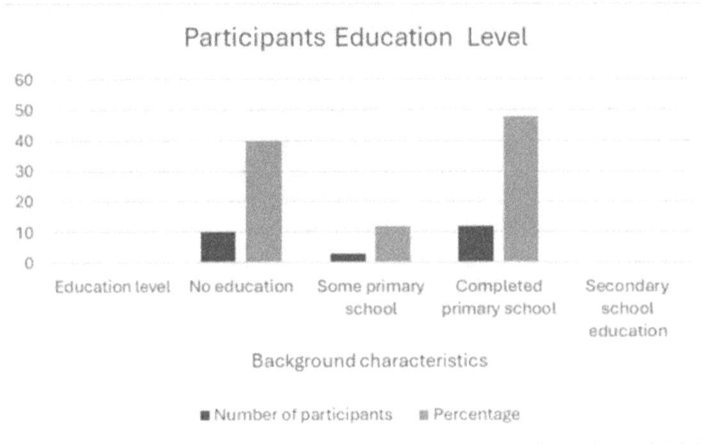

Moreover, rural communities are often culturally diverse, and language barriers further complicate health information dissemination (Mwangakala, 2021). Rural communities' cultural and linguistic diversity poses challenges in effectively communicating health information. Health materials and resources are usually unavailable in rural residents' languages, making it difficult to effectively convey critical pandemic health information. Thus, tailoring health communication to rural communities' unique cultural and linguistic backgrounds is essential for overcoming the barriers.

Timely access to quality healthcare information during pandemic outbreaks can effectively control the spread of the disease and the community's anxiety. However, many rural areas have limited healthcare facilities, and residents have to travel long distances to access healthcare services. In cases such as COVID-19, where a patient needs immediate healthcare, limited access to health facilities contributes to higher mortality rates than what could be avoided. Up-to-date information about specific threats and necessary precautionary measures mitigates public anxiety and reduces morbidity and mortality (Zhao et al., 2020). Further, healthcare facilities tend to have fewer resources and technological capabilities than their urban counterparts. They are usually underfunded and understaffed (as shown in figure 5), which leads to delays in updating electronic health records (EHRs), implementing health information exchanges (HIEs), and adopting advanced healthcare technologies. The shortage impacts the availability of electronic health records (EHRs) and telehealth services, hindering health information communication.

Figure 5. Healthcare Providers Status in the Facilities

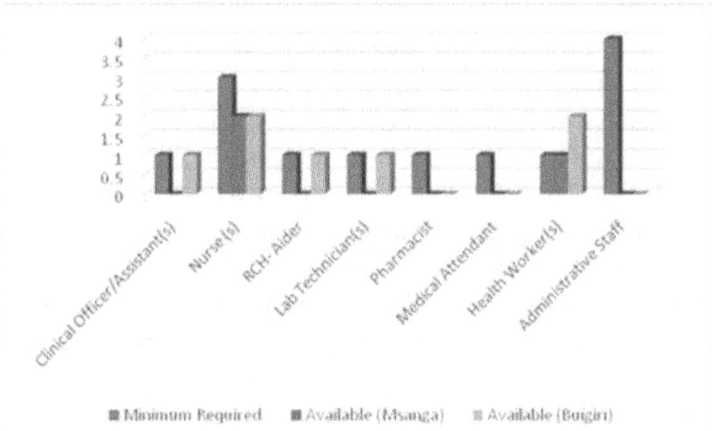

Concerted efforts are needed to address the disparities in access to health information to improve health outcomes for rural populations and achieve healthcare equity. Bridging this divide is a fundamental step toward a more inclusive and healthier society. Healthcare providers must champion health information provisions among the rural population to build a well-informed and knowledgeable society responsible for its health and better-informed health decisions (Mwangakala, 2021).

RECOMMENDATIONS

ICT Potential for Rural Health Information Communication

Health information communication to rural areas is critical to improving community health and promoting healthy living. In the information age, where technology has made it possible to access and share information quickly and easily, rural populations need to take advantage despite the limited resources and infrastructure. Providing access to health information in rural areas requires a combination of strategies that consider the communities' unique challenges. Further, improving health literacy in rural communities requires a multifaceted approach involving functional and interactive health literacy strategies. The proposed solutions need to address the specific challenges faced by rural populations, taking into account their diverse needs, limited access to resources, and potential barriers to health information.

Mobile-Health (mHealth) technologies, Telemedicine, community health workers, radio, television, and printed material can be effectively utilized to empower rural communities to take control of their health and well-being. Furthermore, strategies such as community-based health programs, technology-driven interventions, and partnerships with local organizations could help improve the accessibility of health information in rural areas.

While functional health literacy focuses on basic reading, writing, and numeracy skills required to effectively understand and use health information. In rural communities, where literacy levels vary, there is a need to develop health information materials using plain language, simple visuals, and accessible formats. The printed materials must be available in local languages and use visual aids to enhance understanding. The interactive health literacy involves engaging individuals in the learning process and facilitating active participation in their health. Interactive strategies encourage two-way communication and collaboration. The introduction of digital health tools, such as mobile apps or interactive websites, will provide personalized health information, self-assessment quizzes, and interactive features. The key is to ensure that these tools are user-friendly and accessible to individuals with varying levels of digital literacy.

Studies show that mHealth technologies, such as mobile apps and text messaging services, have successfully provided health information to rural communities (Sokey et al., 2018). In recent years, mobile phones and other mobile devices have increasingly become more affordable and available in rural areas. mHealth technologies enable care providers to provide various health information, including preventive measures, disease management, maternal and child health, nutrition, and treatment options (Haggstrom et al., 2019; Maslowsky et al., 2016). Further, some mHealth applications also connect users with healthcare professionals for consultations and advice. mHealth applications have also been used to send automated patient reminders for upcoming appointments, medication schedules, and follow-up care (Jacobs et al., 2017: Maslowsky et al., 2016). These reminders improve patient adherence to treatment plans and help reduce missed appointments, leading to better health outcomes.

Furthermore, telemedicine uses technology, such as video conferencing, to provide medical consultations to patients remotely. The technology is particularly useful for patients in rural areas who may not have access to medical specialists or have to travel long distances for medical appointments (Scott & Mars, 2015; Scott et al., 2020). It also enables remote consultations between healthcare providers and patients, overcoming geographical barriers and improving access to healthcare services. Further, Telemedicine enables healthcare providers in remote settings to seek second opinions from experts elsewhere, enhancing the accuracy of diagnoses and treatment plans (Pengput & Schwartz, 2022; Bashshur et al., 2014; Jacobs et al, 2017).

Improving access to health information facilitates rural populations to make informed decisions about their health, increases their health literacy, and ultimately leads to improved health outcomes. Thus, policymakers, healthcare providers, and communities must work together to utilize ICT solutions to bridge the health information gap in rural areas and ensure every individual has access to the health information they need during crises, leading a healthy and fulfilling life.

Future Directions and Innovations in Rural Health Communication

Emerging Technologies and innovations are equally critical for rural health communication to improve healthcare access, outcomes, and overall well-being in rural areas. As technology advances and healthcare systems evolve, there are several key areas where emerging technologies can facilitate innovations and developments in rural health communication. Innovations in health communication should focus on improving health literacy in rural communities. Educational programs and resources can be delivered through interactive online modules, webinars, and social media campaigns.

Virtual Reality (VR) can improve access to health information for individuals with disabilities. Customizable interfaces and voice commands can make health information more accessible to those with visual or auditory impairments. Further, VR can simulate medical scenarios and procedures, offering healthcare professionals and students a realistic environment for learning and training. It can train medical staff in surgical techniques, patient care, or emergency response. Additionally, patients can use VR to learn about medical conditions, treatment options, and self-care practices interactively and engagingly.

Telemedicine has already made significant strides in rural healthcare by providing remote access to medical services. However, expanding telemedicine and telehealth services should remain a top priority. Innovations in this area could likely include improvements in telehealth technology, such as more user-friendly platforms, increased connectivity options, and providing rural residents with access to virtual healthcare consultations, remote monitoring, and telehealth platforms for managing chronic conditions and crises (Haggstrom et al., 2020). Telemedicine platforms will become increasingly personalized, tailoring health information communication to individual patients. Using data analytics and artificial intelligence, the platforms will provide customized health information and recommendations based on a patient's medical history, preferences, and current health status. Future telemedicine consultations will be enriched with interactive 3D models, real-time data visualization, and augmented reality overlays. Healthcare providers will be able to use these tools to explain medical conditions and treatment options more effectively to patients during virtual visits.

Advanced AI-driven chatbots and virtual health assistants will play a significant role in health information communication. They will provide immediate responses to health-related queries, offer medication reminders, and deliver personalized health advice, improving health literacy and engagement.

Moreover, mobile health applications and tools are becoming increasingly popular for healthcare management. Advanced mHealth apps will provide highly personalized health information and recommendations based on user's health data, preferences, and goals. These apps will offer tailored content and advice, improving health literacy and engagement. Further, future mHealth apps will feature AI-powered chatbots and virtual assistants capable of answering health-related queries, providing medication reminders, and offering real-time guidance on managing health conditions. These chatbots will enhance communication and provide immediate support. Users will have access to comprehensive health information dashboards on their mobile devices. These dashboards will display real-time data from wearable devices, electronic health records (EHRs), and other sources, empowering individuals to monitor and manage their health proactively.

Additionally, centralized online platforms and health information portals can serve as valuable resources for rural communities, particularly during pandemics. The platforms will serve as centralized hubs for all types of health information, including articles, videos, research findings, and interactive tools. Users can access a wide range of health-related content from a single source, making it convenient to find reliable information. Further, advanced algorithms and artificial intelligence will enable these platforms to provide personalized health content based on users' health profiles, interests, and preferences. Users will receive tailored recommendations and educational materials that align with their unique needs and health goals. Health information portals could also seamlessly integrate with telehealth and telemedicine platforms. Users can schedule virtual consultations, access healthcare providers' profiles and availability, and receive post-visit information and recommendations through the portal. Health information portals could also offer content in multiple languages and culturally sensitive materials to cater to diverse populations. The inclusivity will bridge language and cultural barriers in rural health communication.

Also, empowering community health workers with digital tools and training can enhance rural health communication. These workers can use mobile apps for data collection, health education, and connecting residents to healthcare resources. Innovations in this area may include AI-supported decision-making tools for community health workers. Rural health systems will increasingly use data analytics to identify health trends and allocate resources effectively. Predictive analytics can help anticipate healthcare needs, especially in areas with limited healthcare infrastructure.

More importantly, recognizing the diversity within rural populations, future innovations should incorporate cultural competency training for healthcare providers and culturally tailored health communication materials to serve underserved rural communities better. Governments and healthcare organizations must also continue implementing policies and funding initiatives to support these innovations in rural health communication (Haggstrom et al., 2020; Jacobs et al., 2017). The initiatives could include grants, subsidies, and incentives to expand telehealth infrastructure and promote digital health adoption in rural areas.

In conclusion, the lessons learned from health information communication in rural settings during pandemics have implications beyond crisis response. They underscore the importance of an inclusive approach to healthcare communication that leaves no community behind. They emphasize the value of adaptability and creativity in the face of adversity and illuminate a path forward where technology, community, and culture converge to safeguard the health and well-being of all, even in the remotest corners of our world.

REFERENCES

Anasi, S. N. (2012). Access to and dissemination of health information in Africa: The patient and the public. *Journal of Hospital Librarianship*, *12*(2), 120–134. do i:10.1080/15323269.2012.666647

Babalola, S., Lawal, A. S., Mako, I. V., Rimon, J. G. II, Corso, C., Kiragu, K., & Church. (1993). Mobile family planning drama. *Promotion & Education*, *1*(4), 42–45. doi:10.1177/175797599300100412 PMID:8186944

Bashshur, R. L., Shannon, G. W., & Bashshur, N. (2016). The empirical evidence for telemedicine interventions in primary care: An updated systematic review. *Telemedicine Journal and e-Health*, *22*(1), 37–40. PMID:27336754

Berkman, N. D., Sheridan, S. L., Donahue, K. E., Halpern, D. J., & Crotty, K. (2011). Low health literacy and health outcomes: An updated systematic review. *Annals of Internal Medicine*, *155*(2), 97–107. doi:10.7326/0003-4819-155-2-201107190-00005 PMID:21768583

. Chen, X., Orom, H., Hay, J. L., Waters, E. A., Schofield, E., Li, Y., & Kiviniemi, M. T. (2019). Differences in rural and urban health information access and use. The Journal of Rural Health, 35(3), 405-417. Dalrymple, P. W., Rogers, M., Zach, L., Turner, K., & Green, M. (2013).

Davenport, T. H. (1997). *Information Ecology*. Oxford University Press. doi:10.1093/oso/9780195111682.001.0001

Eysenbach, G., & Kohler, C. (2003). What is the prevalence of health-related searches on the World Wide Web? Qualitative and quantitative analysis of search engine queries on the internet. [American Medical Informatics Association.]. *AMIA Annual Symposium Proceedings - AMIA Symposium. AMIA Symposium, 2003*, 225. PMID:14728167

Ford, N., Williams, A., Renshaw, M., & Nkum, J. (2005). Communication strategy for implementing community IMCI. *Journal of Health Communication, 10*(5), 379–401. doi:10.1080/10810730591009817 PMID:16199384

Gale, N., & Dowswell, G. (2020). Access to healthcare for rural communities: A scoping review of relevant theories and models. *Journal of Rural Studies, 75*, 191–201.

Greenberg, A. J., Haney, D., Blake, K. D., Moser, R. P., & Hesse, B. W. (2018). Differences in access to and use of electronic personal health information between rural and urban residents in the United States. *The Journal of Rural Health, 34*(S1), s30–s38. doi:10.1111/jrh.12228 PMID:28075508

Haggstrom, D. A., Lee, J. L., Dickinson, S. L., Kianersi, S., Roberts, J. L., Teal, E., Baker, L. B., & Rawl, S. M. (2019). Rural and urban differences in the adoption of new health information and medical technologies. *The Journal of Rural Health, 35*(2), 144–154. doi:10.1111/jrh.12358 PMID:30830983

Jacobs, W., Amuta, A. O., & Jeon, K. C. (2017). Health information seeking in the digital age: An analysis of health information seeking behavior among US adults. *Cogent Social Sciences, 3*(1), 1302785. doi:10.1080/23311886.2017.1302785

Kelley, M. S., Su, D., & Britigan, D. H. (2016). Disparities in health information access: Results of a county-wide survey and implications for health communication. *Health Communication, 31*(5), 575–582. doi:10.1080/10410236.2014.979976 PMID:26452300

Lambert, S. D., & Loiselle, C. G. (2007). Health Information—Seeking Behavior. *Qualitative Health Research, 17*(8), 1006–1019. doi:10.1177/1049732307305199 PMID:17928475

Lustria, M. L. A., Smith, S. A., & Hinnant, C. C. (2011). Exploring digital divides: An examination of eHealth technology use in health information seeking, communication and personal health information management in the USA. *Health Informatics Journal, 17*(3), 224–243. doi:10.1177/1460458211414843 PMID:21937464

M'Jamtu-Sie, N. (2003). Disseminating health information in Sierra Leone: The challenge. *Information Development*, *19*(4), 250–254. doi:10.1177/026666690301900404

MacLeod, M. L. P., Kulig, J. C., Stewart, N. J., Anguish, P., Andrews, M. E., Banner, D., & Karunanayake, C. (2020). Rural women's health knowledge: Implications for healthcare delivery in rural communities. *Health & Place*, *65*, 102417.

Maslowsky, J., Frost, S., Hendrick, C. E., Cruz, F. O. T., & Merajver, S. D. (2016). Effects of postpartum mobile phone-based education on maternal and infant health in Ecuador. *International Journal of Gynaecology and Obstetrics: the Official Organ of the International Federation of Gynaecology and Obstetrics*, *134*(1), 93–98. doi:10.1016/j.ijgo.2015.12.008 PMID:27126905

Mwangakala, H. A. (2021). Accessibility of maternal health information and its influence on maternal health preferences in rural Tanzania: A case study of Chamwino District. *South African Journal of Information Management*, *23*(1), 1–9. doi:10.4102/sajim.v23i1.1353

Oliver-Williams, C., Brown, E., Devereux, S., Fairhead, C., & Holeman, I. (2017). Using mobile phones to improve vaccination uptake in 21 low-and middle-income countries: Systematic review. *JMIR mHealth and uHealth*, *5*(10), e7792. doi:10.2196/mhealth.7792 PMID:28978495

Pengput, A., & Schwartz, D. G. (2022). Telemedicine in Southeast Asia: A systematic review. *Telemedicine Journal and e-Health*, *28*(12), 1711–1733. doi:10.1089/tmj.2021.0516 PMID:35417250

Scantlebury, A., Booth, A., & Hanley, B. (2017). Experiences, practices and barriers to accessing health information: A qualitative study. *International Journal of Medical Informatics*, *103*, 103–108. doi:10.1016/j.ijmedinf.2017.04.018 PMID:28550995

Scott, J. T., & Thompson, D. R. (2003). Assessing the information needs of post-myocardial infarction patients: A systematic review. *Patient Education and Counseling*, *50*(2), 167–177. doi:10.1016/S0738-3991(02)00126-X PMID:12781932

Scott, R. E., & Mars, M. (2015). Telehealth in the developing world: Current status and future prospects. *Smart Homecare Technology and Telehealth*, *3*(1), 25–37. doi:10.2147/SHTT.S75184

Scott, R. E., Mars, M., & Bärnighausen, T. (2020). Virtual health interventions during the COVID-19 pandemic: A systematic review. *Journal of Medical Internet Research*, *22*(12), e22796.

Sokey, P. P., Adjei, E., & Ankrah, E. (2018). Media use for health information dissemination to rural communities by the Ghana Health Service. *Journal of Information Science. Systems and Technology*, *2*(1), 1–18.

Szwajcer, E. M., Hiddink, G. J., Koelen, M. A., & Van Woerkum, C. (2005). Nutrition-related information-seeking behaviours before and throughout the course of pregnancy: Consequences for nutrition communication. *European Journal of Clinical Nutrition*, *59*(S1, Suppl. 1), s57–s65. https://www.nature.com/ejcn/journal/v59/n1s/pdf/1602175a.pdf. doi:10.1038/sj.ejcn.1602175 PMID:16052197

Tang, P. C., Newcomb, C., Gorden, S., & Kreider, N. (1997). Meeting the information needs of patients: results from a patient focus group. In *Proceedings of the AMIA Annual Fall Symposium* (p. 672). American Medical Informatics Association.

Warner, D., & Procaccino, J. D. (2004). Toward wellness: Women seeking health information. *Journal of the American Society for Information Science and Technology*, *55*(8), 709–730. doi:10.1002/asi.20016

Zhao, X., Fan, J., Basnyat, I., & Hu, B. (2020). Online health information seeking using "# COVID-19 patient seeking help" on Weibo in Wuhan, China: Descriptive study. *Journal of Medical Internet Research*, *22*(10), e22910. doi:10.2196/22910 PMID:33001838

KEY TERMS AND DEFINITIONS

Community Health Worker: A trained and trusted healthcare professional who works within a specific community or population to promote and improve the health and well-being of its residents.

Gamification: The application of game design principles, mechanics, and elements in non-gaming contexts to engage and motivate individuals, enhance their learning experience, and encourage specific behaviors or actions.

Health Information: These are facts related to various aspects of health and healthcare, including medical records, clinical data, educational materials, and resources that pertain to individual well-being, diseases, medical conditions, treatments, and public health

Health Information Portal: Is A web-based platform or website that serves as a centralized and comprehensive source of health-related information and resources.

Health Literacy: The ability of individuals to obtain, comprehend, evaluate, and use healthcare information to make informed decisions about their health and effectively navigate the healthcare system.

Mobile Health: Also known as "mHealth," is a term used to describe the use of mobile devices, such as smartphones, tablets, and wearable devices, in the delivery of healthcare services, the collection of health-related data, and the dissemination of health information.

Telemedicine: is a branch of healthcare that uses telecommunication and information technology to provide medical services, consultations, and information exchange remotely.

Traditional Birth Attendant: A person who assists the mother during childbirth and initially acquires her skills by delivering babies or working with other TBAs.

Virtual Reality: is a technology that immerses users in a computer-generated, three-dimensional environment, simulating a realistic experience that can engage multiple senses, including vision, hearing, and sometimes touch or motion.

Chapter 4
Use of Digital Technology to Deal With COVID-19

Alaattin Parlakkılıç
https://orcid.org/0000-0002-6834-6839
Ufuk University, Turkey

ABSTRACT

The aim of this chapter is to determine the areas of using digital technology to cope with the COVID 19 pandemic. PubMed and Google Scholar article content analysis was conducted, the governments' good practices were examined and Turkish filiation implementation studies were combined to obtain digital technologies to deal with COVID-19. The areas have been determined as planning and monitoring, contact tracing, infection screening, quarantine and self-isolation, clinical management, and medical procurement. As a result of the investigation, efforts coordinated by governments around the world have focused on successfully isolating and mitigating COVID-19 to varying degrees. Countries that maintain low COVID-19 mortality rates per person are implementing strategies that include early surveillance, testing, contact tracing, and strict quarantine. The low mortality rate in Turkey has been concluded due to Turkey's Filiation application. Turkey quickly locates and isolates the contacts at the rate, of 99.9%, and filiation success is based on the detection of cases through 10 hours.

INTRODUCTION

Governments are scrambling to find new methods of crisis management as COVID-19 continues to endanger public health and the world economy. The propagation of the infection is managed, tracked, and controlled using digital solutions. The patterns

DOI: 10.4018/978-1-7998-9652-4.ch004

include strategies like monitoring the COVID-19 epidemic, warning vulnerable groups, adapting social distance, and staying at home (Oecd, 2020).

Contact monitoring is an important public health measure to control COVID-19. Rapid detection and management of COVID-19 cases makes it easier to identify secondary cases from primary cases. Turkish fillation method is a fast and comprehensive monitoring method for Covid-19 contact tracing. In conjunction with robust testing and surveillance systems, contact tracing and strategies to reduce disease transmission are essential. Therefore, Turkish fillation method is an important effort that successfully reduces the number of cases (United Nations, 2020).

A range of digital technologies are employed to battle the disease. Digital technology can be used to identify and track the virus's spread. Information regarding viruses can be given by means of digital technology acting as virtual assistants. Digital technologies can be used with diagnostic robots to predict severe symptoms that require treatment . In addition, digital technologies are used in crowd monitoring to help enforce social distance rules (Karina, 2020). Monitoring and surveillance methods are also used, such as the use of location data stored or generated by the use of smart phones that monitor public surveillance, scanning public areas for affected persons using infrared cameras, facial recognition and computer monitoring technologies (Sanchez-Comas, Synnes & Hallberg, 2020).

The novel severe acute respiratory syndrome coronavirus 2 (SARS-CoV-2) is the cause of COVID-19, an infectious disease with high contagiousness, a high fatality rate (greater than 1%), and an effective antiviral. The main focus has been to contain and lessen the pandemic because treatment or immunization cannot be given to all societies at once. Pandemic management using mitigating tactics and digital technology that help speed up intervention (Zhu et al., 2020). The following sub-objectives are anticipated as a result of this study's evaluation of the use of digital technology in the fight against disease during the pandemic:

- What are the pandemic's digital technology application areas?
- What are the leading digital technology applications in the world in combating Covid-19?
- How should the digital technologies used in Covid-19 be used?

DIGITAL TECHNOLOGIES IN THE PANDEMIC

Almost all of the methods used to control the COVID-19 are supported by the breakthrough technologies of the 21st century. Digital technologies offer new ways to better detect disease, prevent it, and improve patients. The digitalization process in health, which started in the 2000s, has gained great momentum today. As the World

Health Organization (WHO) underlines, "2020 will be a turning point for digital technologies to transform health systems". The main reason for digital technologies to come to the fore is that the pandemic creates a ball of problems in many areas.

Large-scale natural or biological disasters confront health systems with the necessity of coping with many problems in a short time. While the health system is trying to understand the disease, it is also trying to manage the interventions to control the epidemic. Some of the problems caused by COVID-19 are summarized as follows:

- In coordination between fragmented or dispersed decision-making mechanisms,
- Lack of communication between health decision-making institutions and health facilities,
- Insufficient integration between local and national emergency management systems,
- Insufficient and fragmented data on the patient's location and condition,
- Medical human resources and material stock that is insufficient to respond to sudden increases in demand,
- Lack of instant information about the occupancy rate of the intensive care bed capacity of the public and private sectors,
- Inability to monitor the movements of infected people,
- Insufficient sharing of information about the disease between health professionals and health decision-makers.

Figure 1 illustrates the evaluation of integrated regions and the application of digital technologies in planning, surveillance, testing, contact monitoring, quarantine, and health services as well as pandemic management and response (Ferretti et al., 2020).

Figure 1. Digital technology ecosystem in response to pandemic

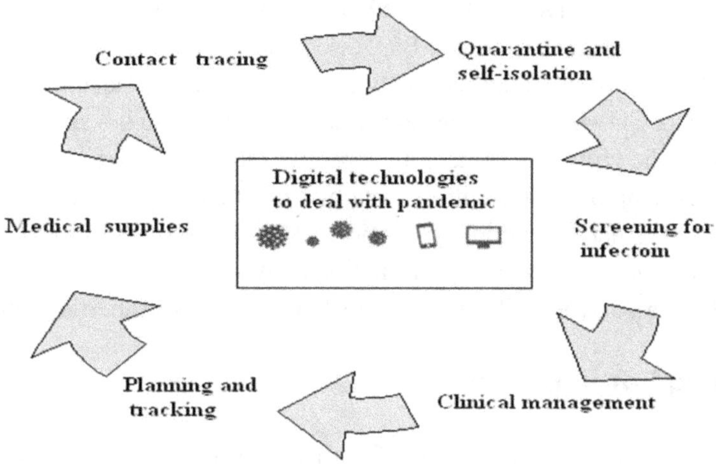

Planning and Tracking

Digital technology's scalability is useful for keeping an eye on all people who pose a high risk for quarantine but aren't serious enough to need medical care. Patients can use digital technologies to assess their fever and send cloud data for analysis to their mobile devices. Currently, patients with chronic diseases like diabetes or hypertension who live at home are monitored remotely. In hospitals, the monitoring of numerous patients with little staff is accomplished by the transfer of biometric measurements such as telemetry, heart rate, and blood pressure from wearable devices to wireless devices for patients. Here, digital technologies can be used to collect more data and increase the productivity of healthcare professionals, using less time to reduce healthcare workers' exposure to infection and their workload (Whitelaw et al., 2020).

To diagnose infected people, thermal cameras and multi-sensor cameras supported by artificial intelligence are used in public places such as airports, hospitals, nurseries (Ribandar, 2020). With these developments, Google and Apple announced that they are collaborating to track COVID-19. The aim of the project they are developing is to examine the person who has been in contact with the smartphone user individuals for a while and who is approaching to detect the coronavirus with BLE (Bluetooth Low Energy) technology. One of the advantages of this project is that users do not need to download any apps from virtual app stores. It is assumed that the devices and existing sensors are used in the application of this method. In doing so, it is aimed to emphasize privacy by not using any location or personal data (Wallis et al., 2020). With the platform developed by Apple and Google, all these third-party applications are gathered under a single structure, aiming to ensure integrity among themselves, and positive results are obtained in the detection of coronavirus in international travels (International Bar Association, 2020).

Big data and artificial intelligence, two examples of digital technology, aid in the preparation for COVID-19 and the monitoring of human behavior and, consequently, the spread of the virus. They may follow people's travels using tools like migration maps, which employ mobile phones, mobile payment apps, and social media to gather real-time data on people's locations. Machine learning models have been created using these data to forecast the regional SARS-CoV-2 transfer dynamics and to direct border controls and surveillance (Americ an Civil Liberties Union, 2021).

Screening For Infection

Infection screening is a field study conducted to determine the disease agent, source, transmission route within the scope of combating infectious diseases and to take protection and control measures after the cases are reported. Those who encounter a case during this research are also included in protection and control measures. When data scientists can track the source of a virus outbreak in time, it is possible to prevent an outbreak. In this context, digital technology can offer a suitable solution as it can accurately detect the contamination site by analyzing the mobile phone data of millions of users. Most users of smartphones depend on the internet geographic information system to track location history. If the majority of infected patients have previously been in the same geographic area, it is likely the point of transmission. Once the origin is determined, the authorities can quarantine the entire area. They can also easily monitor anyone who comes into contact with infected patients and keep them alone (Ekong, Chukwu & Chukwu, 2020).

Early awareness of the potential spread and severity of an infectious disease outbreak, such as COVID-19, can help public health decision-makers take prompt action even while data are still lacking. For example, use mobile phone location data of people in the area who smoke and have hereditary disease. By combining the data of the people, the settlements that may be most affected by the epidemic can be determined. By using new mobile phone location data, the movements of people at high risk of infection can be tracked and precautions can be increased in some settlements .One of the most important decision support tools of health decision makers in pandemics is epidemic prediction models. Models are mathematical formulas that tell when the epidemic will peak and when it can be brought under control, taking into account the rate of spread of the epidemic (Colombia Mailman School of Public Health, 2020)

Models, also referred to as "pandemic science" in some sources, play an important role in COVID-19 outbreak. However, the reliability and adequacy of the datasets on which the models are based is a matter of debate Breakthrough technologies of the 21st century and widespread mobile (Johns Hopkins Center for Health Security, 2020).

It is also argued that the usage of mobile or portable equipment can help predict epidemics before they occur. It is claimed that zoonoses like COVID-19, or animal-borne epidemics, can be forecast in the near future with the use of digital technologies, taking into account factors like climate change and human activities. Algorithms capable of this type of analysis have already emerged. For example, Canada-based start-up BlueDot has predicted the COVID-19 outbreak using natural language processing technology. However, the international community was not warned in time because the magnitude of the danger was not interpreted correctly (Macaulay, 2020),.

It is stated that it is possible to make predictions based on the data of people's social media messages and daily life. These messages can help to create a risk profile of individuals. Analyzing these profiles together with electronic health records may reveal the risk of pandemics. However, performing such analyzes may conflict with the principles of privacy of personal data (Obeidat,2020).

Contact Tracing

The practice of tracking down contacts to stop an outbreak is not new. A tool for infectious disease control against infections is contact tracing. It might not be feasible to halt the COVID-19 virus and go back to normal without applying cutting-edge contact tracing technology (Wang et al., 2020). It has also been suggested to use cellphones and other technology to track down and identify people with such disorders. In addition, contact monitoring technology can speed up the tracking of sick people and play a crucial role in outbreak control even if they do not completely replace humans (Wang, Lin & Wong, 2020).

Life Fits Home (HES -Hayat Eve Sığar) Code is a code that is used to securely share with institutions and individuals whether they carry any risk in terms of Covid-19 disease within the scope of Controlled Social Life, transportation or visiting. Shared HES codes can be queried through the application or through the services provided to institutions. This regulation only aims to lessen the risk of contamination while a person is in areas like public transit vehicles and open spaces (Turkish Ministry of Health, 2021).

Contact monitoring is a fundamental public health response that plays a vital role in controlling COVID-19. The goal is to quickly identify new infected people who may come into contact with existing cases to further reduce transmission. High-risk exposure contacts close to an incident (2 meters or less) or 15 minutes or more in a confined environment and low-risk exposure are dangerous. Guidelines include self-quarantine or physical distancing measures to be informed and informed when COVID-19 symptoms develop. High-risk individuals are then actively followed by daily phone calls, e-mails, and / or text messages until the risk of developing symptoms is over (European Center for Disease Prevention and Control, 2019).

Filiation Application

Covidien-19, a medical term with a long history of filiation with the application, is being used as one of the strategies to fight the pandemic in Turkey. The word "filiation" comes from the medieval Latin fliti, which means "paternity," "father's ancestor," or "ancestry." In the medical setting, it is frequently characterized as "touch" or "unity," and it is also used in slightly different ways in the legal, biological, or theological contexts. Second, it conveys the relationship between objects that are dependent upon or produce one another (Demirtaş and Tekiner, 2020). Filiation is the name given to the process of detecting the reasons for any infectious disease. This term means to find the source of the epidemic and to follow the chain of spread. The Ministry of Health emphasizes that they use this method to prevent the spread of Covidien-19's in Turkey. In other words, filiation is actually a resource search study. These studies provide crucial information, including if the threat still exists and whether additional people are at risk (TRT, 2020).

The field research team identifies potential contact persons. It is learned who the cases are contacted within two days and whether these people show symptoms of the disease is observed. The research team, after listening to the stories of the patients diagnosed with their protective clothing, communicates with the people with symptoms one by one and visits these people in their living areas. In practice, a scan is performed around the patient whose case is seen within 48 hours. Later, the teams in the call center closely follow the people contacted for 14 days. The call center calls people who show symptoms of corona virus or are diagnosed with the disease every day and asks questions such as whether they have complaints and symptoms (TRT, 2020).

During the research process, by scanning the chain of the people with whom the patient is in contact, those people are reached, observed and immediately isolated and the treatments are started. With this method, the most logical way to prevent an outbreak is widespread contact screening and strict follow-up. In many countries of the world, it follows the diagnosis and treatment method on the complaints of the people instead of the case method. Turkey quickly locate and isolate the contacts of the scarcity death rate, with 99.9% of successful results in the fight filyasyo is based on the detection of 10 cases per hour (Anadolu Agency, 2020).

Quarantine And Self-Isolation

Digital technologies can be used to trace the source of an outbreak. If the degree of spread of the outbreak is less, regulatory authorities can use digital technology devices to monitor symptomatic entities for signs of disease. Digital technology-based mobile application development can conduct surveillance activities of suspects to prevent mass spread. In addition, after digital technologies detect infected people as a potential for quarantine, they can be used to determine whether they are complying with measures. Public health personnel screen and quarantine patients and can monitor which patients have violated the quarantine. Digital technology data also helps them keep track of anyone exposed to breach. Digital technology-based surveillance equipment such as remote cameras and drones can effectively monitor whether people are following quarantine protocols (Li and Xu, 2020).

Curfews for infection control may have detrimental socioeconomic effects in some nations. With the help of digital technology, quarantine can be imposed on those who have contracted the virus or have already done so, with fewer limitations on other citizens. For instance, anyone with a QR (Quick Response) code, a COVID-19 health status certificate, and a travel card with color codes for low, medium, and high risk can travel as much as they want, whereas red-coded people are required to stay in isolation (BBC, 2020).

Clinical Management

The biggest challenge for any country during an epidemic is to provide adequate medical facilities to infected patients. If the contamination rate is rapid, sufficient material is needed for new patients as some patients recover. Another major challenge that may arise is the scarcity of test kits and slower detection of the virus. The use of digital technology-based equipment ensures prudent use of existing test kits and helps to plan medical tools. Digital technology-based mobile and wearable applications make it easy to identify people at high risk of infection. Health authorities can make the most of existing test kits by prioritizing testing of high-risk people. Instead of doing daily checks to improve patients, doctors can use digital technology equipment to remotely monitor health conditions. Digital technology-based mobile application development services proactively enable the monitoring and comparison of patients' health data (Caretaker Medical, 2020).

Digital technology's artificial intelligence sector can speed up COVID-19 diagnostic and risk assessment. A cloud-based informatics solution with artificial intelligence support can be utilized to find cases of COVID-19 pneumonia. The diagnostic process is substantially accelerated by this technology, which analyses

CT images quickly and distinguishes COVID-19 from other lung disorders (Chen & See, 2020).

On chest X-rays, COVID-19 cases can be distinguished from other lung diseases fast thanks to COVID-Net, an open source deep convolution neural network architecture that is accessible to clinicians globally. The risk that infected patients would get acute respiratory distress syndrome and a critical illness can be predicted by machine learning algorithms. By identifying areas and hospitals in need of critical care resources and medical supplies, these predictive models help direct clinical decision-making and resource allocation. Patients can lessen their exposure to SARS-CoV-2 in healthcare facilities by employing virtual care platforms that use video conferencing and digital monitoring, which are used to deliver distant healthcare services. However, dangers could also include incorrect diagnoses, equipment breakdowns, privacy violations, and high healthcare system expenses (Wang et al., 2020).

Medical Supply

Healthcare supply chains have been subject to extensive and serious disruptions as a result of the coronavirus (COVID-19) pandemic. Four categories of medical supplies are necessary for treatment and care in the COVID-19 outbreak. These include prescription drugs, PPE, medical equipment, and supplies. Each of these categories has its own supply chain, and if one of these chains fails, the health system could be disrupted (Mirchandani, 2020).

Drugs have extensive supply chains, a lengthy shelf life, and substantial pharmaceutical imports. Only in other countries are many active medicinal components made. China is thought to be the source of almost two-thirds of the active components in generic drugs used in the US. By the dollar amount of US drug imports and the quantity of COVID-19 deaths per capita documented, Italy, Belgium, and the United Kingdom are among the top 10 countries. Pharmaceutical supply networks on a worldwide scale are disrupted by regulatory constraints and virus-related production difficulties (Mirchandani, 2020).

Personal protection equipment is the cornerstone of the protective measures that should be done against COVID-19 to safeguard both patients and healthcare professionals. Particularly when treating COVID-19 patients, healthcare professionals must be completely protected with gowns, gloves, surgical masks, N95/FFP2 masks, goggles, and visors. If there are issues with the material supply, alternatives include disinfecting equipment like eyeglass visors, reusing respirators, or long-term use can be tried. Additionally, using open source software and 3D printers, masks and visors devices can be created (Mirchandani,2020).

Supply networks for medical devices are very tightly controlled. Due to the ambiguity around COVID-19 ventilator effectiveness and the fluidity of the pandemic situation, it is challenging to estimate demand with any degree of accuracy. The absence of brand uniformity makes this issue worse. Increasing capacity is challenging since fans need custom-made components. A smart initial step is to increase capacity by bringing in producers from other industries. It's also important to test out novel techniques, like 3D printing, which is more adaptable and might make use of lab space in academic institutions. In the short term, recent efforts to create open source ventilators may contribute to the establishment of alternate supply chains. Going forward, it must establish a more agile supply chain for ventilators and other critical medical devices by improving product design and providing underlying regulations (Mirchandani, 2020).

Medical Supplies: It consists of medical supplies, test supplies, laboratory and intravenous kits, surgical center supplies, and other supplies and constitute a significant portion of the total expenditure in a healthcare system. Newer testing and alternative testing protocols are currently helping, but creating redundancy and developing emergency plans for medical supplies will help better prepare for the next deadly virus. The effects of COVID-19 on the supply chains for healthcare are significant and far-reaching. To ensure that our supply chains can assist our healthcare professionals both now and in the future, immediate action must be taken (Mirchandani, 2020).

HEALTH LITERACY

Health literacy is expressed as the mental and social skills required for people to access health-related information, understand this information and use it in their health-related decisions. This concept is based on the idea that both health and literacy are critical resources for daily life. Our level of literacy directly impacts our ability to not only act on health information, but also to take greater control of our health as individuals, families, and communities. When we look at the difference between health literacy and literacy; The concept of literacy is traditionally defined as a person's ability to read and write, but being literate does not mean being health literate. Health literacy requires some additional skills. For example, Skills such as knowing a sufficient number of health-related words, finding health information from various contexts, evaluating it and using it harmoniously are required (Truong and Fenton, 2022).

What Does Health Literacy Include?

- Applying the rules that must be followed for health,

- Ability to understand medical education brochures, instructions for prescribed medications, and doctors' explanations,
- Evaluating consent forms in hospitals and tackling complex healthcare systems,
- It includes the ability to access correct information and services and to use this information and services in order to improve one's own and public health. (Shah et.al,2024).

Why Is Health Literacy Important?

You may think that health literacy is not important and that ultimately our doctor makes the decisions for our health. But the truth is that you need to collaborate with your doctor when making health-related decisions. If you do not have the necessary information for this, it may not be possible to realize this cooperation. Health literacy skills enable patients to take control of their own well-being by making sensible healthcare choices, improving their communication with doctors, and giving them the information they need to advocate for themselves in a medical setting (Harding et al., 2022).

In addition, it strengthens people's competence in their own and public health by ensuring the correct use of resources and shaping quality conditions in health services. Because in order to receive quality health care, patients must first understand and express their complaints and symptoms correctly. For this reason, insufficient health literacy negatively affects people's health, as well as their social and cultural development (Harding et al., 2022).

METHODOLOGY

In this study, the terms "coronavirus," "severe acute respiratory syndrome 2," "2019-nCov," "SARS-CoV," and "MERS-CoV" were used, as well as references to academic studies on the COVID-19, digital health, pandemic management, and technology in PubMed and Google. Public disclosures of states were also looked at. By providing a framework for the application of digital technologies, the study evaluated digital technologies for pandemic planning and monitoring, contact tracking, infection screening, quarantine and self-isolation, clinical management, and medical procurement of successful practices (GSMA, 2019).

Initiatives related to digital health have the potential to widen healthcare and socioeconomic disparities. In a limited sense, digital technology comprises the usage of the internet and mobile devices. Despite the fact that 4 billion people would be using the internet globally in 2019, low- and middle-income areas still outnumbered high-income ones disproportionately (82% in Europe and 28% in Africa). Vigilant organizations may not have access to broadband connections, cellphones, or wearable technology like smart watches if they live in low-income neighborhoods or distant locations. To successfully apply digital technology on a worldwide scale, investment is needed in broadband access, technology, and infrastructure (GSMA, 2019).

Subsidized cell phone subscriptions, borrowed gadgets, free Wi-Fi hotspots, and educational initiatives can all help to mitigate these disparities at the local level. Automated apps and gadgets that don't need constant network access should be taken into account in areas where there isn't enough money or infrastructure to provide cellular communication coverage. While some digital health treatments, particularly those that monitor people and impose quarantines, can harm privacy, they also raise the risk for those who are mentally ill or who have poor access to food and water. Additionally, the state's surveillance and control measures have the potential to incite fear and endanger civil freedoms. European officials advise that non-essential digital measures be removed in order to strike a balance between the necessity for contact tracing and privacy by only retaining data for 14 days after the possibility of viral infection and pandemic period has passed (Just Security, 2020).

FINDINGS

To combat the COVID-19 pandemic and deal with a wide range of pandemic-related challenges, governments must fully utilize digital technologies. Governments and communities are being forced by the pandemic to use digital technologies to address the crisis, and it is becoming more and more important for goverments to adopt an open strategy and use digital communication channels to provide accurate information on regional and national COVID-19 developments (Loideain, 2019). Digital technology initiatives and recommendations in combating the pandemic can be stated are as follows:

Planning and execution: Real-time monitoring of disease activity is one of the features. Digital technologies include data dashboards, migration maps, machine learning, real-time data from cellphones, and clothes. The benefits include the ability to see propagation, management of restrictions, direction of resources, and estimation. Additionally, drawbacks include privacy violations, significant expenses, and administration and regulation requirements.

Screening for infection: Functions include disease screening of both individuals and populations. Digital technologies are employed in artificial intelligence, digital thermometers, mobile phone applications, thermal cameras, and web-based toolkits. Information on disease pathology and prevalence is advantageous, and it identifies people for testing, contact tracing, and isolation. Additionally, disadvantages include invasion of privacy, inability to identify persons who are asymptomatic while tracking vital signs or self-reported symptoms, high expenses, need for management and control, and the requirement for tool verification.

Contact tracing: Contact tracing is the process of tracking and identifying individuals who may have had contact with an infected person. Useful technologies include GPS systems, mobile phone apps, mobile device real-time monitoring, and wearable technology. The benefits are Tracks viral spread and identifies exposed individuals for testing and quarantine. The disadvantages include invasion of privacy and the identification of those who have come into touch with it but have not been revealed. It might not be possible to identify exposed people if the app is disabled, there is no mobile device available, or the Wi-Fi or cell connection is poor.

Self-isolation and quarantine: These procedures are used to identify, watch over, and confine affected people. Artificial intelligence, cameras, digital recorders, GPS, mobile phone apps, and quick response codes are some of the digital technologies that will be deployed. It isolates infections, which is a benefit. Travel restrictions and freedom violations are some of the drawbacks. Access to food and other necessities may also be restricted, and the gadget cannot be used to track people who escape quarantine without it.

Clinic management: Clinic management includes identifying infected people; keeping track of the clinical environment; estimating clinical outcomes; and offering telemedicine services and virtual capacity. The technologies include telemedicine systems, virtual care, machine learning, and artificial intelligence for diagnostics. The benefits include facilitating clinical decision-making, diagnosis, and risk assessment; guaranteeing effective service delivery; and enabling patient-based remote care and infection control. The drawbacks include invasion of privacy, inability to diagnose patients accurately, expensive expenses, and potential device failure.

Medical Supply: Pharmaceuticals, personal protective gear, medical gadgets, and material supply are among the responsibilities of the medical supply department. The technologies include source code software, digital supply chain software, worldwide digital standards, and 3D printing production. Fast shipping, affordable manufacture, and bulk orders are benefits. Transportation challenges, a lack of infrastructure, and improper operations by unlicensed institutions are drawbacks.

Health Literacy: Health literacy provides important contributions not only individually but also socially. It is thought that raising public awareness about health literacy and organizing training in this sense will provide positive developments in the health level of the society and the country.

DISCUSSION

Researchers and developers, pandemic built-in digital technology systems disruptions that may occur should keep in mind while developing. However, other built-in digital technology to provide benefits for future are evaluated as follows:

Security and Privacy: The security and privacy of residents is a worry of users who live in intelligent settings and systems. Researchers need to make sure that the relevant data is anonymised in order to profit from digital technology. It should also employ a variety of access control strategies to guarantee the privacy, accessibility, and consistency of data. When people engage with smart settings in the future, a lot of personal data is generated. The creation of security and privacy protection solutions should occur concurrently with the development of these smart environments (Loideain, 2019).

The risks of information systems increase in pandemics. As the OECD warns, the turn of countries towards digital solutions in the fight against the epidemic increases cyber risks (OECD, 2020). At a time when the need for information of healthcare professionals who are heroically fighting the pandemic is at the highest level, cyber attacks pose risks that may lead to loss of life. According to a study, cyber-attacks have increased five times throughout the world during the COVID-19 process compared to the pre-pandemic period (Sharton, 2020).

Video conferencing applications, whose use is increasing as the work increases, are also exposed to a large number of attacks. The primary way to protect healthcare systems from such attacks is to always be prepared for cyber attacks. What to do when exposed to a cyber attack should be planned and recorded in advance. Information should be obtained about current fraud methods and should be announced to employees. Multi-factor authenticator systems should be used. Top management should have alternative communication opportunities. In the COVID-19 crisis as it turns out, security considerations should be increased in video conferencing applications, the use of which has increased due to distance education and working from home (Moseley, 2020).

Blockchain Applications: Blockchain applications are being developed to verify, secure and share data. It is therefore suitable for managing cross-border transactions between multilateral organizations. There is great need. In addition, Blockchain applications can be a good tool to ensure the safe and uninterrupted continuation of the international health supply chain, which has emerged as extremely fragile in the epidemic. Blockchain solutions that have been developed for years have been redesigned and made available to meet the challenges in the COVID-19 crisis. Blockchain applications have also been used in surveillance studies in epidemics. Surveillance information flow is accelerated and secured with Blockchain "wallets". Thanks to secure data transfer, it can help develop new and accurate diagnoses and treatments. This includes drug and vaccine development studies. Blockchain is also an important tool for protecting personal health data. Blockchain can securely manage health records, ensure interoperability without compromising security, and protect patient privacy (Brett, 2020).

Availability and Data: The availability of the necessary data and the volume of data present another difficulty in developing various digital systems. Large amounts of tagged data are necessary for the majority of big data and artificial intelligence applications in the digital environment. Partnerships between the public and private sectors should be established in order to produce datasets that can be utilized to build these smart media models. Special care must be made to guarantee that these models remain impartial and fair when AI-assisted uses are created. Smart systems should be given access to methods that allow for impartial decision-making (Chauhan, Agarwal and Kar, 2016).

Legislation and Policy: For social distances using smart surroundings, privacy is a technical concern; nonetheless, technology options must support the law. Although the development of intelligent environmental technology is accelerating, legislation and policies may remain insufficient for a considerable amount of time. For social distancing, official policies are crucial, and they should at the very least cover topics like secure data gathering, video surveillance, user / resident consent, and trustworthy third parties. Laws must be observed when utilizing smart media technologies. Therefore, the smart ecosystem needs to include research on laws and policies, participation in the formulation of public policy, and technology privacy solutions. In addition to privacy-related legislation, policies that promote innovation, competition, and private investment are needed for social distance sanctions utilizing smart technologies. Such policies ought to emphasize the social advantages of extending social distancing sanctions, partnership between the public and private sectors, the reduction of administrative obstacles, and (Appel, 2020).

Benefit and Cost: Costs for digital systems are significant. In order to connect appliances to electrical public lighting, for instance, it is necessary to isolate them from other crucial systems, which demands a lot of time and effort and raises expenses. Additionally, the amount of data that battery-powered devices can broadcast during their operational periods and battery life is constrained. Since they are frequently installed in great numbers, regular maintenance of such devices can be highly expensive. The expenses also cover operating expenses. The necessity for specific equipment and sensors will drive up the costs listed above as social separation is pushed. Costs connected with other opportunities can be reduced with the use of smart media. Drones that track social distances, for instance, can save law enforcement expenditures and free them up to work on other concerns. Healthcare expenses will be greatly decreased if the COVID-19 pandemic patient population is reduced. Therefore, one crucial area for future research is the creation of a framework that is efficient, timely, and affordable for social distance practice. Cost-benefit analysis studies for smart environments are a significant future research area. For instance, predictive analysis and traffic rerouting in cities can both help to ease congestion. It will save on unnecessary travel costs to busy areas as well as the implementation of social distance limits (Lam, & Yang, 2017).

Awareness and Compliance: Typically, the COVID-19 virus spreads through droplets that are produced when an infected person coughs or sneezes. According to the most recent data, the majority of patients—around 80%—recover from the illness without the need for specialized care. One in six COVID-19 patients has a bad illness and has trouble breathing. The data we have indicates that 2% of people with the condition pass away (Jayaweera et al, 2020).

Cooperation with traditional media organizations and social media platforms is necessary to prevent the spread of messages and comments about the epidemic that may cause panic in the society. WHO has announced that it is collaborating with technology giants to prevent harmful content, which it defines as "fake information epidemic" (Scott, 2020). It has been observed that during the COVID-19 process, media organizations voluntarily participated in public information activities, acting with a sense of social duty. Facebook, for example, is trying to verify facts to prevent the spread of misinformation on media platforms and announced that it took action to control it. Twitter, TikTok, Apple, Amazon, and Google have added COVID-19 notifications to their artificial intelligence assistance services and started to block harmful content. YouTube, on the other hand, has stated that while it directs users searching for COVID-19 directly to content provided by WHO and similar reliable organizations, it deletes videos that provide false information as soon as they are uploade. States have contacted search engines to prevent the proliferation of false claims and to encourage only scientifically sound sources of information (Robertson, 2020).

CONCLUSION

This chapter provides a conceptual overview of current use case studies around the world and provides a basis for a comprehensive research and deployment of technologies based on automated data from smart media and smart systems. In the research, the implementation of best practices with digital technology in practice obtained and Turkish "filiation" analysis of the information gathered about the Covid-19 was revealed. In addition, a conceptual proposal and future directions for the effective use of digital technologies are specified. The specified use cases are predicted to be developed on the basis of the Internet of artificial intelligence-oriented objects to ensure that these applications are more widely adopted in society in the future to ensure that there is no gap between them. One of the few characteristics of nations with flattened COVID-19 incidence curves and low mortality rates may be the integration and response of digital technologies to pandemic strategy. Countries that quickly use digital technology to streamline planning, surveillance, testing, contact tracking, quarantine, and clinical management have been at the forefront of managing the disease burden in the fight to contain the spread of a highly contagious virus. Comprehensive responses from nations that have achieved containment and mitigation success can serve as an example for nations still dealing with a wave of cases.

REFERENCES

American Civil Liberties Union (ACLU).(2021). Principles for technology-assisted contact-tracing. ACLU White Paper. Retrieved from https://www.aclu.org/report/aclu-white-paper-principles-technology-assisted-contact-tracing

Anadolu Agency. (2020). Hidden heroes of the fight against coronavirus: Filection teams. Retrieved from https://www.aa.com.tr/tr/koronavirus/koronavirus-ile-mucadelenin-gizli-kahramanlari-filmasyon-ekipleri/1807025

Appel, G., Grewal, L., Rhonda Hadi, R., & Stephen, A. T. (2020). The future of social media in marketing. [January.]. *Journal of the Academy of Marketing Science*, *48*(1), 79–95. doi:10.1007/s11747-019-00695-1 PMID:32431463

BBC. (2020). Covid-19: China pushes for QR code based global travel system. Retrieved from https://www.bbc.com/news/business-55039662. Posted on October 09, 2020.

Brett, J. (2020). How Blockchain Technology Offers 'Computational Trust' For Tracking The Coronavirus Outbreak", Forbes, https://www.forbes.com/sites/jasonbrett/2020/03/23/how-blockchain-technology-offers-computational-trust-for-tracking---the-coronavirus-outbreak/#c56e0351cd06

Caretaker Medical. (2020). Caretaker Medical News Australia's first 'virtual hospital' for COVID-19 patients use Caretaker Medical wireless patient monitor for remote monitoring and reporting. Retrieved from https://www.caretakermedical.net/australias-first-virtual-hospital-for-covid-19-patients-use-caretaker-medical-wireless-patient-monitor-for-remote-monitoring-and-reporting/

Chauhan, S., Agarwal, N., & Kar, A. K. (2016). Addressing big data challenges in smart cities: A systematic literature review. *Info*, *18*(4), 73–90. doi:10.1108/info-03-2016-0012

Chen, J., & See, K. C. (2020). Artificial Intelligence for COVID-19: Rapid Review. *Journal of Medical Internet Research, 22*(10), e21476. doi:10.2196/21476 PMID:32946413

Colombia Mailman School of Public Health. (2020). Mapping the Areas Most Vulnerable to COVID-19 Hospitalizations. https://www.mailman.columbia.edu/public-health-now/news/mapping-areas-most-vulnerable-COVID-19-hospitalizations

Demirtaş, T., & Tekiner, H. (2020). Filiation: A Historical Term the COVID-19 Outbreak Recalled in Turkey. *Erciyes Med J, 42*(3), 354–358. doi:10.14744/etd.2020.54782

Ekong, I., Chukwu, E., & Chukwu, M. (2020). COVID-19 Mobile Positioning Data Contact Tracing and Patient Privacy Regulations: Exploratory Search of Global Response Strategies and the Use of Digital Tools in Nigeria. *JMIR mHealth and uHealth, 8*(4), e19139. doi:10.2196/19139 PMID:32310817

European Center for Disease Prevention and Control (ECDC). (2019). Infection prevention and control for the care of patients with 2019-nCoV in healthcare settings. Retrieved from https://www.ecdc.europa.eu/en/publications-data/infection-prevention-and-control-care-patients-2019- ncov-healthcare-settings

Ferretti, L., Wymant, C., Kendall, M., Zhao, L., Nurtay, A., Abeler-Dörner, L., Parker, M., Bonsall, D., & Fraser, C. (2020). Quantifying SARS-CoV-2 transmission suggests epidemic control with digital contact tracing. *Science, 368*(6491), eabb6936. Advance online publication. doi:10.1126/science.abb6936 PMID:32234805

GSMA. (2019). The state of mobile internet connectivity. Retrieved from https://www.gsma.com/mobilefordevelopment/wp-content/uploads/2019/07/GSMA-State-of-Mobile-Internet-Connectivity-Report-2019.pdf

Harding, R., Salins, N., Sharan, K., & Ekstrand, M. L. (2022). Health literacy in communication, decision-making and outcomes among cancer patients, their families and clinicians in India: A multicentre cross-sectional qualitative study. *Psycho-Oncology, 31*(3), 532–540. doi:10.1002/pon.5838 PMID:34687573

International Bar Association. (2020). Guidelines and Regulations to Provide Insights on Public Policies to Ensure Artificial Intelligence's Beneficial Use as a Professional Tool. Retrieved from https://www.ibanet.org/MediaHandler?id=f5099a33-1e70-4a32-839d-589236b7568d

Jayaweera, M., Perera, H., Gunawardana, B., & Manatunge, J. (2020). Transmission of COVID-19 virus by droplets and aerosols: A critical review on the unresolved dichotomy. *Environmental Research, 188*, 109819. doi:10.1016/j.envres.2020.109819 PMID:32569870

Johns Hopkins Center for Health Security. (2020), "Modernizing and Expanding Outbreak Science to Support Better Decision Making During Public Health Crises: Lessons for COVID-19 and Beyond". https://www.centerforhealthsecurity.org/our-work/publications/modernizing-and-expanding-outbreak-science-to-support-better-decision-making-during-public-health-crises

Karina, M. (2020). How AI is helping scientists in the fight against COVID-19, from robots to predicting the future. Retrieved from https://www.geekwire.com/2020/ai-helping-scientists-fightcovid-19-robots-predicting-future/amp/

Lam, P., & Yang, W. (2017). A Study of the Costs and Benefits of Smart City Projects Including the Scenario of Public-Private Partnerships. *World Academy of Science, Engineering and Technology, International Journal of Civil, Environmental, Structural. Construction and Architectural Engineering*, *11*, 600–605.

Li, L. Q. L., & Xu, Z. (2020). Artificial intelligence distinguishes COVID-19 from community acquired pneumonia on chest CT. *Radiology*. Advance online publication. doi:10.1148/radiol.2020200905 PMID:32191588

Loideain, N. N. (2019). A port in the data-sharing storm: The GDPR and the Internet of things. *Journal of Cyber Policy*, *4*(2), 178–196. doi:10.1080/23738871.2019.1635176

Macaulay, T. (2020), "AI sent first coronavirus alert, but underestimated the danger", The Next Web, https://thenextweb. com/neural/2020/02/21/ai-sent-first-coronavirus-alert-but-underestimated-the-danger/

Mirchandani, P. (2020). Health Care Supply Chains: COVID-19 Challenges and Pressing Actions. *Annals of Internal Medicine*, *173*(4), 300–301. doi:10.7326/M20-1326 PMID:32369540

Moseley, S. (2020). 5 Steps for Secure Video Conferencing. https://highfive.com/blog/5-steps-for-secure-video-conferencing. (Access Date 12 March 2022)

Obeidat, S. (2020), "How Artificial Intelligence Is Helping Fight The COVID-19 Pandemic", Entrepreneur, (30 March 2020), https://www.entrepreneur.com/article/348368

OECD. (2020). Beyond containment: Health systems responses to COVID-19 in the OECD", (16 April 2020), https://www.oecd.org/coronavirus/policy-responses/beyond-containment-health-systems-responses-to-COVID -19-in-the-oecd/

Ribandar, H. (2020). What COVID-19 teaches us about the way forward for digital health solutions in LMICs.? Retrieved from https://www.linkedin.com/pulse/what-covid-19-teaches-us-way-forward-digital-health-solutions-riband/?trackingId=rlxXqseQ%2BhYmY6b3Yat9kw%3D%3D

Robertson, A. (2020). Facebook will add anti-misformation posts to your News Feed if you liked fake coronavirus news", The Verge, https://www.theverge.com/2020/4/16/21223456/facebook-coronavirus-misformation-fake-news- warning-update-who.

Sanchez-Comas, A., Synnes, K., & Hallberg, J. (2020). Hardware for Recognition of Human Activities: A Review of Smart Home and AAL Related Technologies. *Sensors (Basel)*, *20*(15), 4227. doi:10.3390/s20154227 PMID:32751345

Scott, T. (2020), "Coronavirus: Can artificial intelligence be smart enough to detect fake news?", MarketPlace, https:// www.marketplace.org/2020/02/12/coronavirus-can-artificial-intelligence-be -smart-enough-to-detect-fake-news/

Security, J. (2020). Can governments track the pandemic and still protect privacy? Retrieved from https://www.justsecurity.org/69549/can-governments-track-the-pandemic-and-still-protect-privacy/

Shah, P., Thornton, I., & Turrin, D. (2024). Informed Consent. In: StatPearls [Internet]. Treasure Island (FL): StatPearls Publishing; 2024 Jan-. Available from: https://www.ncbi.nlm.nih.gov/books/NBK430827/

Sharton, B. R. (2020). How Organizations Can Ramp Up Their Cybersecurity Efforts Right Now. Harvard Business Review, (May 1, 2020), https://hbr.org/2020/05/how-organizations-can-ramp-up-their-cybersecurity-efforts -right-now?ab=hero-subleft-3.

TRT. (2020). What is fillation? How does filyasyo process in Turkey? Retrieved from https://www.trthaber.com/haber/infografik/filyasyon-nedir-turkiyede-filyasyon-sureci-nasil-isliyor-476210.html. Posted on June 17, 2020.

Truong, M., & Fenton, S. H. (2022). Understanding the Current Landscape of Health Literacy Interventions within Health Systems. *Perspectives in Health Information Management*, *19*(Spring), 1h. PMID:35692852

Turkish Ministry of Health. (2021). What is HPP Code? Retrieved from https://hayatevesigar.saglik.gov.tr/hes.html

United Nations. (2020). Digital technologies critical in facing COVID-19 pandemic? Retrieved from https://www.un.org/development/desa/en/news/policy/digital-technologies-critical-in-facing-covid-19-pandemic.html

Wallis, L., Blessing, P., Dalwai, M., & Shin, S. D. (2017). Integrating mHealth at point of care in low- and middle-income settings: the system perspective. *Global health action*, 10(sup3), 1327686. . doi:10.1080/16549716.2017.1327686

Wang, C., Horby, P. W., Hayden, F. G., & Gao, G. F. (2020). A novel coronavirus outbreak of global health concern. *Lancet*, *395*(10223), 470–473. doi:10.1016/S0140-6736(20)30185-9 PMID:31986257

Wang, L., Lin, Z. Q., & Wong, A. (2020). COVID-Net: A tailored deep convolutional neural network design for detection of COVID-19 cases from chest X-ray images. *Scientific Reports*, *10*(1), 19549. doi:10.1038/s41598-020-76550-z PMID:33177550

Whitelaw, S., Mamas, M. A., Topol, E., & Van Spall, H. (2020). Applications of digital technology in COVID-19 pandemic planning and response. *The Lancet. Digital Health*, *2*(8), e435–e440. doi:10.1016/S2589-7500(20)30142-4 PMID:32835201

Zhu, N., Zhang, D., Wang, W., Li, X., Yang, B., Song, J., Zhao, X., Huang, B., Shi, W., Lu, R., Niu, P., Zhan, F., Ma, X., Wang, D., Xu, W., Wu, G., Gao, G. F., & Tan, W. (2020). A Novel Coronavirus from Patients with Pneumonia in China, 2019. *The New England Journal of Medicine*, *382*(8), 727–733. doi:10.1056/NEJMoa2001017 PMID:31978945

KEY TERMS AND DEFINITIONS

Blockchain: In its most general definition, blockchain; It can be defined as a technology protocol that enables data sharing with trust-based transactions such as identification and authorization in a decentralized-distributed network environment without the need for approval or control of a central authority.

Contact Tracing: Contact tracing is the process of identifying, evaluating and managing people who have been exposed to the virus to prevent person-to-person transmission of the virus. Contact tracing has been used by health departments for decades to slow or stop the spread of infectious diseases.

Coronavirus/ Covid-19: The novel coronavirus, also known as the unofficial Wuhan coronavirus, as it was first seen in the Wuhan region of China in early

December 2019 and was identified by the authorities in that region, is a contagious virus that causes respiratory tract infection and can be passed from person to person.

Digital Health: Digital health is the use of information and communication technologies in the diagnosis and treatment of patients, monitoring the health and risk status of individuals who are not sick, training health system workers, and monitoring and improving public health.

Digital Technology: It includes all electronic tools, automatic systems, technological devices and resources that produce, process or store information. Digital technology has facilitated and accelerated production, distribution and consumption. Products are produced on machines, distributed and consumed via the public network. People buy products without going to stores.

Filiation: This term means finding the source of the epidemic and following the chain of its spread. In other words, filiation is actually a source search exercise. As a result of these studies, important information is obtained such as whether the danger still continues and whether other people are at risk.

Health literacy: Health literacy is a concept that increases in importance day by day with the developments in the field of health and the increasing awareness level of health users.

Life Fits Home: With the "Life Fits Into Home" App, citizens are able to see the risk status and incidence rate in the area they live in or they want to travel on the map and in addition to the incidence rate, places to bear in mind in case of emergencies such as hospitals, pharmacies, supermarkets and bus stops are also marked on the map for citizens.

Chapter 5
An Analytical Review of the Roles of Digital Media and Health in India During the Pandemic of COVID-19

Subir Sinha
https://orcid.org/0000-0001-7578-9809
Dum Dum Motijheel College, India

ABSTRACT

The 21st Century has experienced a global pandemic caused by a highly infectious viral disease called COVID-19. It spread globally and put a wide impact on human civilization. In India, the scenario of the pandemic was not different. The Indian government took several serious steps to resist the COVID-19 and several other health issues during the pandemic. India initially focuses on the health literacy, information dissemination and awareness programme to resist the spread of infection. Digital media played some significant roles in it. The article entitled "An Analytical Review of the Roles of Digital Media and the Health in India during the Pandemic of COVID-19" analysed five case studies and justify significances. The article reflected how digital media disseminates information on Corona virus and the diseases called COVID-19, creates awareness among the public and helps to resist the spread of infection. During the pandemic, digital media also acts as a platform which provided comfort to mental stress and support in the vaccination process.

DOI: 10.4018/978-1-7998-9652-4.ch005

INTRODUCTION

The dawn of 21st century has shown a massive health crisis with the arrival of Corona virus disease commonly called COVID-19, the highly infectious viral disease that spread globally and infects millions of people from across the globe. The rapid pace of the infection rate attracts the attention of the globe and keeps the health system busy of almost every nation. India was not remained aloof from the rest of the world. It also reflected a similar scenario which the rest of the world has shown. In India the impact of COVID-19 was tremendous. It infects thousands of people every day and killed several. It creates turmoil and confusion throughout the nation. In the introduction of the book *'The Pandemic Notebook: A handy guide from The Hindu on understanding the coronavirus pandemic and staying protected against COVID-19'* published by the Indian media group The Hindu it was mentioned as:

"Since then, more than 6000 deaths have been reported due to COVID-19 across the world till March 20, 2020. Cases have been reported from more than 180 countries, including India. Lockdown, curfews, massive airport screenings, quarantine, and social distance have become the norm across the globe." – (Prasad. Et.al, 2020)

Along with the COVID-19 several other health issues also shows its coexistence during the pandemic period. It reflected a massive health crisis but Indian government took several vital steps from the initial days of its arrival to resist the COVID-19 and to deal with the other health issues. To deal with health crisis India mainly concentrates on the medical treatments but it also gives focuses on the health literacy through proper information dissemination and awareness campaign. However digital media has proved significant in health literacy and performed several essential roles during the pandemic of COVID-19. It helps to disseminate information widely and create awareness among the public which revealed highly beneficial to resist COVID-19 and other health issues during the pandemic. Along with the information and message, the digital pictorial presentation also helps to understand several aspects related to corona virus and the disease COVID-19. The digital based application also helps to detects COVID-19 infected persons and their families which make the public aware and tried to keep the society safe. The roles of digital media in supporting the mental health, delivering health advices and maintaining the connectivity were also significant. Along with all these essential roles digital media also shows its essentiality in vaccination dive and tried to records an accurate data related to vaccination which runs throughout the India.

OBJECTIVES OF THE RESEARCH

COVID-19 arrived in the 21st Century and become a serious life threatening issue which critically hampers and devastated the health system of almost every nation of the globe. In India the scenario was almost same but Indian government took several responsible measures to resist the infection of COVID-19. Along with medical treatment it gives a huge focus on health literacy through information dissemination and various campaigns. However it was reflected that the digital media plays a significant role in strengthening the overall health system and in awareness campaign. The multidimensional roles of digital media during the pandemic of COVID-19 make it as a vital subject of research. It becomes essential to find out various impacts and significances of digital media on the health system. However the article entitled *'An Analytical Review of the Roles of Digital Media and the Health in India during the Pandemic of COVID-19'* reflected a wide scope of research and was conducted to find out the correct explanation while focusing the following objectives:

- Significance of digital media during the pandemic of COVID-19.
- How it helps to create health awareness among the public during the pandemic
- How Indian government and other organisations uses various platforms of digital media during the pandemic of COVID-19

METHODOLOGIES

The article entitled *'An Analytical Review of the Roles of Digital Media and the Health in India during the Pandemic of COVID-19'* is mainly based on case study research analysis. It analyses five case studies and several data and contents published in books, journal and websites to focus on the essential roles played by digital media in India during the pandemic of COVID-19.

CASE STUDIES AND ANALYSIS

Case 1: Web Portal of The Ministry of Health and Family Welfare – Government of India

Case 1 analyse various data and the structure of the web portal of the Ministry of Health and Family Welfare, Government of India. The web portal provides a full data of COVID-19 in India. In the upper section of the front page of the web portal provides toll free helpline number and revealed the percentage and figure of 'Active

Cases', 'Discharge' and 'Death'. In the middle section of the web page it provides 'Latest Update', 'COVID-19 State wise Status' and 'Resources' where as in the lower section it provides with 'Awareness' and 'FAQ'.

The upper section provides full detail in figure and percentage of active cases of COVID-19 in India, figure and percentage of discharge from hospitals and the mortality rate and figure. These figure and percentage revealed the summary of COVID-19 in India. Along with these data the upper section also provide toll free helpline number for help and assistance.

The middle section provides all latest update on COVID-19 which mainly deals with all government announcements related to COVID-19, stories of research and research finding, National and international guidelines, Pandemic and the harmful effect of Tobacco use, etc. The middle section of the page also provides full detail of state wise COVID-19 status. The lower section is full of some social awareness message on COVID-19 and Frequently Ask Question (FAQ) and their answers.

The web portal gives full details information of COVID-19 in India, international rules and regulations on COVID-19 and various awareness messages which can be viewed through various platform such as Computer desktop, laptop, advance mobile set, and tablet.

Case 2: NPH India – National Health Portal

The Ministry of Health and Family Welfare, Government of India has set up the National Health Portal in pursuance to the decision of the National Knowledge Commission to provide health care related data and information. The activities of the National Health Portal are managed by the Centre for Health Informatics which was established by The National Institute of Health and Family Welfare (NIHFW). The National Health Portal is a digital web portal of Ministry of Health and Family Welfare which provides enormous valuable authentic data and information related to health and health awareness which in several cases acts as health advice. The information and data are highly beneficial for the citizen, healthcare professional and research scholar who are researching on health topics.

The upper section of the front page of the National Health Portal provides a sub heading Health Tips followed by What's New?, Directory Service, e-Booklet and Online Service MoHFW. The middle section of the portal provides the link with the caption AYUSH / NATUROPATHY /SPIRITUALITY AND HEALTH and the lower section of the front page provides the captions Major Health Initiatives.

The upper section with the caption 'What's New?' provides latest news related to health and health service in India. During the Covid-19 pandemic this section provides valuable news related to COVID-19 along with several other news related to health. The section 'Directory Service' provides contacts and details of Ambulance,

Helpline and Hospital. The section 'e-Booklet' provides a booklet on IT initiatives of National Health Mission and the section 'Online Service MoHFW' shows all the online facilities provided by Ministry of Health and Family Welfare.

In the middle section under with caption 'AYUSH /NATUROPATHY/ SPIRITUALITY AND HEALTH' the icon first come is 'Ayurveda' followed by Yoga, Unani, Siddha, Homeopathy, Naturopathy, Health and spirituality. This section does not nurture with allopathic treatment rather it discuss various alternative medicine system with historical roots from Indian subcontinent. The lower section of the front page of the National Health Portal provides the caption 'Major Health Initiatives' which provides the link of various health initiatives of India taken by Government of India. The section provides initiatives link like 'Disease A-Z', 'Online Registration System', 'mCessation Programme', 'NHP Voice Web Application', 'Pradhan Mantri Surakshit Matritva Abhiyan', ' Mera Aspataal', 'eRaktKosh', ' My Health Record', 'Family Planning', ' mDiabetes', ' eSanjeevani National telemedicine Service', etc.

Case 3: Web Portal of the Ministry of Health and Family Welfare – Resources: Behavioural Health

Mental health was become a major serious issue in India during the pandemic of COVID-19. Government of India has taken several initiatives to tackle the situation. The Ministry of Health and Family Welfare put in their web portal a section called "Behavioural Health" to deal with the issues of mental health. The section is not big enough but provided various valuable information and data on mental health in the form of written documents and video. The quality of the data and information are wide and highly beneficial to deal the mental health.

On 28th March 2020 it has uploaded and linked in the 'Behavioural Health' section of the portal a short video programme of Ministry of Health and Family Welfare, Government of India with title 'Various Health Experts on how to manage Mental Health & Well Being during COVID-19 outbreak'. The video provided experts opinion on mental health during the pandemic. On 31st March 2020 the portal uploaded a three pages written document with title 'Minding our minds during the COVID-19'. The three pages written document focus on understanding the importance of the nationwide lockdown, handling social isolation, reject rumours, handling emotional problems, recognising mental health problem in near and dear one, etc. On 31st March the Ministry of Health and Family Welfare uploaded and linked again a short video in its web portal with title 'Video on Practical tips to take care of your Mental Health during the Stay In'. Where Dr. Pratima Murty, Professor of Psychiatry and Head Department of Psychiatry, NIMHANS delivered a short lecture on what to do and what not to do during the pandemic and the lockdown stay in.

In the month of April 2020 the Ministry of Health and Family Welfare uploaded sixteen items in the 'Behavioural Health' section of it web portal. On 1st April they uploaded in the 'Behavioural Health' section three items with titles 'Psychosocial issues among migrants during COVID-19', 'Taking care of mental health of elderly during COVID-19', 'Taking care of mental health of children during COVID-19'. These three topics mainly deal with migrant, elders and children. On 5th April two video items were uploaded with title 'Lockdown to Knockdown COVID-19' and 'Lockdown to Knockdown-additional tips'. The topic deals with stress and depression during the outbreak of COVID-19 and their solutions. On 8th April they uploaded four items with titles 'Video on meditation for stress management (Hindi)', 'Video on Yoga for stress management (English)', 'Addressing Social Stigma Associated with COVID-19', and 'Video on Addressing Social Stigma Associated with COVID-19'. These four items deal with stress management and social stigma associated with COVID-19. On 10th April they uploaded three items with title 'Video on Addressing Social Stigma Associated with COVID-19 (Hindi)', 'Audio Visual on Managing Mental Stress and Depression during Lockdown', 'Audio Visual on How to Safely Stop Drinking During Lockdown'. These three items deals with social stigma associated with COVID-19, mental stress and its solution and negative effect of alcohols and its avoidance during COVID-19 pandemic. On 11th and 13th April they again uploaded item related to meditation and yoga for stress management. On 15th April they uploaded an audio visual document with title 'Audio Visual on How to safely Quit Tobacco during Lockdown (Hindi)'. It deals with the negative effects of Tobacco and how to quit tobacco. On 20th April they again uploaded an audio visual on stigma related to COVID-19 with titled 'Audio Visual on Addressing Stigma Related to COVID-19'. In the month of June 2020 they uploaded a single audio visual title 'Video on Addressing Psychosocial Concerns of Healthcare Workers'. The video was concerned with the psychosocial issues of the healthcare workers.

In the month of July 2020 they uploaded four items in their web portal with titles 'Mental Health in the times of COVID-19 Pandemic- Guidance for General Medical and Specialised Mental Health Care Settings', 'Caring for Health Care Warriors- Mental Health Support During COVID-19 (Jointly prepared by Department of Health & Family Welfare, Government of Karnataka and National Institute of Mental Health and Neurosciences, Bengaluru)', 'COVID-19 Pandemic and Tobacco use in India', and ' A/V on "Mental Health Matters..Let's Talk"'. The first on with the title 'Mental Health in the times of COVID-19 Pandemic- Guidance for General Medical and Specialised Mental Health Care Settings' is a guideline in the written form, where as the second one with title 'Caring for Health Care Warriors- Mental Health Support During COVID-19 (Jointly prepared by Department of Health & Family Welfare, Government of Karnataka and National Institute of Mental Health and Neurosciences, Bengaluru)' is a highly valued document on mental health related to health care professionals. The documents with title"COVID-19 Pandemic and Tobacco use in India" deals with the negative effect of tobacco and the documents 'A/V on "Mental Health Matters..Let's Talk"' is a video based on byte taken from effected persons.

On 1st November 2020 they uploaded a single documents related to the guideline on mental health. It was uploaded with the title "Guideline on Managing Mental Illness in Hospital Setting during COVID-19". The Behavioural section of the web portal of The Ministry of Health and Family Welfare continuously uploaded the documents to support the mental health of the citizen.

Case 4: Aarogya Setu App

Aarogya Setu App or application is an Indian COVID-19 contact tracing, syndrome mapping and self-assessment digital mobile application that was developed by the National Informatics Centre under the Ministry of Electronics and Information Technology. The Aarogya Setu was launched by Government of India in public private partnership mode on 02nd April 2020. The App was developed in 21 days, to respond to the exigencies of the pandemic with lockdown restrictions. The objective was to build a made in India contact tracing app to detect COVID-19. The app was designed to inform its users a number of important details regarding risks, best practices and relevant advisories pertaining to the containment of Covid-19. The Aarogya Setu app uses Bluetooth and location generated social graphs to trace the movement of users and track whether they have come in contact with a Covid-19 positive person.

Aarogya Setu, application arrived in India in a first track basic but it has become the most downloaded app in the recent times and as a testimony to citizen's innate belief in the power of technology to inform, guide and protect them from unwanted consequences in the times of public health emergency. *Almost 98% of Aarogya Setu users are on Android platform. The app reached 50 million subscribers in 15 days and 100 million subscribers in 40 days. - (E.T. Goverment, 2020)*

The Home page of the application mainly provide four options – 'Your Status', 'Media', 'COVID Update' and 'CoWin'. Your Status will give the evaluation of the user risk status. Media provides various information and news. COVID Update provides the updates of nationwide as well as state wise update of the COVID-19 cases and the CoWin provides the updates of Vaccination information, Vaccination Certificate and Vaccination Dashboard.

The data collected by the Aarogya Setu app is broadly divided into four categories — demographic data, contact data, self-assessment data and location data. These are mainly response data. Demographic data includes information such as name, mobile number, age, gender, profession and travel history. Contact data is about any other individual that a given individual has come in close proximity with, including the duration of the contact, the proximate distance between the individuals, and the geographical location at which the contact occurred. Self-assessment data are the responses provided by that individual to the self-assessment test administered within the app. Location data comprises the geographical position of an individual in latitude and longitude.

Case 5: News Article Published by 'Firstpost' on Its Web Portal With Headline "Media Usage During COVID-19 Lockdown: Indian Users Flock to FB and Whatsapp; General News Sites See Numbers Rise"

'Firstpost' is a well renowned Indian news and media web portal that published and posted a news article on its website on April 09, 2020 with a headline "Media usage during COVID-19 lockdown: Indian users flock to FB and WhatsApp; general news sites see numbers rise". The article described how social media were used by the Indian during the lockdown. In the initial part of the article, it was clearly mentioned that in the initial days of the COVID-19 crisis the public use social media more and more for the news and communication. They revealed certain part of Hammerkopf Consumer Survey report where it was mentioned that in the first week of lockdown citizen spend more than four hours on social media a day:

"Since India went into lockdown on 24 March, it seems more and more of the public are turning to social media to consume news and communicate with their friends and loved ones. The first week of the lockdown saw citizens spend more than four hours a day on social media — an 87 percent increase compared to the previous week, as per a poll conducted by Hammerkopf Consumer Survey" - (Firstpost, 2020).

The first half of the article also revealed the analysis of the American media measurement and analytic company 'Comscore' they examine the impact of the lockdown on digital content consumption in India. They revealed after the first week traffic to websites and mobile apps related to 'general news' category was increased

The middle section of the news article came with a sub headline 'Google Trend paint a picture' where it was clearly mentioned the interest for searching "corona virus cure" increased on 19 March and it reached zenith on 23 March the day after 'Janta Curfew' was declared by the Prime Minister of India.

It is clear from this news article that Indian citizen used social media which is also a part of new media for the gain of information and data during the pandemic crisis caused by the COVID-19.

DISCUSSION

The 21st Century has seen a global pandemic caused by a highly infectious viral disease called Corona virus disease. It spread rapidly around the globe and put a wide impact on our modern society. It tried to stop every system and to cripple the entire human civilization. Health system of almost every nation was devastated. In the introduction of the book *'The COVID-19 Pandemic: The Deadly Coronavirus Outbreak'* it was mentioned:

"Corona virus infection not only has caused disease and death but has also affected almost every aspect of human life. It has resulted in the disruption of daily lives with cities and countries under lockdown, with many international sporting events, social events, marriage, and other ceremonies being postponed or cancelled, triggering a global economic crisis. Almost every industry has been affected throughout the world. Stock markets have crashed. Airlines, the hospitality industry and the travel and tourism sector have been crippled. It has also led to widespread job losses across sectors." – (Koley and Dhole, 2021)

However India, with its vast population of around 1.3 billion also faced several problems during the pandemic period of COVID-19.The rapid escalation in the number of COVID-19 patient turn a major issue while on the other several regular non communicable diseases also shows its coexistence during the days of pandemic crisis. Indian government took the COVID-19 and other health issues very seriously and planned several actions to resist COVID-19 and to deal with other health issues. Along with medical treatments, Indian government focused on the health literacy. They started to disseminate information widely and focused on the awareness campaign as a major tool to fight against COVID-19 and other health issues.

However in India, during the pandemic of COVID-19, digital media performed several significant roles to support the health systems, health literacy and to resist the spread of COVID-19. Digital media were widely used to disseminate information and instruction related to Novel Corona Virus, the viral diseases called COVID-19 and various other health issues. It played a major role in the awareness campaign and propagated various health tips related to health awareness among the public. The role of digital media in detection of COVID-19 patient was highly important. The Indian digital application 'Aarogya Setu' shows remarkable result in detection of COVID-19 cases. The role of digital media in connectivity was no less important. Several platforms of digital media try to connect the COVID-19 patients with their families, relatives and their loved one. Digital media not only maintains connectivity among patients and their families but also they helped to maintained connectivity among the doctors and the medical practitioners. In India during the days of pandemic and lockdown, digital media also shows a significant role in dealing with the mental health. Government of India uses their web portals to disseminate various written documents, video and animation to support the mental health. Along with these all essential roles, digital media also proved highly essential in vaccination drive. The 'CoWin' application was introduced by the Ministry of Health and Family Welfare, Government of Indian for COVID-19 vaccination registration. The application portal helps to register the names of the candidate who are going to be vaccinated, provide appointment details and after the vaccination it provide a certificate of COVID-19 vaccination to the vaccinated candidate.

Digital media played a significant role in the health system and performed several essential functions regarding the issues of health and COVID-19 during the pandemic. The massive use of digital technology in the health system during the pandemic intensified the concept of 'Digital Health' in India which ultimately benefitted the citizen in numerous ways. Digital media and the digital technology supported the citizen and the government in its own way and simultaneously show the vitality of Digital Health during the pandemic of COVID-19.

INDIA DURING THE COVID-19 PANDEMIC

COVID-19 has become one of the most serious health issues of the 21st Century and the cause of one of the greatest pandemic that world has ever seen. The diseases called COVID-19 caused by a highly infectious virus Sar-Cov-2 or Novel Corona Virus. The virus put an effect on almost every nation of the globe, and it infects and killed millions of people from across the globe. The spread of COVID-19 affected almost every sectors of our modern society. However in India, Covid-19 first shows its existence in Thrissur district of Kerala. The first case were come to light on 30th January as The Ministry of Health and Family Welfare issued a statement which highlight the first patient of India was a student of Wuhan University of China. The case was confirmed to the government by National Institute of Virology. India was highly conscious and kept all the essential service on high alert from the initial days of its arrival, but COVID-19 slowly stretches its legs within the society and become a major health issue of the nation.

Indian Government took the issue of Corona virus disease very seriously from the very beginning of its arrival. On 22nd March 2020, Prime minister Shri. Narendra Modi gave a clarion call for the citizen of India where he urged for a fourteen hours nationwide 'Janta Curfew'. It was just the beginning of a long battle against Corona Virus and the disease called Covid-19. On 24th March 2020 Government of India took a vital decision of 'Lockdown'. Honourable Prime Minister Shri Narendra Modi declared 21 days lockdown that began from 25th March 2020 to 14th April 2020. It was the first phase of lockdown. The lockdown extended in several phases which continue for several months. The intension of the lockdown was to save the public from the spread of infection of Corona virus. Lockdown in India shows shut down of all factories, government office, schools, colleges, universities, transportation and communication system but all essential services like hospitals, banking sectors, police system, food and agricultural transportation and high ranking government office were all excluded from the lockdown.

However in India, during the pandemic period of the COVID-19 and within the lockdown, maintaining the public health was becomes a major health issue. COVID-19 shows the face of brutality as it infects and killed thousands of people every day while on the other side several other health issues have also shows its coexistence. Mental stresses were highly common among most of the public. Within this horrific condition digital media along with various other forms of mass media become highly active and gave its best efforts to secure human life from corona virus and other health issues.

In India the significance of the digital media while dealing with the COVID-19 and other health issue during the pandemic cannot be ignored. The wide networks of the digital media show its capability during the pandemic and perform various significant roles in a wonderful way. Most prominently digital media shows its efficiency in information dissemination and instruction propagation among the public which was highly necessary to resist the spread of infection during the initial period of COVID-19 pandemic. Along with the information dissemination and instruction propagation, digital media also proved success in fighting against the disturbance of mental health and in the propagation of various health advices during the pandemic when most of the citizen resides in their residence. The roles played by the digital media in detection of COVID-19 cases through digital application during the pandemic of COVID-19 are no less important than the essential medical service. Digital media also proved a great success in the vaccination drive which runs across the nation. In India, digital media shows its best effort to combat the COVID-19 and other health issues during the pandemic in its own way.

DIGITAL MEDIA AND THE DISSEMINATION OF INFORMATION RELATED TO COVID-19

In the opening chapter of the Johns Hopkins Project on Ethics and Governance of Digital Contact Tracing Technologies with title "Digital Contact Tracing for Pandemic Response" it was clearly mentioned:

"Information about COVID-19 patients' signs, symptoms, and course of illness is important to public health because it provides a basic for refining clinical case definitions and informing heath care providers and the general public (CDS2020c)"-(Kahn, 2020)

The statement clearly mentions the significance of information for refining clinical case definitions, and for informing health care providers and the general public.

In India during the days of COVID-19 pandemic the dissemination of right and accurate information was highly necessary. The digital media which is one of the latest forms of mass media has taken an active part in the information dissemination process during the period of COVID-19 pandemic. The wide use of internet through personal computer, smart mobile phone and tablet provided a wide digital media platform to the user. Digital media successfully penetrates deep into the heart of the society and disseminates information to a wide audience from across the nation. Several platforms of digital media help in wide dissemination of information related to health and COVID-19 and proved successful.

From the initial days of the pandemic, Central Government of India, State Governments, several news organisations along with the citizens frequently use various platforms of digital media to disseminate information. The main objectives is to propagates right information related to COVID-19 and Corona virus and to eliminates false news or hoax from society to avoid chaos, confusion and misconceptions. The Central Government of India as well as Indian State Governments continuously provided valuable information related to COVID-19 through newspaper, radio, television and various forms of the digital media. They use various platforms of digital media for the wide dissemination of various data and information for the benefit of public interest. The data mainly revealed daily rate of infected person, active cases, recovery rate, mortality rate, helpline numbers etc.

Health and Family Welfare Department, Government of India regularly updated various data and information related to COVID-19 and its awareness on their web portal. The web portal of Ministry of Health and Family Welfare of Government of India highlight all the details related to COVID-19 in India. In the upper section of the website it provides toll free helpline number and revealed the percentage and figure of 'Active Cases', 'Discharge' and 'Death'. In the middle section of the web page it provides 'Latest Update', 'COVID-19 State wise Status' and 'Resources' where as in the lower section it provides with 'Awareness' and 'FAQ'. Through the use of web portal the ministry easily disseminate the entire information and message of social awareness on COVID-19 not only with in the nation but also across the globe. The ministry is using wonderfully the digital media platform for the welfare of the nation.

During the pandemic of COVID-19 most of the Indian news organisations are also used digital media to propagate various news and information related to COVID-19. They used their web portal and various social media to disseminate wide variety of information mostly related to COVID-19, its testing, hospital activities, vaccine developments, and government curriculum. These information and news were highly significant to resist the spread of infection of COVID-19 and to support the moral of public during the pandemic period.

In this pandemic situation the role of social media in information dissemination process cannot be ignored. Social media is another platform of digital media, which help to connect the entire world through its social networks during the pandemic. Social media easily exchanged information or any form of data from one corner of the world to another within a very short span of time. It connected the users to the world and provided information about the Corona virus, COVID-19, government activities within the pandemic crisis, hospital and medical facilities and all that happened around us. Social networking sites like Facebook helps to connect with various news portals and blogs from across the globe just by clicking the 'Like' button user can access information which make them well informed about various detail related to COVID-19.

DIGITAL MEDIA AND THE AWARENESS RELATED TO COVID-19

The development of social awareness related to COVID-19 among the public and practicing them regularly was highly necessary during the pandemic. In India there is a wide campaign on awareness programme through digital media. Along with the traditional methods, the messages of the awareness campaign were propagated mainly through various official websites and web portals which were highly authentic and effective during the crisis of COVID-19. The vast domains of the digital media helped several organisations to propagate the messages of social awareness on Corona virus and COVID-19 among a large number of receivers. As the digital media has the capacity to give a mass appeal and its impacts are also much higher so the government organisations, Municipal Corporation and several non-governmental organisations (NGO) used the platforms of digital media for the propagations of social awareness message related to COVID-19, health, hygiene and sanitation during the pandemic period. After the outbreak of COVID-19 in India, Government of India and Telephone Regulatory Authority of India took a unique technique of awareness creation. Whenever a phone caller gives a phone call to any one, before the ring tone is heard there is a unique awareness message on COVID-19 which the caller will listen. The message rapidly gives COVID-19 awareness instruction along with toll free helpline number. The technique widely use throughout India just to make public aware about COVID-19 and its precautions.

Other than the official websites and web portal, various platforms of social media also played a significant role in awareness creation. An article entitled *'Impact of social media advertisements on the transmission dynamics of COVID-19 pandemic in India'* mentioned in the initial part about the government use of social media for the awareness campaign as:

"The government is also continuously using various media and social networking websites to aware the citizen regarding the current scenario of disease threats and their control mechanisms. They are employing different modes of propagating information including social media, TV, radio, internet using various types of slogan such as "Stay home, Stay safe", "Be clean, Be healthy", "Jab Tak Dawai Nahi, Tab Tak Dhilai Nahi" (No carelessness till a medicine is found), "Do Gaj ki Doori, Mask Hai Jaroori" (Mask and maintaining distance of two yards is necessary), etc. The main motive of such social media campaign is to stimulate people to adopt healthy sanitation practices, frequent hand washing, use of mask, sanitizer, maintaining social distance, avoid touching eyes/nose/mouth etc."- (Rai, Et.al, 2021)

The user of social media randomly scattered and disseminated information related to Corona Virus and the diseases caused by Corona Virus called COVID-19. This information were mostly related to social awareness like maintaining social distancing, use of mask, washing hand with soap at regular interval, use of hand sanitizer for hand sanitization etc. These messages through social media played a crucial role in the development of awareness creation among the public.

DIGITAL MEDIA AND THE DIGITAL PICTORIAL PRESENTATION

Digital media performed several vital roles and helped the Indian society in numerous ways during the pandemic of COVID-19. Digital media represent it's contain through digital presentation. During the pandemic of COVID-19 it presents several digital images and video which help the Indian society in numerous ways. The digital images and video were widely disseminated for the purpose of knowledge propagation and awareness creation about the unknown infectious virus called Novel Corona Virus. The images and video of the microscopic structure of Novel Corona Virus, how it enter and affects human body, along with several other images related to COVID-19 which available in various website and which are circulated through various social media help the nation to understand the structure and character of Novel Corona Virus. The pictorial presentations proved highly beneficial for the scientist, microbiologist, pharmacist, and doctor as they gain clear knowledge about the virus which spread fear and frustration along with the infection around the globe.

The digital info graphical images of the symptom create more impact and help everyone to understand more easily the symptom of COVID-19. They were disseminated through various platforms of digital media and help the citizen to understand more clearly than the only written words. The Info graphical images also provided a clear view of how to wash hands, how to use mask, how to sanitise hand, etc. The pictorial presentation proved the phrase "a picture tells a thousand words" during the pandemic period of COVID- 19 as it performed several roles and one can easily decode in their own way without any hesitation.

DIGITAL MEDIA AND THE DETECTION OF COVID-19 PATIENT THROUGH DIGITAL APPLICATION

The digital Aaragya Setu App or the application promotes the initiatives of Digital India nationwide. During the COVID-19 pandemic, Indian government turned toward digital technology driven solution to curve the rapid growth in the spread of COVID-19 infection. India use digital media and digital technology in the detection of COVID-19 patients. National Informatics Centre (NIC) under Ministry of Electronic and Information Technology developed a COVID-19 contact tracing, syndrome mapping and self assessment digital mobile application called 'Aarogya Setu App'. The Application based on fully digital technology that was initially released during the month of April 2020 with an objective to detect COVID-19 patients through their contact and to provide various data related to COVID-19. Within a very short span of time its shows a huge popularity, the app reached 50 million subscribers in 15 days and 100 million subscribers in 40 days. The user can access the app in eleven different languages but English were mostly preferred.

The Aarogya Setu app supports the concept of Digital Health in India. The app helps the health department to locate COVID-19 cluster areas which they marked as 'Containment Zone'. The application utilizes the data provided by the users via Bluetooth and generated social graph based on location to track those who may have come in close contact with COVID-19 positive person. The application developed on a platform that can provide an Application Programme Interface (API), so that other computer programmes, mobile application, and web services can make use the data available in the Aarogya Setu for the betterment of the future. The App was one among many uses of digital-surveillance technologies that the central and state governments were pervasively deploying in their efforts to stop the spread of COVID-19. The application was based on digital technology which supporting not only the health department but also every Indian during the pandemic crisis.

Through this app National Informatics Centre use digital technology to check and resist the spread of infection. It becomes a tool to defeat COVID-19.

DIGITAL MEDIA AND THE MENTAL HEALTH

The spread of COVID-19 and the declaration of lockdown by the government of India to save the citizen mainly put restriction on the free movement of the public in the public place. People were restricted to stay within their residence which keeps them aloof from their friends, colleagues, relatives and their loved one. This aloofness for many becomes the cause of the disturbance in the mental health. Anxiety, anger, depression, stress, insomnia, etc, were highly common among various people. People started to feel uncomfortable within their residence due to the long home stay. In India, the issues of mental health become common during the pandemic of COVID-19. The role of digital media in this context was significant.

Digital media proved highly beneficial while dealing with the issues of mental health. The platforms of digital media were used by the government to upload several remedies and advices related to mental health. The web portal of The Ministry of Health and Family Welfare put a section called "Behavioural Health" to deal with the issues of mental health. The platforms of digital media also provide satisfaction, comfort and amusements to the public during the period of COVID-19 pandemic. Digital media platform like web pages provides various valuable information, news, stories, funny comics etc which the viewer can select and read according to their own choice and time. Youtube provides various video which are digital in nature and accepted as a vital source of infotainment as it provide information as well as entertainment. Along with this information based video, Youtube also provides songs and music which are highly entertainment based. These videos are beneficial for giving comfort to the mental stress and anxiety. Along with these online webcast video streaming provider such as Hotstar, Netflix, Amazon Prime Video, etc also became a vital source of entertainment during the period of pandemic crisis. They provide various web series and films to the audience. These web series and film provided by streaming provider viewed through various platforms such as desktop, laptop, tablet, and advance mobile set

Instant messaging social media apps like Facebook, WhatsApp are another platform of digital media which also play a significant role in dealing with the issues of mental health. The pandemic crisis makes the Indian highly conscious, and forces them to stay wilfully within their house for their own safety and for the safety of the others. Most of the time in their house during the pandemic, they stick to their mobile phone and laptop through which they use to communicate with their relatives and close one. The communication with their close one through social media helps the

Indian to remove mental stress which caused due to social distancing. The Chatting and talking through social media refresh most of the Indian and provide them mental support during the pandemic crisis. Through chatting they shared several information and data which was necessary not only for COVID-19 awareness creation but also in various other fields which were highly necessary in their professional and social life. In India it was revealed by various researches that there was a sharp rise in the user of social media during the period of COVID-19 pandemic. However digital media provide a wide mode of entertainment to the Indian during the lockdown period and support in the removal of the disturbance of the mental health.

DIGITAL MEDIA AND THE HEALTH ADVICE

In India the pandemic of COVID-19 continued for a long period. With the arrival of the COVID-19 government of India declared lockdown to resist the spread of the viral infection. The lockdown continued in several phases for several months. During the period of lockdown most of the people resides within their home, less involved with works and physical activities and turn lazy in nature which show in several cases negative effect on health. However during the pandemic period maintaining health is a major issue of concern. Health departments of Central and State Governments of India, International organisation like World Health Organisation (WHO), various universities, NGO's along with various news media organisations propagates various valuable advices on health. Most of them used digital media along with media like radio and television for the propagation of health advices.

Digital media has become a tool for the propagation of health advices. Digital platforms like mobile phone, computers, internet, web pages, and various forms of the social media were widely used to transmit digital data related to health advices. Thorough the use of digital media they propagates various valuable advice related to healthy food habits, significance of quitting smoking and drinking during the period of COVID-19, benefit of conducting regular exercises, yoga and physical activities.

Social media also becomes a valuable tool which disseminates various message and information on health issues during the pandemic period. Public along with various health organisations used social media to upload and share various data and information related to health. The health's advices disseminate by social media create awareness among the public about various health issues. There is no doubt that the social media plays a significant role in the dissemination of health advices during the pandemic of COVID-19.

DIGITAL MEDIA AND THE CONNECTIVITY

Digital media from the very beginning of its arrival played a significant role in the connectivity and communication process where as during the pandemic crisis of COVID-19 it shows its vitality and efficiency. In India, connectivity and communication was highly necessary during the days of COVID-19 and digital media plays a significant role in it. On the one hand it connect the individual with his or her family, relatives and the loved one while on the other it connects doctors and health workers with their colleagues, which was essential during the pandemic period of the crisis. The role of connectivity and communication plays a major role in combating against the spread of COVID-19 in India.

During the pandemic crisis of COVID-19 millions of people get infected by novel corona virus, a new strain that has never been identified before. Most of the infected people went to the hospital and stayed under medication for weeks. During this circumstance, social media which are forms of digital media help them to remain in touch with their close one. Social media help to maintain connectivity and to communicate with their families and relatives. The connectivity with the families and their loved one give them a touch of comfort during the critical circumstances of COVID -19. It gives them a moral support which boosts their courage to fight against the COVID-19.

Connectivity and communication through the use of digital media platforms also become helpful for the doctors and healthcare personals. Digital media platform like various social media apps became highly beneficial in connectivity among the doctors and healthcare personnel. They can easily connect with their fellow colleagues through various instant messaging apps like Facebook, Messanger and Whatsapp whenever they feel necessary. These digital apps were also used to share various video and health related data for the medical purpose. However connectivity through digital media proved highly beneficial during the pandemic of COVID-19 in India.

DIGITAL MEDIA AND THE VACCINATION DRIVE

India begins its vaccination process in the first half of January, 2021 as the Drug Controller General of India (DCGI) approved the use of Oxford- Astra Zeneca vaccine with trade name 'Covishield' and Bharat Biotech BBV152 vaccine with trade name 'Covaxin' for the protection against the viral disease COVID-19. However in the process of vaccination digital media take an active part. The Ministry of Health and Family Welfare of Government of India introduced a digital application called 'CoWin' to register the name of the candidate who is going to take the vaccine. The vaccination drive runs throughout the nation with the help of this digital application.

The application not only registers the name of the candidate but also makes the candidate aware about the vaccination date, the centre or the allotted hospital for the vaccination and the name of vaccine through a document called 'COVID-19 Vaccination Appointment Details' and after the vaccination the CoWin portal provides certificate of vaccination to the vaccinated candidate. The process is completely digital in nature which not only helps the public but also support the Ministry of Health and Family Welfare by providing an authentic data related to the vaccination.

In India, digital media proved highly beneficial in the vaccination derive. Digital media also helps in the promotion of vaccines and vaccination process. It disseminates various information about vaccination process, how the vaccine works to resist COVID-19, where to get the vaccine, how the vaccine process get start, when the second dose is to be taken, who are the producer of the vaccine, etc. This information through various form of digital media encourage the public and motivate them to take vaccine. The role of digital media in the vaccination process of India is enormous and significant.

CONCLUSION

The analysis of the case studies and the entire discussion in the article justified and highlight the significance of the digital media in dealing with the highly infectious viral diseases COVID-19 and various other health issues in India during the pandemic crisis. The digital media proved its efficiency in information dissemination and awareness campaign during the days of COVID-19 pandemic. Wide dissemination of valuable information about Novel Corona Virus, the diseases COVID-19, the modes of the spread infection and the safety precautions while dealing COVID-19 patients, through websites and social media platforms proved highly beneficial to resist the spread of infection. Along with the information dissemination, pictorial and info-graphical presentation through digital media were also seems exclusive. The pictorial presentation propagated by the digital media provides various magnified microscopic image in a wonderful manner which help to understand the structure of the Novel Corona Virus and how it affect the human body. The informative data along with the combination of pictorial presentation disseminated through digital media shows higher impact and turned highly beneficial in resisting the COVID-19 in India.

The significance of digital media while dealing other health issues and mental health during the period of COVID-19 was enormous. The valuable health advice provided by various platforms of digital media proved highly beneficial and life saving in various occasion during the pandemic. It spontaneous effort to refresh the melancholic stressful mood, anxiety, and other minor mental issues with various amusing programme and music was also excellent. It acts as a medicine which heals mental issues and maintains the mental health.

The role played by the digital media in connectivity during the pandemic period in India was also significant. The use of digital media for the connectivity reached the zenith during the pandemic period of COVID-19 and within the lockdown. It becomes an excellent medium through which every Indian connects with their loved one. The victims of COVID-19 who were shifted to hospital mainly used digital media to connect with their families, relatives and loved ones. Doctors and health workers also used digital media platforms to connect with their colleagues to discuss various issues related to profession. During the pandemic of COVID-19 and the lockdown in India, digital media shows no match with any other forms of media while dealing with the connectivity. In India the significance of digital media during the pandemic period is significant. Most of it roles are vital and beneficial for the human race. Digital media help the Indian society during the pandemic in a multi dimensional way. It present itself as a gift of science and technology that support to resist the spread of infection of COVID-19 and help to maintain health awareness and connectivity.

REFERENCES

Agarwal, S. (2020). *'Aarogya Setu app launched by GoI in public-private partnership mode'*. The Economic Times. Retrieved from https://economictimes.indiatimes.com/tech/information-tech/aarogya-setu-app-launched-by-goi-in-public-private-partnership-mode/articleshow/78916970.cms

David. R. (January 2020). *'India Confirm its first corona virus case'*. CNBC. Retrieved from https://www.cnbc.com/2020/01/30/india-confirms-first-case-of-the-coronavirus.html

Department of Health and Family Welfare, Government of Karnataka. Department of Psychiatry National Institute of Mental Health and Neurosciences, Bangaluru. (2020, July). Caring for Health Care Warriors Mental Health Support during. *COVID*, 19.

Firstpost Staff. (April 09, 2020). *'Media usage during COVID-19 lockdown: Indian users flock to FB and WhatsApp'*. Firstpost. Retrieved from https://www.firstpost.com/health/media-usage-during-covid-19-lockdown-indian-users-flock-to-fb-and-whatsapp-general-news-sites-see-numbers-rise-8242811.html

Goverment, E. T. (2020). *'Digital India: Govt braces for robust, secure tech solutions as Aarogya Setu App opens up source code'*. ET Government.Com. Retrieved from https://government.economictimes.indiatimes.com/news/digital-india/digital-india-govt-braces-for-robust-secure-tech-solutions-as-aarogya-setu-app-opens-up-source-code/76059270

'Guidelines on Managing Mental Illness in Hospital Settings during COVID19'. (n.d.). Ministry of Health and Family Welfare, Govt. of India. National Institute of Mental Health and Neurosciences, Bangaluru.

Kahn, P. J. (2020). *Digital Contact Tracing for Pandemic Response*. Johns Hopkins University Press. doi:10.1353/book.75831

Koley, T. K., & Dhole, M. (2021). [*Pandemic: The Deadly Coronavirus Outbreak'*. Routledge. Newyork Ministry of Health and Family Welfare, Government of India. Retrieved from https://www.mohfw.gov.in/]. *COVID, 19*

Mukul. P. (May 14, 2020). *'Aarogya Setu: Who can access your data, and when?'*. The Indian Express. Retrieved from https://indianexpress.com/article/explained/coronavirus-aarogya-setu-who-all-can-access-your-data-and-when-6407175/

NHP INDIA -National Health Portal. Retrieved from https://www.nhp.gov.in/

Prasad. R, Bindu Shajan Parappadan, Shelar Jyoti, Koshy Jacob; (Edited by George. P.J); The Hindu (2020); *'The Pandemic Notebook'*. Retrieved from https://www.thehindu.com/news/resources/the-hindus-e-book-on-covid-19-in-multiple-indian-languages/article31174374.ece

Qu, J. M., Cao, B., & Chen, R. C. (2020). 'COVID-19: The Essentials of Prevention and Treatment'. Shanghai Jiao Tong University Press, Published by Elsevier Inc.

Rai, R. K., (2021). 'Impact of social media advertisements on the transmission dynamics of COVID-19 pandemic in India'. Journal of Applied Mathematics and Computing. Springer. Retrieved from: https://link.springer.com/content/pdf/10.1007/s12190-021-01507-y.pdf

Sharan, S. (2020). *Lockdown: India Under Siege From Corona*. Published by RosettaBooks.

World Health Organiation. (April 2020). *'Doing What Matter in Time of Stress: An Illustration Guide'*. Retrieved from https://www.who.int/publications/i/item/9789240003927?gclid=EAIaIQobChMIyPG8ueOB7wIVgjMrCh1iRQnJEAAYASAAEgJFNvD_BwE

World Health Organisation. *'Healthy at Home'*. Retrieved from https://www.who.int/campaigns/connecting-the-world-to-combat-coronavirus/healthyathome#:~:text=The%20COVID%2D19%20pandemic%20means,during%20this%20period%20of%20confinement

KEY WORDS AND ITS DEFINITIONS

Awareness Campaign: A process or a campaign to make the people aware.

Connectivity: The state of being connected or interconnected.

COVID-19: A highly infectious viral disease caused by SARS – CoV 2 or novel corona virus.

Digital Apps: The application that runs digitally.

Digital Media: The media which is digital in nature.

Health Advice: Advice on health issues.

Information Dissemination: Propagation of Information.

Mental Health: Healthy state of mind; A state or a condition of well being in which the individual realise his or her own abilities and feel good to think and act in a ways to achieve a better life.

Pictorial Presentation: Presentation with the help of picture or diagram.

Vaccination: The act of vaccinating or giving vaccine.

Chapter 6
Inductive Ontology for Specifying the Contexture of Web Health Information Systems

Minaxi Parmar
School of Library and Information Science, Gandhinagar, India

ABSTRACT

Inductive ontology helps to describe the algorithm of process, application, architecture, plan, design, etc. It is easily pertinent for elaborating the concept. An ontology creator shows all connectivity of the core concept to another concept, procedures, and application with the five fundamentals i.e., properties, matter, energy, space, and time; hence, it made broader the idea plan of its users/reader enables to find out various connected elements relevant to the query on the direct and indirect way. The services sector has two main property-level functions first to develop/produce the service and second to provide the service. Both the property has specific phases of multiple processes i.e., creating services, owner/authority functions, user functions, identity, process, etc phase can be easily described in a graphical way. Here, a researcher describes the ontology for web-based health information systems (WHISs) by explaining two websites namely Web MD, and drugs.com. Both the WHISs are rich in information and data relevant to mankind's health, lifestyle.

DOI: 10.4018/978-1-7998-9652-4.ch006

1. INTRODUCTION

Ontology is fortified to elucidate logical, predictable, and conceptual connections among entities and their association with the universe. As a result, it has found applications across various disciplines in the realm of knowledge. Its foundational principles facilitate the systematic mapping of entities, novel concepts, and processes for diverse applications. Consequently, it is employed here to delineate the contextual framework of a web-based health information system, designed to cater to global citizens without being confined by geographical boundaries. This system encompasses the structure of the human body, its functions and organs, diseases, remedies, symptoms, precautions, medications, expertise on diseases, and related medical professionals along with their locations. It also includes information on medicines with user-specific dosage recommendations, nutritional requirements for different body structures, and more. Through this approach, individuals gain a comprehensive understanding of the significance of health and are empowered to combat common ailments. Importantly, ontology plays a pivotal role in managing life-threatening diseases. Its utilization spans across all subjects within the knowledge world, encompassing various branches and sub-branches. Human health, including anatomy, skeletal structure, diseases, treatment modalities, lifestyle, behaviors, and technology, is a comprehensive domain. Furthermore, it comprises specific disciplinary subjects within the medical branch and its associated sciences, as illustrated in Figure 1.

Figure 1. Subject Branches of Medical and its Relevant Sciences

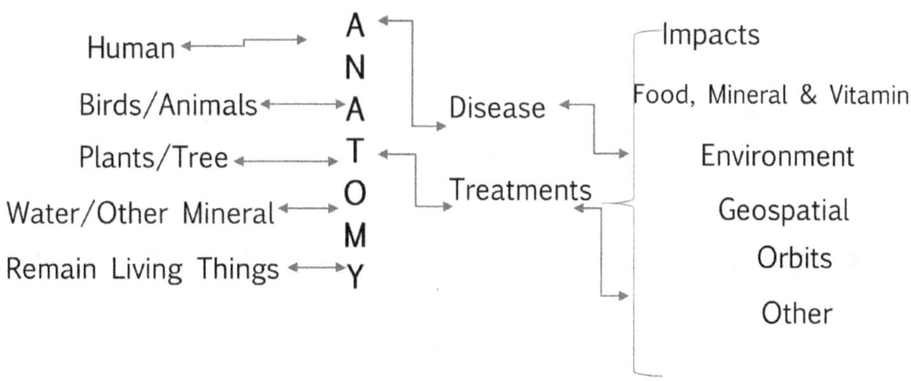

All living organisms exhibit distinct anatomical features that can significantly influence their internal and external environments, thereby warranting thorough exploration within their respective disciplines. The study of anatomy, treatment modalities, and their interdisciplinary impacts cannot be compartmentalized; rather, they are intricately interconnected. This holistic approach has been prevalent since ancient times, with investigations conducted in diverse branches such as medical science, Ayurveda, Homeopathy, and other specialized fields.

The advent of Information and Communication Technology (ICT) has ushered in transformative changes, particularly in the accessibility of information. The continuous development of ICT facilitates the dissemination of information to a broader audience. Numerous web tools and techniques have streamlined the research process, enabling experts, professionals, and the general public to acquire information more efficiently.

In the field of medicine, the need for health-related information, common precautions, and understanding of various syndromes is crucial. Web-based technological tools have significantly eased this process. Platforms such as WebMD and Drugs.com serve as web-based health information systems, offering comprehensive details ranging from normal to critical medical conditions, treatments, related drugs, nutritional advice, symptoms, infections, and lifestyle guidance. These valuable resources are easily accessible on web pages, with both WebMD and Drugs.com being among the most widely used platforms.

2. AIM OF THE STUDY

This study has been done to justify the following three specific aims.

- To check and compare the web healthiness of selected WHISs.
- To present an inductive ontology model that connects both WHISs from a users' perspective.
- To present an inductive ontological graph that illustrates the features of both WHISs concerning users' individual perspectives.

3. REVIEW OF LITERATURE: ALSHAMMARI, THAMIR A. (2014)

Approved drugs undergo a rigorous evaluation process, prioritizing safety initially and subsequently assessing their effectiveness. Regulatory standards are continually evolving to ensure that these drugs maintain a positive benefit-risk balance. The consideration of personalized medicine becomes crucial when administering medications to patients, as the pharmacokinetic processes within the body vary not only from patient to patient but also across different disease states. Consequently, researchers emphasize the importance of obtaining comprehensive information about drugs and their relevance to individual patients. This underscores the need for thorough reviews encompassing the unique aspects of drug response in diverse patient populations and disease conditions. Rade, Babic, Zoran Milosevic & Gordana Stankovic Babic (2012) publish a professional article entitled " Web Technology in Health Information System" Here they give compendious information about some web-based health information systems i.e. teleradiology, radiological information system, modern medical information system, PACS (Picture archiving and communication system), and DICOM (Digital imaging and communications in medicine). The architecture of PACS they describe as various elements, modalities, resolutions, Palette of colors, uncompressed file size, etc., Here, a writer has seen the implementation of web technology and web services in the medical discipline. Web technology has been triumphantly enabled in this discipline. Today, The three-wing of medicine i.e. medicine, treatment, and diagnosis had been enabled to work on web tools and techniques. During the literature finding process, a writer noted that much research had been done on web medical, web-based MD services, Web drugs, web technology on medical discipline, etc., hence this topic is totally new for the literature world of medicine, where the two different websites of the medical field have been explained through ontology concept. Williams, P., Nicholas, D., Huntington, P. and McLean, F. (2002), research entitled "Surfing for health: user evaluation of a health information website. Part one: background and literature review" here they presented the electronic health system of the United Kingdom of http://www.surgerydoor.co.uk/. It is a web-health information system provided by the government of the UK. The researchers conducted a users study of real and potential users with inspection methods including website evaluation content quality, reliability, accuracy, scope and depth of content, page design, the currency of information and frequency, authors' disclosure, authority, reputability, navigability, links, quality, documentation, references, etc., attributes were added in a checklist. Hence, many studies have been done on health information systems with different perspectives, but the ontological presentation is entirely new

4. RESEARCH QUESTION

How does the ontology amplify the healthiness of chosen Web-based Health Infomation Systems?

5. METHODOLOGY

Here, two distinct domains, namely Ontology-graph and Web Health Information System (WHIS), are interconnected to address the research question and provide justification for the objectives. The researcher employed mixed methods, incorporating web-case study and ontological graph presentation. The ontological graph illustrates the presence of features on WHIS pages along with their connections to users, elucidating the web-healthiness described in the web report.

The ontology concept is utilized to depict the relationships among various attributes in specific ways, such as broad, core, and sub-attributes of selected WHISs, namely Web MD and Drugs.com. It is assumed that all the checkpoints in the site audit describe results with more than 50% similarity. The conceptual framework of selective websites is aligned based on the merit of user-friendly reference language which may standard vocabulory in technical standard of web assessment tool.

The web-health report for WHISs is generated using a specific web tool called "scrawler." Among the various available crawlers, the researcher chose "THE HOTH" scrawler for its equal diagnostic process, analogous to human diagnosis by doctors using a stethoscope. The Hoth provides several features for web page diagnosis, with one-page SEO results, keywords, links, usability, and web performance forming the diagnosed health report of WHISs. Some attributes of The Hoth are also focused on users' activities, potentially influencing the usability of web-based health information systems, which could be enhanced based on the site audit results.

WHISs are designed for diverse user services, accompanied by disclaimers emphasizing individual responsibility for the use of web information. The actual application of information should be confirmed by relevant practitioners. Both WHISs exclusively offer health-related information, promoting awareness among users. Practitioner, patient, and professional interviews were conducted to understand the justification of the research question. Feedback from relevant users, including doctors, patients, medical representatives, nurses, and laboratory professionals, was gathered. The researcher met with an MD-Orthopedic, pharmacist, and a cervical cancer patient with ten years of suffering, all having experience with both WHISs. Medical practitioners access WHISs independently, while the researcher explains the content to patients. The experiences of all three samples are detailed in the study.

5.1 Limitation

The sample Web-Based Health Information Systems (WHISs) are selected by the researcher based on their personal experiences. Both systems are developed by individuals from the USA and Oceania continents, resulting in certain features that are specifically designed for a geotag, such as the 'Allergy Tracker' module from

WebMD, which is intended to function exclusively in USA regions. The researcher aims to assess the applicability of WHISs among Indian medical and non-medical practitioners using applied ontology principles. However, a notable contention in this study arises from the global visibility of WHISs, while the respondents providing feedback on usability are primarily from the Indian population.

6. HISTORICAL BACKGROUND OF SELECTIVE WEB-BASED HEALTH INFORMATION SYSTEMS

Web Health Information Systems (WHIS) operate with a distinct emphasis on user services. Certain systems prioritize users' health by incorporating essential features such as patient records, multi-directional communication, information on various diseases, treatments, procedures, and more. This necessitates the establishment of a communication hub among individual users. Additionally, some systems concentrate on promoting awareness of healthy lifestyles to users. In this context, WHISs play a crucial role in disseminating medical-related information throughout society, fostering a greater understanding of health-related topics.

6.1 Web MD

The Web MD was started in 1996 by internet entrepreneur Jeff Arnold as an American corporation for primary works of online publishing of news about mankind's health and wellbeing. Later a year it had been merged with Healtheon, Netscape Communication. It is network operated health system, where a gathering of Medscape, Medicine Net, eMedicine, eMedicineHealth, RxList, OnHealth, and the heart, etc., is noted impotence health service providers.

The Web MD is a huge website about health information. It proclaims the linked information through the skeleton of a human being by highlighting all body parts with related medical terminology. Hence, maximum information shows off on the website in the form of hyperlinked sources that users can access through infographics and text. It is working in a multidimensional way, so, it also offers more than two procedures simultaneously. For Example, if users would like to find doctors, the Web MD gives them various clues as to an advanced search.

The Web MD provides a variety of access points to users i.e., finding out doctors, symptoms, remedies, precautions, medicine, related drugs, side effects, required nutrients and minerals, procedures of remedies, etc., therefore, the multidimensionality way to access the information is the real essence of Web MD, where non-medical discipline people can easily access the better information for better health. It has an active blog where new information always has been posted related to health.

The coronavirus update tab also describes detailed information about itself up to a worldwide level. Here, the COVID 19 confirmed cases and death numbers are also highlighted through the GPRS system. It is to be noted that the Geo-Spatial Tab for searching doctors must be working in specific continents.

Figure 2. Search Ontology of Web MD created by author.

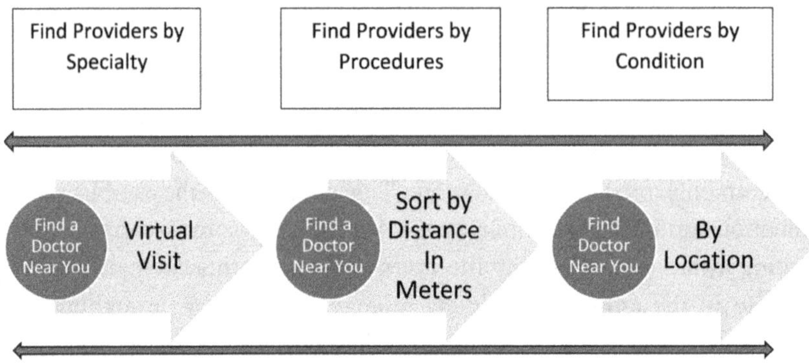

Figure 3. Ontological Graph of Web MD created by author.

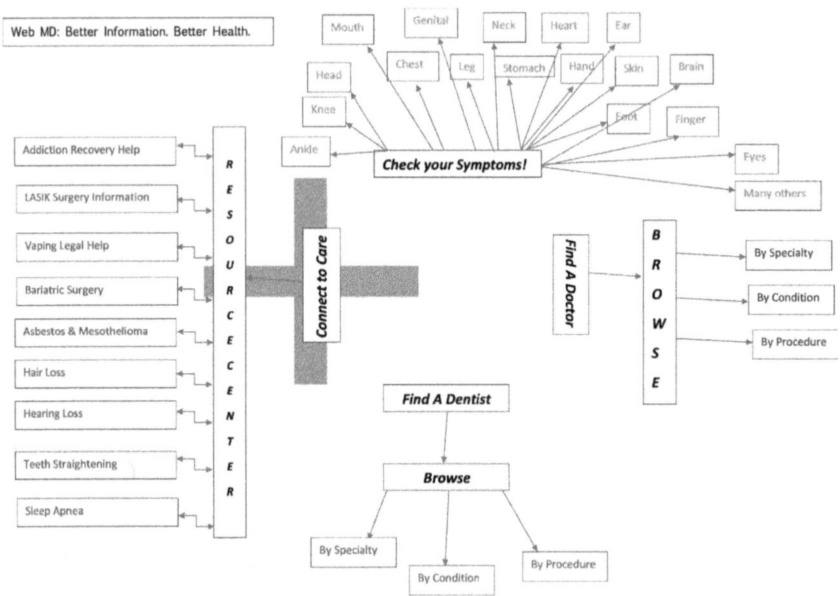

6.2 Drugs.Com

It is a website, official launch in September of 2001, now it is administered by a trust namely "Drugsite" whose operators are two pharmacists Karen Ann and Phillip James respectively belong to New Zealand and Toronto. It was opened with one mission statement "To empower patients with the knowledge to better manage their healthcare and to improve consumer safety by assisting in the reduction of medication errors." It is medical information database where many individual providers i.e., American Society for Health-System Pharmacists, Cerner Multum, and IBM Watson Micromedex caregivers a lot on the site.

According to the health information system, namely Medline Plus "Drugs are chemical substances that can change how your body and mind work. They include prescription medicines, over-the-counter medicines, alcohol, tobacco, and illegal drugs". It plays a vital role in the mediation process and the health of mankind. This website describes the details of the drugs in a specific head i.e., generic name, brand name, dosage form, drug class, uses, warnings, precautions before taking it, probable questions for the doctors, probable impact on the patient when missing it out while overdosing, etc. The Pill Identifier is the uniqueness of the website which MAC mobile application is also available on the site, where users can identify the pills through the acceptance of the wizard. The descriptions of the pill i.e., its' color, shape, relevant drug name, national drug code, imprints with manufacturing place and company, and disclaimer are shown. The web page also gives a tab about professional resources relevant to the drugs, medicine, diseases, drug impact, manufacturing companies, and place, i.e., a ship AHFS DI Monograph, FDA Professional drug information, drug interaction checker, IBM Watson Micromedex patient care notes, Harvard Health topic, natural product information, etc. The other tab gives information about consumer drugs, interactive tools, and resources for both patients and professionals. This tab also shows the way of various medical services and their related references. For example. Pharmaceutical Companies Directory. More than a hundred companies' web link is listed alphabetically. Hence, the users either professionals or patients may find out the medication description from the identification tab while enabling access to the companies' original website.

Figure 4. Ontological Graph of Drug.com created by author

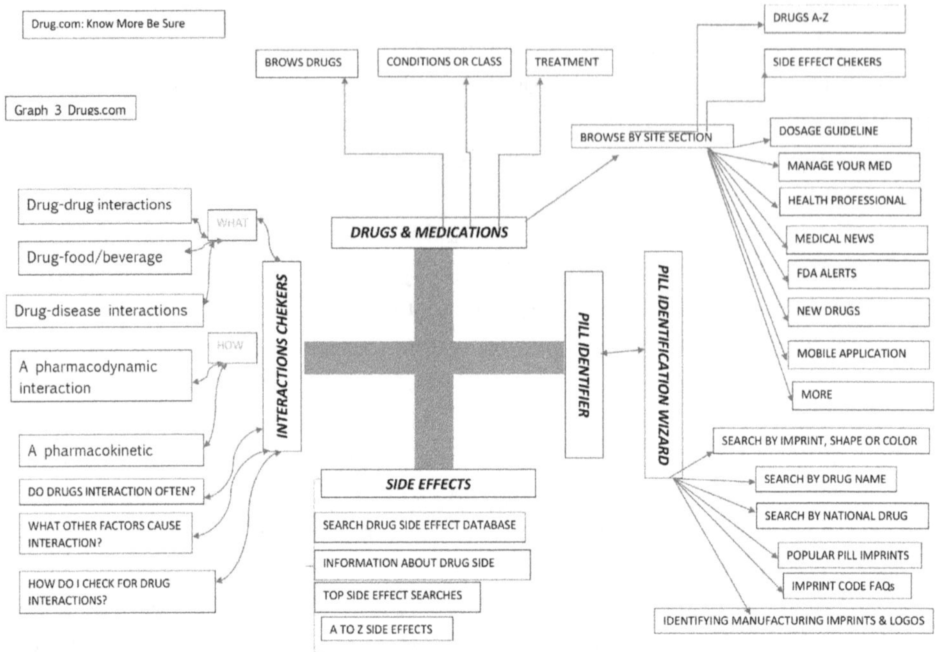

7. OBJECTIVE ANALYSIS

It is a crucial aspect of research, as it helps establish connections between nodes to emphasize the relationships between variables and objectives. This involves analyzing both quantitative and qualitative data to gain a comprehensive understanding.

7.1 Objective 1

This study has been done with majorly two objectives. The first objective of the study, to check and compare the healthiness of selected WHISs. The below table shows the web-health of WHISs with specific features that should establish the connection in both direct and indirect ways to the users.

Table 1. Comparative SEO Audit of WHISs

Sr. No.	Particular	WebMD	Drugs.com
1.	**On-Page Search Engine Optimism Report**	B	A
2.	**Keyword Consistency Top 8 words listed with the highest page frequency of both the WHISs**	Word F: drugs (30)	Word F: Health (31)
3.	**Phrases**	Phrase: see all (06)	Phrase: today medical (11)
4.	**Estimated Traffic (With Frequency)**	738197208	96580330
5.	**Links (With Frequency)**		
	External	222.3M	22.6M
	Referring	870.6K	127.4K
	Moz Domain Authority	94	83
6.	**Usability**	B-	C-
7.	**Email Privacy**	No email addresses have been found in plain text	No email addresses have been found in plain text
8.	**No. of Resources: Total Objects**	641	719
	No. of HTML pages	119	139
	No. of Java Scripts Resources	122	73
	No. of Images	230	196
	No. of CSS resources	5	7
	Other resources	243	226

The web-health report indicates a commendable search engine optimization level, with a grade B for WebMD and an A for Drugs.com. Keyword consistency analysis reveals that the term "health" has the highest frequency, occurring 31 times on WebMD, while "Drugs" follows closely with a frequency of 30 on Drugs.com. Examining the most accessible phrases on the selected Web Health Information Sources (WHISs), "see all" and "today medical" stand out. Additionally, the estimated traffic within WHISs demonstrates a robust frequency. The links are categorized into three parts: external, referring, and Moz domain authority, all of which exhibit favorable frequencies for both WHISs. Furthermore, the web resources on WHISs manifest in various forms, including HTML pages, JSR, images, CSS, and others. The corresponding frequencies are detailed in the table, underscoring the growing digitization of the medical science field.

Inferences:

The inference drawn from the table above suggests that the SEO grades of both entities could be enhanced by adjusting the search options, taking into account the experiences of information uploaders on the WHISs. On the other hand, user feedback enhances the consistency of keywords. Consequently, the provision of vector search should be enabled on WHISs for both medical and non-medical practitioners.

7.2 Objective 2: Users Perspective Inductive Ontological Model

The philosophy of ontology involves the identification of five primary and secondary categories for modeling ontology, a framework utilized in this study. The research endeavors to establish cohesion between two distinct Web Health Information Systems (WHISs) with the explicit goal of developing an inductive ontology model from the user perspective. Both WHISs under consideration offer distinct features and services, treated as substances in this context. Consequently, users gain the capability to identify diseases based on symptoms, access relevant medication information, precautions, and foundational knowledge from WebMD. Specifics regarding medication, such as drugs, effects, warnings, and classes, are sourced from drugs.com. Consequently, the ontologist leverages two distinct sources for identifying substances, each of which serves multiple purposes, catering to diverse user needs. The ensuing discussion outlines the procedural steps within each category, aligned with the chosen WHISs."

Figure 5. Inductive Ontological Model

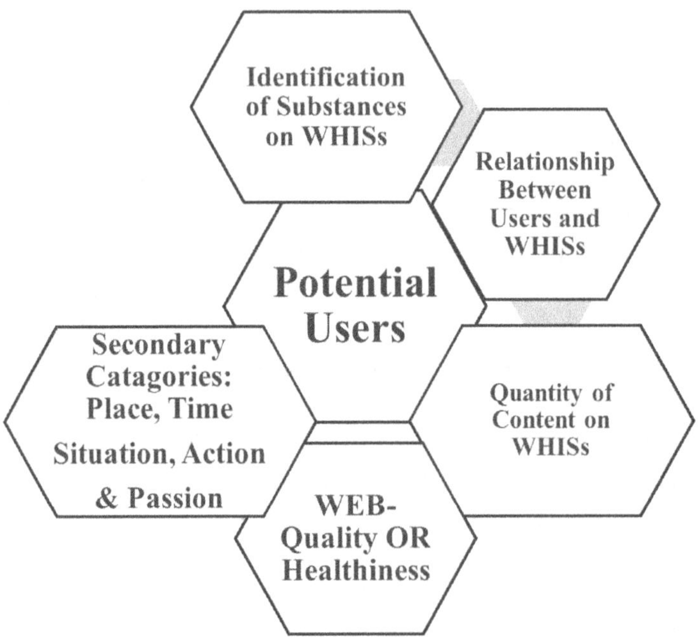

7.2.1 Identification of Substances on WHISs

WebMD and Drugs.com offer a diverse range of information categorized into different sections. On WebMD, these sections encompass top stories, patient conditions, health news, expert insights, newsletters, skeletal atlas, diseases, symptoms, various animal health tools, and food & nutrition. In contrast, Drugs.com provides information on drugs, conditions, treatments, drug interactions, drug-food/beverage interactions, drug-disease interactions, pharmacodynamics interactions, dosage, side effects, and more. Medical practitioners utilize these platforms to connect globally with peers, staying informed through blogs, videos, newsletters, and other resources. Non-medical practitioners, on the other hand, access these platforms for general health information, symptom checking, and identification of medicines and drugs. Both platforms offer extensive information, allowing users to tailor their exploration based on their specific interests. Patients may navigate the platforms with varying perspectives, focusing on specific diseases, updates, dietary information, medications, new developments, side effects, and more. Therefore, all the content on these platforms can be categorized into four main hierarchies: medical practitioner, non-medical practitioner, patient, and general user. This classification helps users find relevant information according to their unique needs and perspectives.

7.2.2 Relationship Between Users and WHISs

As the discussion centers around Web Health Information Systems (WHISs), it is crucial to examine the relationships between information providers (uploaders) and information seekers (downloaders) with WHISs individually. In this context, direct relationships are considered only for authorized practitioners within the medical domain, who may also assume responsibility for content updates and deletions. Authorized medical practitioners have the privilege of contributing to and managing content on WHISs. However, non-medical practitioners' users must adhere to the disclaimers provided by WHISs. For instance, if a patient searches for information on the medicine 'Pembrolizumab,' they can access existing information related to its colors and shape. However, they are not permitted to contribute new details about the medicine or save such information on WHISs. Users, in dual roles as both information uploaders and downloaders, are encouraged to engage in self-review and interpretation within these relationships.

7.2.3 Quantity of Content on WHISs

Here, only accessible information can be listed; therefore, it is essential to check all substances with their corresponding frequencies/quantities. This evaluation will determine the scope of Workplace Hazardous Information Sheets (WHISs). Utilizing this data will also contribute to assessing the overall health and safety of WHISs.

7.2.4 Web – Quality and/or of Content on WHISs

Both WHISs are accompanied by a depth disclaimer, indicating that the content may be subject to plagiarism, repetition, inaccuracies, ethical concerns, and lack of responsibility. No information is guaranteed for users. While the platform aims to provide authentic awareness, it is important to note that the platform has limitations. Therefore, it is crucial to seek proper diagnosis from a qualified medical practitioner before utilizing or following any content.

7.2.5 Secondary Categories

Place, time, situation, condition, action, and passion are secondary categories in the ontology procedures of the Web-based Health Information System (WHIS). Given its web-based nature, all these categories are exclusively utilized in digital form. The 'place' of WHIS is defined on the web, with its users dispersed globally. The 'time' attribute, particularly concerning the uploaded information, is primarily relevant for researchers. Other users can access information at their convenience. 'Situation' refers to the user's context; users accessing the platform should be cognizant of their circumstances to ensure a satisfactory experience. An overly dynamic situation may not meet user expectations.

7.2.6 Justification of Inductive Ontological Model by Connecting Both WHISs Concerning Users' Perspectives

In this study, the researcher intentionally selected two health information sources (WHIS), namely WebMD and Drugs.com. WebMD provides comprehensive primary information on the human skeleton, including details about various parts, joint functions, symptoms of diseases, the patient's condition as diagnosed by doctors, and potential medications. On the other hand, Drugs.com specializes in medication-related information, covering details such as drugs, dosage, effects, side effects, and more. Both platforms cater to a diverse audience, including patients, doctors, and medical representatives, offering a holistic view of medical information. Participants in the study shared their experiences and insights on both WHISs, providing a thorough understanding from both medical and patient perspectives.

Figure 6. Respondents Feedback of WHISs

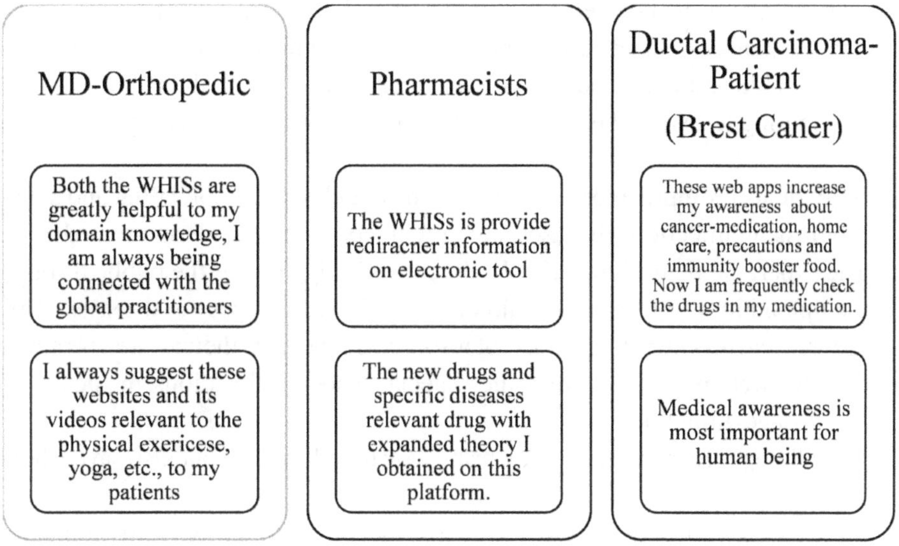

All three respondents shared their experiences with WHISs; thus, it is evident that the inductive ontological model serves as a comprehensive framework for specifying the user perspective and contextual intricacies of WHISs. Consequently, tailored to individual needs and the diverse user base, a deep ontology model can be developed to enhance medical awareness and positively impact end users.

7.2.7 Role of Web-based Health Information Systems in Holistic Well-Being

Holistic well-being encompasses a myriad of concepts, and Choudhary, Satabdi Roy, and Barman, Arup (2014) shed light on the subjective model in their research titled 'Holistic Model of Subjective Well-being: A Proposed Model and Exploration of Contents.' In their study, they present a subjective well-being model that includes four approaches: spiritual well-being, physical well-being, social well-being, and psychological well-being. In the contemporary landscape, numerous electronic platforms are purposefully addressing and succeeding in enhancing various aspects of well-being. Consequently, the maintenance of a healthy physical body has emerged as a vital component of holistic well-being. Web-based health information systems play a pivotal role in raising awareness about health among individuals. While medical terminology has traditionally remained on the outskirts for the general population, excluding those in medical disciplines, web-based Health Information Systems

(HIS) have effectively bridged this gap by providing dictionaries and other language tools. The advent of web-based HIS brings several benefits to society, including resolving challenges related to understanding health information. These systems serve as valuable resources, not only offering clarity on medical terminology but also contributing to overall health awareness in the broader community."

a. Individuals promptly receive information about both fast-spreading and slow-progressing infectious diseases, along with corresponding home remedies.
b. The expert medical team at the WHIS consistently updates the public through the uploading of video and audio content addressing specific diseases. This ensures that people have a variety of resources to increase their awareness about diseases, treatments, home remedies, specialist doctors, locations, medications, and dosage guidelines.
c. Visualizing information not only brings joy to individuals but also saves them valuable time.
d. Pre-existing knowledge about health, treatments, and symptoms aids humanity in preparing for mental well-being.
e. Web-based information is commonly perceived as a means of promoting awareness, playing a pivotal role in the lives of individuals. Considering the impact of information on lives, it is imperative for medical experts to verify its authenticity and accuracy.

7.3 Objective 3: To Present an Inductive Ontology Graph by Connecting Both WHISs Concerning Users' Perspective

A researcher prepared figure 3 & 4 of ontological graph to show of the chosen WHISs web platform; which is called main domain in technical terminology of ontology, therefore here the chosen WHISs are calling "Main Domain" in the following explanation.

7.3.1 Main Domain: WEB MD: Better Information. Better Health

Sub Classes: The WEB MD have sub classes with their own specific features.

Sub Class 1: Connect To Care – This subclass encompasses numerous core classes, incorporating diverse sources of information related to various health concepts. These include topics such as addiction recovery assistance, LASIK surgery details, legal guidance on vaping, bariatric surgery, asbestos and mesothelioma information, hair loss remedies, hearing loss solutions, teeth straightening options, sleep apnea insights, and more. This class is dedicated to analyzing the users' perspectives, aiming to reconnect them with their distinct desires for seeking information.

Sub Class 2: Check Your Symptoms! – This class is designed according to human anatomy, emphasizing observation. The content is comprehensive, covering symptoms related to diseases or specific body parts such as the mouth, head, knee, etc.

Sub Class 3: Find A Doctor - This category encompasses various properties, specifically the classification of medical doctors based on their specialties, patient conditions, and the procedures involved in their treatment, including phases such as primary diagnoses, operations, etc.

Sub Class 4: Find A Dentist – This category features a distinct attribute, specifically the 'Dentist' property. It processes information in accordance with Subclass 3, but commences with the primary term 'Dentist.'"

7.3.2 Main Domain: Drug.com: Know More Be Sure

Sub Classes: This domain provides information about various drugs, their applications for specific conditions, treatments, and related features.

Sub Class 1: Drugs & Medications – This category encompasses various sub-properties, including browsable drugs, conditions, treatments, and a 'By Site Section' feature. The 'By Site Section' property is enriched by diverse sources such as drug guidelines, health professional directories, medical news, FDA alerts, and more.

Sub Class 2: Pill Identifier – This unique class provides information about pills, including details about their colors, shapes, and imprints. Its wizard categorizes drugs by their name, manufacturer, code, colors, and more.

Sub Class 3: Side Effects: It has a unique database about drugs and its side effects with advance search options i.e. drugs side, top side effects, and A-Z side effects.

Sub Class 4: Interactions Chekers – This class provide the inforamtion about drugs with different sub domains i.e. food & beverage, disease interaction, pharmacodynamic interaction, and other factors.

Inferences: The Ontological Graph of selected Web-Based Health Information Systems (WHISs) represents a foundational level graph, potentially characterized as a progressive ontology. This framework provides a comprehensive overview of WHISs, serving as robust platforms for addressing various 'WH' questions (What, Why, Where, Who, Whom) posed by users, accommodating both diverse medical professionals and non-professional users. The section titled 'Relationship Between Users and WHISs' elaborates on how different professionals and non-professionals (patients) benefit from these platforms. Consequently, it can be argued that the inductive ontology presented here represents the initial phase, while the detailed ontology and the ontological graph constitute the primary level of research to be undertaken.

8. ANSWER TO RESEARCH QUESTION

The primary question that arose in the researcher's mind was: "How does ontology amplify the healthiness of selected Web-Based Health Information Systems (WHISs)?" Throughout the investigation, it was discovered that the amplification of healthiness involves elements that can be easily assessed on the web. These elements can be broadly classified into two parts:

8.1. Technical Elements

In this category, elements encompassing improved search and retrieval, decision support, personalized health information, data integration, quality assurance, interdisciplinary collaboration, and data analytics are included. The effectiveness of these elements is largely contingent on the hosting decisions made by the platform owner. Consequently, the evaluation of all the listed elements can be facilitated through the web stethoscope, specifically "Scrawler," along with other relevant tools.

8.2. Non-Technical Elements

Evaluation of essential elements within the chosen Web-based Health Information Systems (WHISs) involves an examination based on user and researcher experiences. These elements encompass: Semantic Interoperability: Ensuring precise and meaningful information presentation with a reduced risk of misinterpretation. User and researcher experiences affirm that the information available on the platform accurately informs users about their health conditions, relevant medicines, and treatments. Standardized Vocabulary: Both user and researcher experiences indicate that both platforms employ a standardized vocabulary in the medical domain. Hyperlinked Graphical Symptom Checker: The graphical symptom checker on WebMD, with hyperlinked features, could establish itself as a standard graphical vocabulary for non-professional users.

In summary, the optimization of health-related information within these WHISs involves technical elements, influenced by platform owner decisions, and non-technical elements, assessed through user and researcher experiences. Tools like "Scrawler" and the incorporation of standardized vocabulary and graphical features contribute to the overall healthiness of these web-based health information systems.

9. SCOPE

This chapter primarily outlines the ontological framework of the WHISs platform, focusing on its 'WEB' aspect. Encompassing numerous sub-domains, the platform facilitates interdisciplinary research from scientific and societal perspectives. It embodies a progressive ontology, illustrating interconnected nodes with diverse subjective relationships. Exploring aspects such as 'People's Health,' 'User Satisfaction Levels,' 'Professional and Non-Professional Users' Objective Perspectives,' 'Medical Education,' 'Medical Profession,' 'Medical Service for Chronic and Long-term Users,' and the intersection of 'Medical & ICT,' the comprehensive approach allows for a thorough examination of the platform's impact across multiple dimensions.

10. CONCLUSION

The concept of ontology has been employed by various disciplines to illustrate inter and multi-subjective branches. In this study, a researcher probes the Medical domains through WHISs, highlighting their multifaceted attributes catering to various user types. The amalgamation of ICT and Medical domain expertise manifests through an inductive ontological model's explanation, demonstrating the significance of information volatility and competency. The uniqueness of the medical domain, encompassing terminology, concepts, explanations, and practices, is supported by ICT, benefiting both domain experts and users. The study assesses two chosen WHISs through an inductive ontological presentation, checking their healthiness with "The HOTH" web tool. The site audit reveals key attributes, indicating the vitality of the webpage. Recommendations for improvement, such as reducing days to report to developers and enhancing keywords for a more accessible website, are highlighted. While the study provides valuable insights, it acknowledges that further research is needed to comprehensively explore WHISs services, web-based performance, and users' experiences, given the vast information provided by these systems. The LIS profession may consider adopting WHISs as new awareness services, and the study suggests exploring WHISs information seekers' behavior as another branch within the LIS domain.

REFERENCES

https://www.drugs.com/ (Accessed: 8th May to 26th July 2023)

https://www.webmd.com/ (Accessed: 8th May to 26th July 2023) https://en.wikipedia.org/wiki/WebMD (Accessed: 8th May to 26th July 2023)

https://en.wikipedia.org/wiki/Drugs.com (Accessed: 8th May to 26th July 2023)

https://www.thehoth.com/hoth-x/ (Accessed: 8th May to 26th July 2023)

Alshammari, T. (2014). Drug safety: The concept, inception and its importance in patients' health. *Saudi Pharmaceutical Journal*, *24*(4), 405–412. doi:10.1016/j.jsps.2014.04.008 PMID:27330371

Choudhary, S. R. & Barman, A. (2014). Holistic Model of subjective well-being a proposed model and exploration of contents. *Zenith International Journal of Multidisciplinary research, 4*(3), 259-278.

Open, A. I. (n.d.). ChatGPT: Improving Grammar and Statements. https://chat.openai.com/c/fccd4b4f-78bc-44f8-9f8e-734ba032ea62

Rade, Babic, Zoran, Milosevic & Gordana, (2012). "Web technology in health system" Acta facultatis medicae naissensis. UDC: 616-073:621.3929 (2):81-87. DOI: doi:10.2478/v10283-012-0011-9

Williams, P., Nicholas, D., Huntington, P., & McLean, F. (2002). Surfing for health: user evaluation of a health information website. Part one: background and literature review. *Health Information and Libraries Journal*, *19*(2), 98–108. doi:10.1046/j.1471-1842.2002.00374_2.x PMID:12389607

Zhang, J. K., & Xu, W. (n.d.). Web Service-based Healthcare Information System (WSHIS): A Case Study for System Interoperability Concern in Healthcare Field. *2006 International Conference on Biomedical and Pharmaceutical Engineering*, Singapore, 2006, pp. 588-594.

Chapter 7
Predictive Analysis of Consumers' Immunity Literacy Towards Immunity Products:
A Statistical Study Using Discriminant Method

Poonam Arora
https://orcid.org/0000-0001-8578-3638
SKIPS School of Business, India

Nidhi Arora
Full Stack Technology LLP, India

ABSTRACT

The outbreak of COVID-19 pandemic and the subsequent recurrences have profound effect on psychological, social and physical health of people. The fear of Corona virus has posed unexampled stress on all the population segments of country. The perceived threat has made people more conscious about their health and immunity. This has triggered a significant change in consumer buying behaviour towards immunity products. This study attempts to analyse the factors influencing immunity literacy among people and to determine predictor variables for people's immunity consciousness. A sample of 391 respondents was collected and analyzed using descriptive and determinant analysis. The findings of the study highlight important factors behind consumers' literacy and their buying behaviour towards immunity products. In conclusion, a high variance is observed on the basis of the length of time, use of products and money spent in buying immunity products. A function mapping based on their buying intention towards immunity products categorized people as immunity aware or immunity ignorant.

DOI: 10.4018/978-1-7998-9652-4.ch007

1. INTRODUCTION

Developing immunity against viruses has become the greatest challenge in recent times. Since the outbreak of COVID-19 in India, there have been around millions of people who got infected with the Corona virus. The fear and anxiety of the increasing number of cases has transformed people to become immunity aware to protect themselves against the virus. To control the spread of the virus, Government of India has taken proactive vaccination drives across the nation. The biggest and most successful vaccination drive in India is one of the major reasons due to which people are now immune in the world (Business Standard, 2022). It has been observed that COVID-19 vaccines are effective in preventing mortality and play a significant role in reducing the risk of spread and deaths associated with the COVID-19 (Kaunain, 2021).

Each immunity aware individual contributes to the safety of other people in their closed coterie thereby minimizing the spread of it. This has caused decrease in the number of people being infected in late 2021. Understanding and devising the consumer behaviour based on demographic factors and needs of people is vital during pandemic. Government can utilize the conclusions drawn from such researches to enhance immunity literacy among people. At the same time companies dealing in immunity booster products can better plan their targeted customers.

Who is not conscious about their health? Be it a professional, businessman, housewife, retired individual or a student, whether male or female, working or non-working people. The findings of our last statistical analysis on the monthly consumption of people on immunity products points to the fact that most of the working people are conscious about their health which makes them spend on immunity products (Arora, Mehta & Arora, 2021). Some people are more conscious, while some are carefree. This can be rephrased in the other way also; those who have better buying capacity are ready to spend on their health as compared to others who are ignorant to improve their immunity. Our second study, created a novel categorization based on people, their health awareness and priorities towards immunity. The research coined the concept that people who take regular measures to stay healthy are called immunity aware and those individuals who do not spend on their health as healthy immune system is not their priority fall in immunity ignorant category (Arora & Arora, 2023). Both these terms are coined with substantiate review and study undertaken by authors in previous researches.

An individual's behavior is impacted by directly or indirectly observing others in their social proximity. There are many theories that connects people conscious decisions with their health behavior. Fishbein and Ajzen in 1975 found out that an adequate social cognitive health behaviour predicts an individual's health behaviour and also promotes the change in health consciousness and behavior (Fishbein &

Ajzen, 1975). The social cognitive behaviour provide strong health related intentions in people (Norman & Conner, 2005). Also, behaviors are the end products of beliefs. One of the psychological theory says that the three factors of attitude, subjective norms, and perceived behaviors designs an individual's health behaviors and hence the actions. People becoming conscious or neglecting their health, this intention is shaped by their attitude towards importance of health. Ajzen in his research coined that intention of people to behave in a particular manner can be accurately predicted via their attitude towards that particular behavior, their values and norms affecting the outcome and the perceived behavioral control. All these intentions, account for the variation in an individual's actual behavior (Ajzen, 1991).

There are numerous research evidences that suggests that people make contributions in their own health and overall well-being by accepting certain good hygienic health behaviors while avoiding other compromised behavior which may impact their health adversely. Identification of such good health behaviors has become a focus in psychological research (Adler & Matthews, 1994). These researches are the results of the motivational desire to change the prevalence of these behaviour which may produce improvements in an individuals' health. Right interventions may also help individuals in gaining an understanding of the reasons of why an individual perform in a specific way (Adler & Matthews, 1994).

There are numerous variables, from different models, worked on by researchers that relate to the performance of health behaviour of individuals. Cummings et al. (1980) studied 109 variables to predict health behaviour. Most of the researches on health behaviors have considered few of the following six variables of accessibility of health care services, attitudes towards health care, perceptions of disease threat, knowledge about diseases, social network characteristics and demographic factors (Norman & Conner, 2005). Four out of the five factors relate to the social cognitive theory and have been central to a number of models of the determinants of health behaviour. These factors are responsible for paving characteristics of the individual and make their health behaviour These variables are subject to change and variations in them represent and label routing influence on health indicators and performance of individuals (Norman & Conner, 2005).

Lot of studies exist in literature in which researchers have worked on analysis related to COVID-19. Zintel conducted a study to analyse the COVID-19 vaccination intentions basis gender differences (Zintel, Flock & Arbogast, 2022). According to a previous research work conducted by Bish et al. on other vaccines there are gender differences in vaccination favoring men on their intentions (Bish, Yardley, Nicoll & Michie, 2011). This study can be considered to determine the immunity literacy and awareness of people towards COVID-19 broadly pertaining to their work status. Moving forward, similar surveys were reported by researchers during pandemic years which points to varied intentions of people for COVID-19 vaccination (Galanis,

Vraka, Fragkou, Bilali & Kaitelidou, 2021). It is believed that household women in India are not very particular about their health. Although they play a central role in ensuring the best health of their family, they don't intend to spend on their health unless necessary. As stated by a group of researchers, a balanced nutritional diet, including variety of vitamins and micro nutrients, may play an essential role in maintaining health of people. Their study was aimed at discussing the role of vitamins and minerals in the treatment of COVID-19 (Kumar, Kumar, Bedi, Gupta, Kumar, Jaiswal, Rahi, Yedke, Bijalwan, Sharma & Jamwal, 2021). This is evident from the studies that either through social media, television, news articles, experience of elders or by word of mouth, people have become conscious about their immunity. This has resulted into a higher purchase towards immunity products.

Certain products which are easily available either online or on pharmacy stores, and can be purchased without a prescription are termed as Over The Counter medications. There have been studies related to consumption of Over the Counter (OTC) products and Ayurvedic products by people during this time. Landge and Petare (2021) underwent a study on consumer buying behaviour towards Over the Counter (OTC) products during the COVID-19 pandemic. The outcomes of the study revealed that consumers above age 20 years use the Over the Counter (OTC) products against most common diseases like cold, cough and fever. Of all the products, allopathic medicines were found to be more acceptable for curing the above diseases (Landge & Petare, 2021). Suganya and Hamsalakshmi (2017) found that people are not only brand specific and also prefer immunity products which are chemical free (Suganya & Hamsalakshmi, 2017). This is the reason why consumers of age group 36-45 years are more interested to buy Traditional medicinal products. In another study on post COVID-19 trends in consumer buying behaviour of pharma Over Counter products, it was found that there was an increase in self-health awareness among consumers (Tomar & Krishnamoorthy, 2021). In response to their self-health awareness, the consumers were found to consume immunity booster products for positive impact of COVID-19. This study also pointed out the most of the consumers were brand conscious to buy products with Ayurvedic ingredients rather than buying unknown brands.

On one hand, where people have been observed to be too conscious about their health during Corona virus pandemic, some other group of people have been found to be hesitant to consume additional supplements to keep their immunity high in addition to their regular medicines. Number of different factors increased hesitancy including negative perception of vaccine efficacy, convenience, and safety. Some of the consistent socio-demographic groups that were identified to be associated with increased hesitancy included: women, younger participants, and people who were less educated, had lower income, had no insurance, living in a rural area, and self-identified as a racial/ethnic minority (Cascini, Pantovic, Al-Ajlouni, Failla &

Ricciardi, 2021). In contrast, some people are inclined towards Ayurveda products because of general belief that they are safe. Mohamed carried out a study to analyse the awareness of people on Ayurveda as an option of boosting their immunity. The study concluded that during this pandemic outbreak most of the people are aware of the role of Ayurveda in immunity boosting (Mohamed & Gheena, 2020).

A similar study aims to assess the awareness of people with no medical background about COVID-19 and the preventive strategies against the same. The people targeted in the study were people including students, homemakers, employees and entrepreneurs. (Patkar & Berry, 2020). They found that most of the people have good awareness about the preventive measures but some important factors like mask disposal technique, over the counter medication, affection of pets etc. needs to be considered as additional measures against COVID-19.

This work is undertaken in continuation with our work on immunity consciouness in which we concluded that working people consume more immunity products monthly than non-working people as they are more immunity conscious. We also found that the amount spent by working people towards the purchase of immunity products is more than non-working people pertaining to their health consciousness. The present study is aimed at determining the effects of the COVID-19 pandemic on buying behaviour of people especially their immunity literacy and awareness. The changes in behaviour of people during COVID-19 and factors influencing their consciousness are examined. The two-fold objectives of the study are to analyse the factors influencing immunity literacy and awareness among people and to determine predictor variables for people's immunity consciousness. The study comprises of a three-stage analysis aims at assessing the literacy and awareness of COVID-19 among people. At first stage, data exploration is done to understand the inclination of the respondents. Descriptive analysis is performed over the collected data to study the impact of immunity on consumer behaviour at second stage. At last, discriminant analysis is undertaken to test the significant difference between the two groups of consumers and to evaluate the accuracy of classification between ignorance and awareness.

2. MATERIALS AND METHODS

2.1. Data Collection

The specific focus of the current work is on the spending choice among different categories of people with the belief of keeping themselves protected against the virus. The data for this study was collected through a structured multiple-choice questionnaire during the months of September to December 2022. The data was collected from 391 respondents from Gujarat State of India to conduct an in-depth analysis of people distributed over various age groups belonging to different employment categories. The respondents from working and non-working categories of people were asked questions on the number of immunity booster products they are consuming, the length of time for which they are consuming immunity products and the amount of money they are spending per person per month. The respondents were also asked questions to determine the factors affecting their buying behaviour towards immunity products during COVID-19 pandemic.

2.2. Data Analysis

As pointed out from the results drawn from our previous work (Arora, P. et al., 2021), working people spend more on buying immunity products which makes them more immunity aware as opposed to non-working people who are ignorant towards their immunity. The factors affecting the consumer buying behaviour are analyzed as follows:

Figure 1. Consumption of Immunity Products due to Relapse of COVID-19

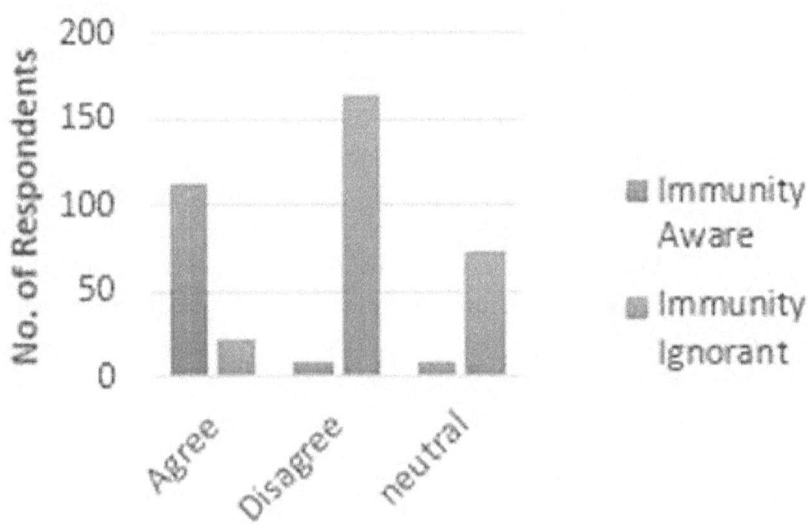

Figure 2. Consumption of Immunity Products to keep Immune System Strong

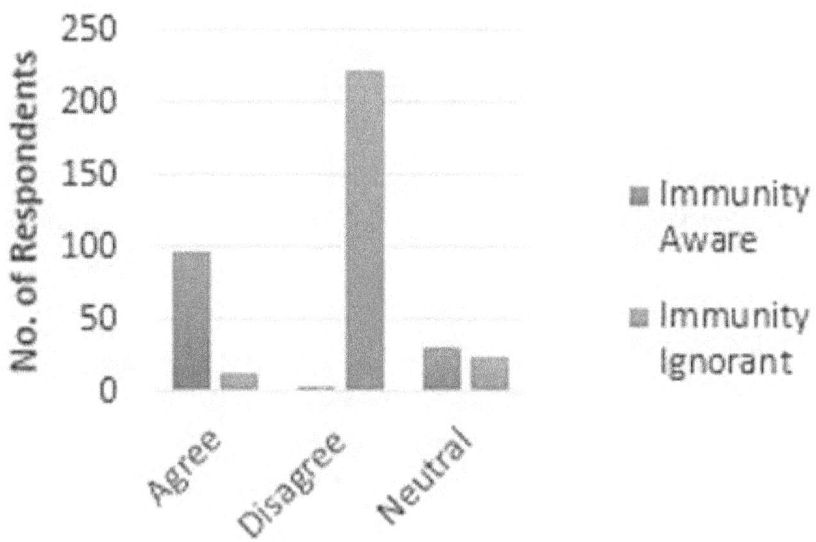

To understand the consumer buying behaviour, respondents were asked about the factors behind their consumption of immunity products. As seen from figure 1, the survey revealed that majorly immunity aware people started consuming the products as the COVID-19 relapsed in September 2021, while immunity ignorant people dominantly disagreed the relapse as the reason. Even the factor of keeping the immune system strong could not motivate them to start using immunity products and alter their consumption behaviour as they highly disagreed on this as well shown by figure 2. For immunity aware respondents this factor was also seen as one of the reasons of their change in behaviour.

Figure 3. Consumption of Immunity Products due to Suggestions/Awareness from Social Media

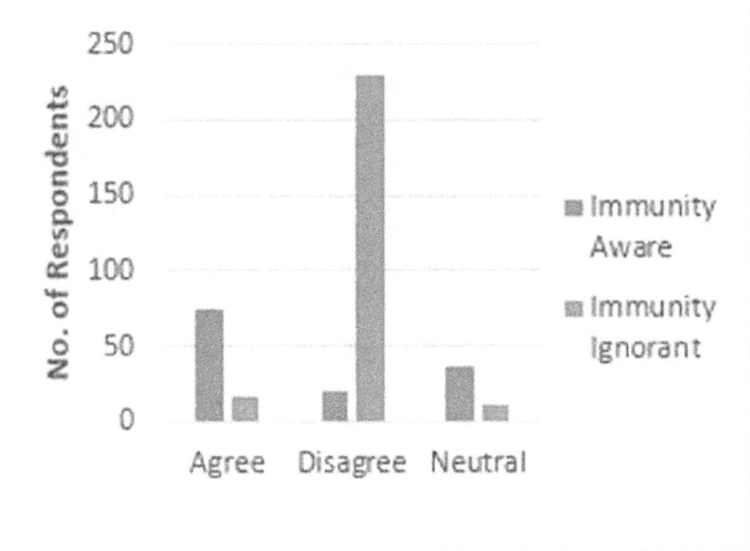

Figure 4. Consumption of Immunity Products due to Anxiety and Fear

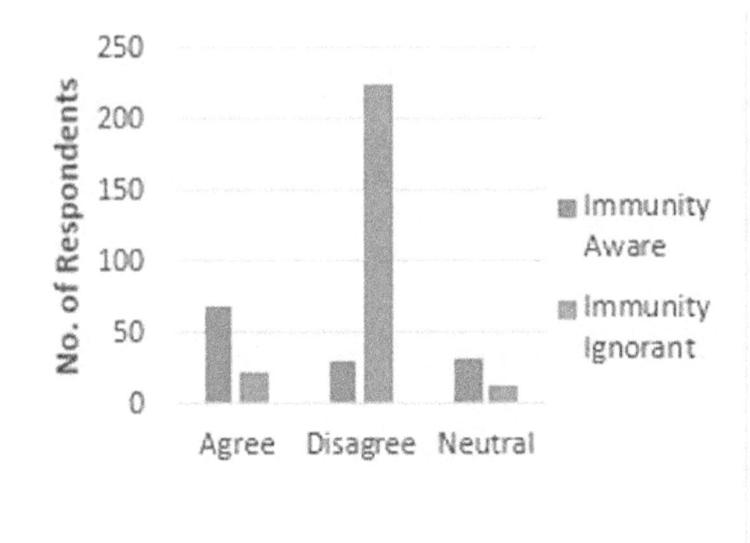

Two more factors on which people were asked to respond were: suggestions from social media and fear and anxiety because of the spread in the country. To this, immunity aware category of people highly agreed, refer figure 3. They stated that one of the reasons of their consumption is suggestion they got from social media regarding the products to be consumed. An important factor was found to be the fear of getting infected and the high spread in the country, the behaviour of immunity aware people saw a change as depicted in figure 4. The immunity ignorant category of respondents disagreed on both the factors reason being the spread could not affect them as they did not venture out mostly during the pandemic.

Figure 5. Consumption of Immunity Products due to Family Medical History

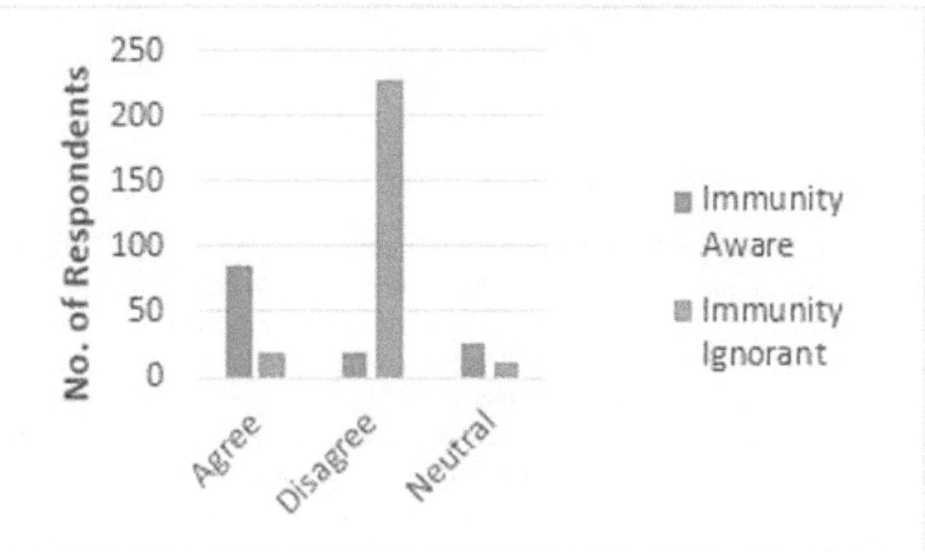

Figure 6. Consumption of Immunity Products due to Doctor Recommendation

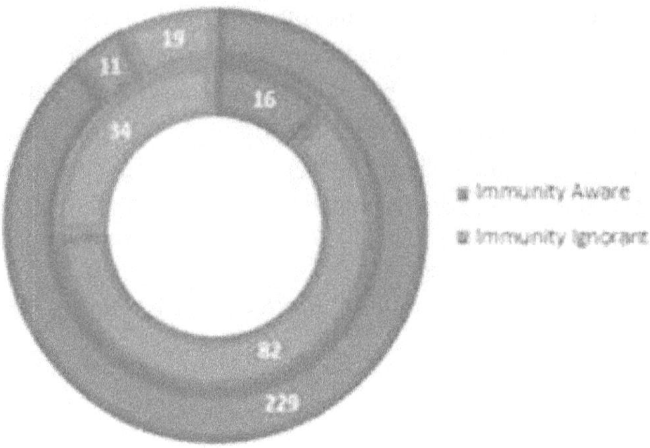

Looking at figures 5 and 6, the other factors state that majority of immunity ignorant respondents also disagreed to the fact that the family medical history made them change their buying behaviour. They started consuming these products only when the recommended by doctor. This is how they brought immunity products in their daily routine consumption pattern. Out of 391 respondents, 229 immunity aware respondents consider doctor's recommendation as crucial factor for using the health products and 82, a big number of immunity ignorant respondents agreed with immunity aware people, while the remaining people stood neutral.

The research is also aimed at analyzing the differences in the intention of people based on consumption of immunity products over length of time in months, number of immunity products consumed and money spent on immunity products per person per month with respect to immunity consciousness with three independent and one dependent variable. First, the descriptive statistics of the variables were calculated in order to understand and summarize the variable set.

Table 1. Group Statistics

Immunity			
Consciousness		Mean	Std. Deviation
Immunity Ignorant	Consumption of immunity products over length of time	9.97	2.672
	Number of immunity product consumed	1.60	.554
	Money spent on immunity product	1844.67	919.817
Immunity Aware	Consumption of immunity products over length of time	11.69	5.204
	Number of immunity product consumed	5.03	.823
	Money spent on immunity product	8235.29	1969.883
Total	Consumption of immunity products over length of time	10.50	3.712
	Number of immunity product consumed	2.65	1.708
	Money spent on immunity product	3789.64	3229.680

As can be seen from Table 1, the mean of all the three variables for immunity aware category is higher than the immunity ignorant category which means all the variables have positive impact on immunity consciousness. Discriminant analysis was used to estimate the relationship between the categorical dependent variable and the metric independent variables. The analysis was taken to check whether significant difference exist among the two groups and also to evaluate the accuracy of categorization.

Table 2. Box M's Test Results

Test Results		
Box's M		219.677
F	Approx.	36.232
	df1	6
	df2	93992.499
	Sig.	.523

Tests null hypothesis of equal population covariance matrices.

The significance value of Box's M test in Table 2 is 0.523 > 0.05 which shows that there is no difference in the group variances and the population covariance.

Table 3. Eigen Values

Eigenvalues				
Function	**Eigenvalue**	**% of Variance**	**Cumulative %**	**Canonical Correlation**
1	11.074[a]	100.0	100.0	.958

a. First 1 canonical discriminant functions were used in the analysis.

The canonical correlation in Table 3 shows that 91.7 per cent (square of canonical correlation = 0.958) of variance is explained in the model containing one criterion variable and three independent variable and the eigen value; 11.074 confirms that the function discriminates between the groups.

Table 4. Wilk's Lambda Test Result

Wilks' Lambda				
Test of Function(s)	**Wilks' Lambda**	**Chi-square**	**df**	**Sig.**
1	.466	965.298	3	.000

As seen from Table 4, the sig value in Wilk's lambda, which is a test of significance shows that the overall model is significant as the p value comes out to be .000 < .05.

Table 5. Standardized Canonical Discriminant Function Coefficients

Standardized Canonical Discriminant Function Coefficients	
	Function
	1
Consumption as length of time	.132
No. of products consumed	.450
Money spent on immunity product (Per person per month)	.912

Table 5 depicts the importance of each predictor variable on criterion variable. Here, among all the three coefficients of standardized canonical discriminant function, the coefficient of money spent on immunity products is 0.912, which implies that money spent affects the degree of literacy and awareness and ignorance; the highest followed by number of products (0.450) consumed and length of time (0.132). So, based on the importance of prediction, the following relation is identified.

Money spent on immunity products > No. of products consumed > Consumption as length of time

Table 6. Canonical Discriminant Function Coefficients

	Function
	1
Consumption as length of time	.027
No. of products consumed	.466
Money spent on immunity product (Per person per month)	.011
(Constant)	-1.679

Unstandardized coefficients

The above table gives the discriminant score using the coefficients of canonical discriminant function. Here

D= (-1.679) + 0.027 * length of time + 0.466 * no. of products consumed +0.011 * money spent

This equation will predict the immunity consciousness of people by putting the actual scores of all the three independent variables. If the value of D is more than 0.5, then the person is immunity aware, otherwise the person is immunity ignorant.

Table 7 shows the hit ratio and shows that 93.8 per cent of original grouped cases correctly categorized.

Table 7. Classification Results

Classification Results					
		Immunity Consciousness	Predicted Group Membership		Total
			0	1	
Original	Count	Immunity ignorant	259	13	272
		Immunity aware	11	108	119
	%	Immunity ignorant	95.2	4.8	100.0
		Immunity aware	9.3	90.7	100.0
Cross-validated[b]	Count	Immunity ignorant	259	13	272
		Immunity aware	12	107	119
	%	Immunity ignorant	95.2	4.8	100.0
		Immunity aware	10.1	89.9	100.0

a. 93.8% of original grouped cases correctly classified.

b. Cross validation is done only for those cases in the analysis. In cross validation, each case is classified by the functions derived from all cases other than that case.

c. 93.6% of cross-validated grouped cases correctly classified.

3. RESULTS AND DISCUSSIONS

Among the factors affecting buying behaviour of people, immunity aware category of people agreed to all factors that affected their consumption and expenditure on immunity products. These factors are: relapse of COVID-19, objective of keeping Immune system strong, suggestions from social media, anxiety and fear, family medical history and doctor recommendation. The most dominant reason among all the six was found to be the relapse of COVID-19, which motivated them to start consuming the products to increase their immunity on their own. The second highest factor that impacted was to keep people's immune system strong so that even when they are at work, their immunity is strong enough to fight against the foreign virus. The least number of people stated doctor's recommendation as the factor as they had proactively started the consumption of immunity products. Immunity ignorant respondents agreed only to the factor of doctor's recommendation that made them consume the immunity products. This brought a change in their buying behaviour. They disagreed to all the other five reasons ignoring the importance of immunity.

Discriminant analysis was used to conduct a multivariate analysis of variance to test the hypothesis that immunity aware and immunity ignorant people differ significantly on a linear combination of three variables i.e., consumption as length of time, number of products consumed and money spent on immunity products. The discriminant function accounted for nearly 92 per cent of variance in immunity consciousness of people. The overall chi-square test was significant (Wilk's lambda= 0.466, chi square = 965.298, df= 3, canonical correlation = 0.958, $p < 0.001$) and so the overall model was significant. From the Box M test, the null hypothesis that there is no difference among the groups is found to be true. Among the independent variable, money spent on immunity products is the best predictor. The discriminant function is: D= (-1.679) + 0.027 * length of time + 0.466 * no. of products consumed + 0.011 * money spent.

4. CONCLUSION

The goal of the research was to review the results of our previous study, investigating whether there are any systematic differences in the immunity consciousness of people. The survey clearly concluded that working people are immunity aware while non-working category comprising of retired people, housewives and students learning from online classes are immunity ignorant. The study focused on finding the factors affecting the decision of people in spending and changing their buying behaviour towards immunity products. Immunity aware people are found to spend on immunity booster products due to fear and anxiety to keep their immune system strong following suggestions from social media looking at family medical history with relapse of COVID -19. On the contrary immunity ignorant people consumed immunity products because of doctor's recommendation. For immunity aware category, the most dominant reason among all was found to be the relapse of COVID-19 followed by the factor of keeping their immune system strong. The least number of people stated doctor's recommendation as the factor. Immunity ignorant respondents agreed only to one factor i.e., doctor's recommendation that made them consume the immunity products. The study significantly proves the fact that this category is immunity ignorant as they are not affected by any of the factors. On the other hand, people who understand the need to keep their immune system strong, got influenced by social media and their family history brought a change in their consumption pattern. These people are found to fall in the immunity aware category.

The study also showed that a high variance is created by the length of time, use of products and money spent in immunity consciousness of people and hence are categorized as immunity aware or immunity ignorant. The analysis concluded that around 94 per cent of the respondents are correctly classified in immunity aware and immunity ignorant categories based on the predictor variables. Out of all the three independent variables, money spent on immunity products is the best predictor of consumer intention and the change in their buying behaviour. The immunity consciousness function was also modelled depending on the predictor variables viz. consumption as length of time, number of products consumed and money spent on immunity products. The function empirically categorizes a person as immunity aware or immunity ignorant based on their differences in buying intention towards immunity products. The study results can be used by the government bodies to educate the people about benefits of keeping oneself strong and enhancing the immune system to prevent the infection of the Corona virus. More literacy and awareness can be spread among people to include immunity booster products in their daily consumption. Central and State health departments can use the function modelled in this study to identify the immunity ignorant class of people and can target these people to spread more literacy and awareness to make the country more responsive against the upcoming waves of COVID-19.

5. FUTURE IMPLICATIONS

The study used various variables to forecast buying behaviour of people and categorize them. The study uses the primary source and the data has been registered from a specific number of respondents. More elaborated work can be undertaken segmenting people based on the area of living. Also, other variables of social cognitive theory can be taken to predict specific behavior of people towards their health and detailed methodologies and health interventions can also be studied. How people may switch from one health category to another can be the future scope of this study. More health literacy theories impacting health behaviors can be applied on people from varied stated to add more evidence to effective research. The detailing on the linkage of theory and usage can be advanced as health literacy is definitely a stepping stone to determine significant change in health behaviors, but the groundbreaking ways through which the theories and framework impacts people's health behaviors is not clear nor completely consistent.

REFERENCES

Adler, N., & Matthews, K. (1994). Health psychology: Why do some people get sick and some stay well? *Annual Review of Psychology*, *45*(1), 229–259. doi:10.1146/annurev.ps.45.020194.001305 PMID:8135503

Ajzen, I. (1991). The theory of planned behavior. *Organizational Behavior and Human Decision Processes*, *50*(2), 179–211. doi:10.1016/0749-5978(91)90020-T

Arora, P., & Arora, N. (2023). People, Immunity and Nutrition: A Categorization. *International Journal of Innovative Science and Research Technology*, *8*(4).

Arora, P., Mehta, S., & Arora, N. (2021). Effect of Consumers' Immunity Consciousness on Monthly Consumption of Immunity Booster Products.

Bish, A., Yardley, L., Nicoll, A., & Michie, S. (2011). Factors associated with uptake of vaccination against pandemic influenza: A systematic review. *Vaccine*, *29*(38), 6472–6484. doi:10.1016/j.vaccine.2011.06.107 PMID:21756960

Cascini, F., Pantovic, A., Al-Ajlouni, Y., Failla, G., & Ricciardi, W. (2021). Attitudes, acceptance and hesitancy among the general population worldwide to receive the COVID-19 vaccines and their contributing factors: A systematic review. *EClinicalMedicine*, *40*, 101113. doi:10.1016/j.eclinm.2021.101113 PMID:34490416

Fishbein, M., & Ajzen, I. (1975). *Belief, Attitude, Intention, and Behavior*. Wiley.

Galanis, P., Vraka, I., Fragkou, D., Bilali, A., & Kaitelidou, D. (2021). Intention of healthcare workers to accept COVID-19 vaccination and related factors: A systematic review and meta-analysis. *Asian Pacific Journal of Tropical Medicine*, *14*(12), 543. doi:10.4103/1995-7645.332808

India's COVID vaccination programme one of world's most successful: Govt. (2022, January 2). *Business Standard*. Retrieved March 18, 2022, from https:// www.business-standard.com/ article/ current-affairs/ india-s-COVID- vaccination-programme- one-of-world-s-most- successful- govt-122010200558_1.html

Kaunain Sheriff, M. (2021, September 10). Explained: What latest govt data reveals on COVID-19 vaccine effectiveness, preventing mortality. The Indian Express. https:// indianexpress.com/ article/ explained/ govt-data- COVID-19- vaccine- effectiveness-preventing- mortality-7499460/

Kumar, P., Kumar, M., Bedi, O., Gupta, M., Kumar, S., Jaiswal, G., Rahi, V., Yedke, N. G., Bijalwan, A., Sharma, S., & Jamwal, S. (2021). Role of vitamins and minerals as immunity boosters in COVID-19. *Inflammopharmacology*, *29*(4), 1001–1016. doi:10.1007/s10787-021-00826-7 PMID:34110533

Landge, R. R., & Petare, P. (2021). Study on Consumer Behaviour in COVID Pandemic with respect to OTC medicine. *International Research Journal of Humanities and Interdisciplinary Studies*, *2*(5), 104–113.

Mohamed Arsaath, N., & Gheena, S. (2020). Awareness on the possible role of Ayurveda as an immunity booster in the covid19 pandemic. *International Journal of Research in Pharmaceutical Sciences*, 567-574.

Norman, P. A. U. L., & Conner, P. (2005). Predicting health behaviour: a social cognition approach. Predicting health behaviour, 1(478), 17-8.

Patkar, A., & Berry, A. K. (2020). Awareness of COVID-19, preventive strategies for the same and factors affecting immunity in adult community dwellers with no medical background-a questionnaire based study. *International Journal of Health Sciences and Research*, *10*(7), 287–295.

Suganya, R., & Hamsalakshmi, R. (2017). A study on customer buying behaviour of selected Ayurveda healthcare products. *International Journal of Advanced Research and Development*, *2*(2), 13–18.

Tomar H., Krishnamoorthy B. (2021). Post-COVID Emergent Trends in Consumer Buying Behaviour for Pharma-OTC Sector. Advanced Journal of Graduate Research, 1-60.

Zintel, S., Flock, C., Arbogast, A. L., Forster, A., von Wagner, C., & Sieverding, M. (2022). Gender differences in the intention to get vaccinated against COVID-19: A systematic review and meta-analysis. *Journal of Public Health*, 1–25. PMID:35018277

Chapter 8
Navigating Mental Health Crises:
Understanding Pivotal Phases, Health Campaigns, and Community Resilience for Recovery and Reform

Rita Komalasari
https://orcid.org/0000-0001-9963-2363
Yarsi University, Indonesia

ABSTRACT

This study delves into personal narratives of mental health crises and psychiatric treatment, comparing them with an extended Caplan's Crisis Theory. The objective is to unravel identifiable phases and turning points in these narratives, challenging traditional diagnostic categories and advocating for a paradigm shift in crisis intervention strategies. Through meticulous analysis, distinct phases of mental health crises emerged, showcasing the impact of interventions on recovery trajectories. Proposed alternative crisis categories highlighted the universal quest for safety and professional care, countered by social barriers. The study calls for a paradigm shift in mental health services, emphasizing psychosocial factors and community support. Through empathetic understanding and strategic interventions, mental health services can be restructured to be more responsive, fostering recovery and resilience among individuals facing mental health crises.

DOI: 10.4018/978-1-7998-9652-4.ch008

INTRODUCTION

This research delves into the personal narratives of individuals experiencing mental health crises and undergoing psychiatric treatment, comparing these accounts with an extended application of Caplan's Crisis Theory. The primary objective is to identify distinct phases and turning points within these narratives, challenging conventional diagnostic categories and advocating for a paradigm shift in crisis intervention strategies. Through meticulous analysis, the study reveals discernible phases in mental health crises, illustrating the influence of interventions on recovery trajectories. Proposed alternative crisis categories underscore the universal pursuit of safety and professional care, hindered by prevailing social barriers. Individuals may see mental health crises and breakdowns as tragic events, but they also provide chances for personal development and transformation (Lawrance et al., 2022). According to statistics, the number of cases of mental health crises has been rising globally in recent times (Holmes et al., 2020). This empirical data highlights a crucial problem that demands quick action, affecting an estimated 450 million people (World Health Organization, 2022). In addition, research by Jordanova, (2021) shows that people from different socioeconomic backgrounds have very different access to crisis care, which makes things even more difficult for them both during and after a crisis. The widespread dissatisfaction with post-crisis care demonstrates a serious flaw in the current system (Williams et al., 2021). More efficient, fair, and all-encompassing mental health services are required, especially in the wake of catastrophes, and these patterns indicate a real and doable issue.

There are four parts to this chapter. The research and its methods are introduced in the first part. Section two presents the study's findings, which are structured around the following themes: the crisis's psychosocial origins, the crisis's stages, the point at which the individual begins to recover or becomes a long-term mental health patient, and the effect of the crisis on the individual's social status, employment prospects, and self-sufficiency. Section three talks about how these discoveries may be used to treat and prevent mental health crises. At the end of the chapter, in Section four, the key themes will be reviewed and suggest where the future study should go. This chapter argues that more effective and suitable preventative and treatment programs may be developed by listening to the stories of people who have been through mental health crises and breakdowns. Researchers concluded that crisis services should prioritize self-advocacy, active listening, and community support based on a psychosocial model of crisis.

This research explores the complex terrain of mental health crises through the insightful stories of people who have survived devastating breakdowns. After reviewing the literature extensively, the author based our investigation on Caplan's Crisis Theory and will show how it applies to crisis situations' psychological and social aspects (Baumgardt & Weinmann, 2022). As we traverse through the structure of this chapter, we unravel the threads of personal narratives, proposing alternative crisis categories that challenge traditional diagnoses. Our narrative journey navigates the crucial quest for safety, the yearning for professional care, and the resilience found within communities. The contours of social class impact crisis care access, but our focus extends beyond the aftermath, where dissatisfaction with care emerges as a common refrain (Erchul & Schulte, 2019). Loss of social standing and opportunities becomes a shared experience, met with ingenious coping mechanisms within community engagement, enjoyable activities, and activism.

This introductory chapter lays the groundwork for a transformative discourse, advocating for a shift in mental health services. The knowledge and information yielded by this research can be instrumental for various individuals and groups involved in mental health care, policymaking, and advocacy. There are specific stakeholders who can benefit from the findings: Psychiatrists, psychologists, counselors, and other mental health professionals, all of which can use the insights gained from this research to refine their understanding of mental health crises. Recognizing identifiable phases, turning points, and the impact of interventions can inform more targeted and effective therapeutic approaches. Government agencies, policymakers, and mental health organizations can use this research to shape mental health policies and services. The emphasis on psychosocial factors, community support, and self-advocacy could guide the development of more comprehensive and accessible crisis care programs. Local community groups and organizations engaged in mental health support can leverage the study's findings to enhance their programs. Those who have experienced mental health crises and received psychiatric treatment can benefit directly from this research. The validation of diverse crisis experiences, the identification of common challenges, and the emphasis on community support can empower individuals in their recovery journeys. Hospitals, clinics, and healthcare providers involved in mental health care can incorporate the research findings into their practices. Understanding the factors influencing crisis care access and the aftermath of mental health crises can contribute to more patient-centric and effective healthcare delivery. The knowledge generated by this research has the potential to catalyze positive changes across multiple sectors, fostering a more empathetic, inclusive, and effective approach to mental health care and support.

BACKGROUND

Individuals, families, and communities are greatly impacted by mental health crises and breakdowns, which pose a substantial public health risk (Morganstein & Ursano, 2020). One in four people may have a mental health illness in any given year, and the incidence of these diseases is growing globally (World Health Organization, 2022). Moreover, mental health disorders are associated with a substantial economic burden, estimated at US$1 trillion annually in lost productivity and healthcare costs (Health, 2020).

There is mounting evidence that a large percentage of people who go through mental health crises eventually make a full recovery. According to research by Naushad et al. (2019), after a year of experiencing a mental health crisis, almost 70% of people had a favorable result. Similarly, Pavli et al. (2021) discovered in their meta-analysis that people with severe mental illness showed considerable increases in their ability to operate and integrate socially as time went on. Notwithstanding these encouraging improvements, the need for better crisis care services are becoming more acknowledged. Nearly 20% of people who go through a mental health crisis do not get assistance from a professional, according to research by Stuijfzand et al. (2020). Similarly, Radez et al. (2021) discovered that people with mental illness are more likely to get improper or insufficient treatment when compared to those with other types of health issues. The results shed light on the lived experiences of those who have gone through mental health crises and breakdowns, which adds to our knowledge of these topics. The study's results stress the need for improved mental health crisis prevention and treatment programs.

This study contributes significantly to improving the mental health profession and the broader field through several key avenues. Mental health professionals will benefit from a nuanced understanding of identifiable phases and turning points in mental health crises. This insight allows for more tailored and informed therapeutic approaches, enhancing the effectiveness of interventions and promoting quicker paths to recovery. Policymakers and mental health service providers can utilize the study's findings to refine existing mental health policies and services. The emphasis on psychosocial factors, community support, and self-advocacy aligns with a holistic and person-centered approach, paving the way for more comprehensive and accessible mental health care services. The study challenges traditional diagnostic labels by proposing alternative categories of crisis experiences, contributing to destigmatization efforts. A more welcoming and empathetic attitude may result from this, which can improve communication and understanding in the field and beyond. Advocates for mental health and community groups may use the study's findings to inform community involvement efforts. Creating successful grassroots programs and support networks may be initiated by appreciating the significance of community assistance in managing mental health crises. The study's focus on self-advocacy gives those who have been through it more agency. Empowering individuals to take an active role in their rehabilitation promotes a paradigm shift from a state of passive acceptance to one of full mastery over their mental health condition.

The suggested alternative crisis categories provide a foundation upon which academic institutions and scholars might expand their investigation of novel methods of instruction. As a result, mental health education is always improving, and the next generation of experts will be better prepared to deal with mental health emergencies. The call for a paradigm shifts towards psychosocial factors, good listening, and community support can drive systemic changes in mental health care. This includes reevaluating existing crisis services and focusing on prevention, ultimately fostering a more resilient and supportive mental health system. This study has the potential to catalyze positive changes within the mental health profession and the broader field by providing actionable insights that align with evolving perspectives on mental health care. It encourages a more holistic, person-centered, and community-oriented approach, contributing to the ongoing improvement and transformation of the mental health profession.

METHOD

The methodology employed in this study centers on a comprehensive literature review strategically chosen to unravel the intricacies of mental health crises. The study examines personal narratives from scholarly works post-2018, aligning them with an extended Caplan crisis theory. Rigorous data analysis involves categorizing crisis experiences, identifying phases, and identifying turning points. This methodology ensures a nuanced exploration, allowing for the emergence of alternative crisis categories and highlighting the psychosocial dimensions crucial for reshaping mental health services. The following figure 1 illustrates the specific method.

Figure 1. The Specific Method

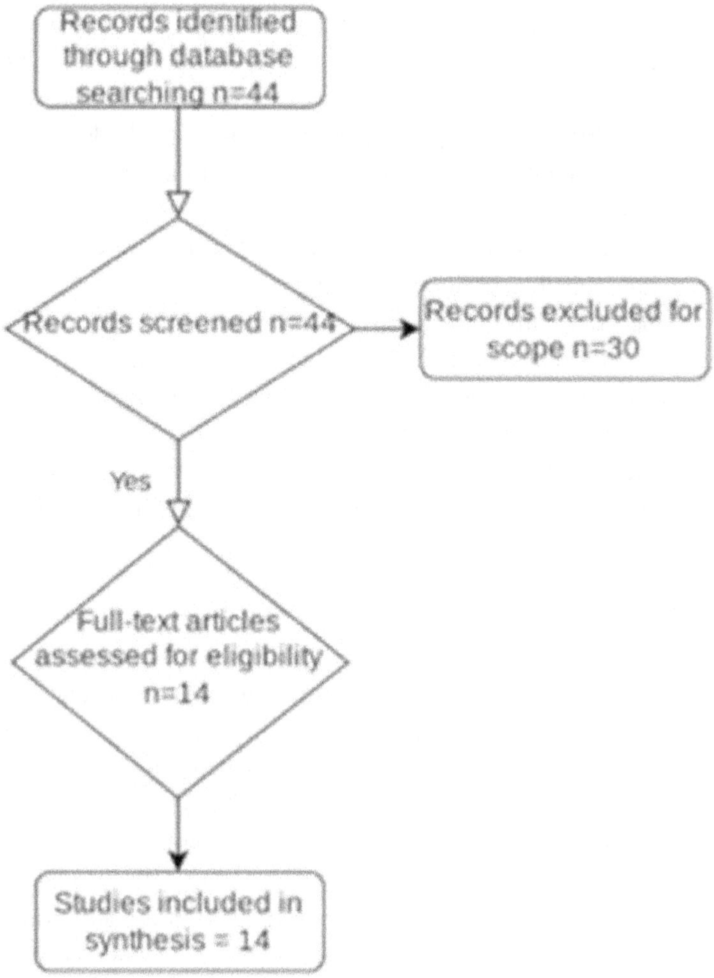
Records identified through database searching n=44
Records screened n=44
Records excluded for scope n=30
Yes
Full-text articles assessed for eligibility n=14
Studies included in synthesis = 14

Literature study is a powerful lens, illuminating diverse narratives and enriching the understanding of mental health crises beyond conventional frameworks. This review's inclusion and exclusion criteria were meticulously designed to ensure a comprehensive yet focused examination of the literature on mental health services, specifically in the aftermath of crises. This evaluation relies heavily on Google Scholar, which provides access to various scholarly literature. Studies published between 2019 and 2023 were included in the inclusion criteria, guaranteeing that the most recent study results will be included. For linguistic consistency, the language requirement was limited to English and Indonesian. To conduct a focused investigation on the efficacy and equality of mental health services, the population of interest was patients. The conceptual framework highlighted the need for mental health services to be comprehensive, equitable, and effective, especially in the aftermath of a disaster. Academic journals and freely available full-text publications were given precedence for accessibility, although all sorts of research were taken into consideration. While adhering to academic norms of methodological rigor, this inclusive approach sought to get detailed knowledge of mental health treatments in crisis circumstances.

The Ecological Systems Theory provides an appropriate paradigm for thoroughly examining mental health services' efficacy, equality, and comprehensiveness, especially in the aftermath of a catastrophe (Sharma & Thapa, 2023). From the microsystem (one's immediate circle of friends and family) to the macrosystem (one's larger community and culture), according to this idea put forth by Urie Bronfenbrenner, people exist within a web of interrelated systems. With this approach, the author can look at mental health care as a whole and see how different ecological elements affect the fairness and efficiency of treatment during and after a crisis.

CRISIS INTERVENTION

The term 'crisis' is often used synonymously with the concept of a nervous breakdown, which is a mental illness or disorder that prevents a person from functioning normally (Lindholm & Wickström, 2020). This concept originates in Western psychological discourse, with Caplan describing the existence of normative developmental crises throughout life (Bernstein & Kaplan, 2022). However, the concept of a developmental crisis did not transfer readily from psychology to psychiatry, and the work of psychiatrists exploring trauma-induced crises has never become mainstream. Crisis intervention and emergency psychiatry were not regarded as a specialty to be developed and investigated, as little was written in psychiatric textbooks about how doctors and nurses should respond to or treat people in states of emergency (Mitchell, 2021).

Environmental stress causes psychological disequilibrium, often lasting from a few days to a few weeks, and is hence referred to as a crisis. A person may begin a short treatment called a crisis intervention to help them recover to their pre-crisis level of adaptive functioning as soon as feasible after a crisis has occurred. The first time such a crisis occurred, it became a psychiatric emergency to find out what impact psychiatric intervention, given at that point, had on the subsequent trajectory of the individual concerned (Cappelletty, 2022). Research on acute wards has shown that the biomedical model approach to crises produces a service in which little attention is given to patient's psychosocial needs (Morant et al., 2021). Existing services are overstretched, making it more difficult for staff to find time to deal with patients' problems (Beech et al., 2023). There is little therapeutic or social interaction-oriented activity in acute wards, and patients may be at risk of self-harm or violence (Sampaio & Bispo 2021). It is not clear whether the provision of more beds and more staff would result in better service, in which patients' psychosocial needs would be addressed, or whether the failure to address these needs is inherent in psychopathology. The discourse of psychopathology, formed in the mid-19th century, has been criticized for its paternalism and lack of dialogue with patients (Barkataki & Ross, 2019). The biological method continues to dominate crisis care, even if novel shock therapies and medications have emerged. No evidence exists that acute care helps individuals in crisis, and community services seldom intervene early on.

Government initiatives and policies have attempted to address these problems, but some commentators see the problems worsening due to shortages of staff and beds. Research shows that half of all mental health emergencies occur outside of normal working hours (Harris et al., 2023). Most patients in first-time crises have psychosocial problems, but most staff do not have the skills to address psychosocial needs. The risk of violence and suicide has been widely publicized as a reason for hospital treatment, but services are not addressing these problems well. Research has shown that Accident and Emergency Units (A&E) are often inappropriate places for dealing with people in crisis due to staff shortages and lengthy waiting times before seeing a mental health specialist (Maconick et al., 2023). This highlights the need for out-of-hours services, as many people in a crisis seek or are brought into emergency services outside the 9–5 hours that most CMHTs operate within. Research has shown that a high proportion of people using emergency services are experiencing their first episode of crisis, usually based on psychosocial problems (Chan et al., 2019). Many people go to emergency services, but the evidence is inconclusive; it appears that A&E units are not providing a rapid and appropriate response to people in crisis, though this might be better in specialized psychiatric emergency clinics where these exist. Research on self-harm and dangerousness among patients has found that 40% of psychiatric referrals at A&E were for deliberate self-harm, and 35% were for taking an overdose of over-the-counter drugs (Bowden & Abdulrahim, 2020). People with psychoses made up the majority of CMHT referrals to the mental emergency clinic; around half of these patients were aggressive or otherwise disturbed, and it seemed like the clinic served as a haven for evaluation prior to admission. Research indicates a need for out-of-hours services, quick responses from staff, and access to specialist services for those in crisis (Edwards et al., 2023). Self-harm is a high risk among people in crisis, but self-harm is often given a low priority in A&E units. Acute wards are overcrowded, understaffed, and non-therapeutic, with patients often waiting for acute beds or being referred to another area.

Patient satisfaction surveys and research have highlighted patients' concerns about problems with services for people in crisis (Dalton et al., 2021). Studies have shown that patients consider having an interested person to talk to more helpful than 'treatment-oriented care,' such as drugs (Evans et al., 2023). Patients are not familiar with the benefits of psychotropic medication and often express their difficulties in vague and imprecise terms. Research has shown that psychiatrists are the least liked of the professionals involved in their treatment, with only 11% regarded as the most helpful aspect and 21% as the least helpful aspect (McGorry et al., 2022). Nearly half of those taking antidepressants reported side effects, and 85% had been offered no alternative form of treatment (Guy et al., 2020).

This chapter explores the personal narratives of people who have experienced mental health crises and breakdowns and who have received psychiatric treatment. Examining these stories through the lens of an expanded version of Caplan's Crisis Theory, the chapter concludes the psychological origins of crises and the phases and turning points that lead to recovery or long-term mental patient status.

The Evolution of Mental Health Crises

Far from being isolated events solely under the control of psychopathology, mental health crises emerge as complex phenomena intricately entangled with psychosocial factors (Barrett, 2022). An exhaustive literature review illuminates a consensus among scholars that understanding these crises necessitates a departure from traditional psychiatric frameworks. Studies consistently affirm that life events, nuanced social dynamics, and individual coping mechanisms wield substantial influence over the initiation and evolution of mental health crises (Robin et al., 2023). The literature reveals a wealth of evidence supporting the psychosocial complexity inherent in mental health crises. From 2018 onwards, research papers have continuously stressed that these crises are not only the result of abnormal processes inside a person's mind (Thomsen et al., 2023). On the contrary, they are highly dependent on the interaction of psychosocial elements, such as triggers in one's life, the complex dynamics of one's social environment, and the many coping techniques used when distressed. Recognizing the far-reaching effects of living circumstances on mental health, these investigations broaden the scope beyond diagnosable mental diseases. Tragic life circumstances, such as the death of a loved one, difficulties at work, or major life changes, may trigger mental health crises. In addition, these crises occur against the social environment's background, which includes relationships, support systems, and societal expectations. The variety of coping tactics used during these types of crises, from healthy habits to unhealthy ones, only goes to show how complicated these situations can be.

According to crisis treatment and services studies, most individuals do not get the necessary assistance in the early stages of their crisis (Savalescu et al., 2020). It is often considered that crisis inpatient services are in bad shape, with patients frequently reporting that the treatments they get are inadequate and that facilities and personnel are overworked. Services provided by acute care facilities are often dangerous and lack therapeutic rigor because of staffing shortages. Factors contributing to the strain on acute services were as follows: inefficient bed management practices, probable increases in psychiatric morbidity, and ineffective discharge arrangements between social services and health (Duggan et al., 2020). The provision of a safe refuge for people experiencing mental health crises has long made hospitals an integral aspect of mental health care. Unfortunately, many patients believe that nurses do not assist them enough because they do not comprehend their demands or cannot provide the required assistance. The concentration on disease mode by the hospital regime is at odds with people's expectations, which is why this is happening. Because of problems with communication, denial of citizenship, prejudice, humiliation, and gloomy settings, inpatient care in hospitals often falls short of these expectations. As doctors and nurses do not appear to grasp how bad patients' conditions are, patients often feel alone and scared (Aukerman et al., 2022).

Acute crisis hospitalization has long-term consequences, such as reducing patients' agency and choice (Chuang et al., 2023). There is often a lack of empathy and understanding among hospital staff when people are receiving treatment for mental health issues. In order to guarantee their patients' well-being while in the hospital, healthcare practitioners must address these concerns and provide appropriate treatment services. Seclusion, repetitive procedures, and feelings of alienation are common among patients in acute mental facilities (Hennessy et al., 2023). The atmosphere is terrible, and the nurses do not spend enough time chatting with the patients, so they do not hear or comprehend their pain (Baker et al., 2019). It is important to acknowledge that seclusion is inherently harmful and to take measures to reduce its effects. Research shows that patients do not feel their long-term underlying needs, particularly social needs, are being met during acute hospital care (Montenegro et al., 2023). More than half of patients do not consider they are receiving enough information about their illness and treatment choices, and there is little therapeutic contact with staff. Patients are bored, and one in five liked nothing about their stay. Nearly a quarter found nurses and other staff helpful, but only 40% undertook social or recreational activities. Patients in acute psychiatric hospitals face challenges such as isolation, poor communication, and treatment that can be traumatizing.

Women in acute services have been acknowledged for their needs, but they are often less satisfied with acute ward environments than men. The National Health Service (NHS) established a women's crisis home to provide a haven for women experiencing an emergency rather than a hospital stay. Systemic, family therapy-based crisis resolution incorporates medicine, complementary treatments, group and individual therapy, and other forms of treatment. Research on women in crisis has shown that there are particular issues for women in acute wards, such as safety and privacy (Pilav et al., 2022). Where women-only wards or crisis houses have been evaluated, they show increased satisfaction levels and a better ability to address women's social needs.

Acknowledging the psychosocial complexity of mental health crises calls for a paradigm shift in our understanding. This insight not only calls into question the prevailing psychopathology narrative but also highlights the need for a comprehensive approach that considers the larger setting in which these crises emerge. By recognizing the intricate interplay of psychosocial factors, mental health professionals can move beyond symptom-centric approaches, fostering more comprehensive and effective interventions that address the root causes and contributing elements of mental health crises. This section lays the groundwork for a more nuanced understanding of these crises beyond traditional diagnostic frameworks by examining the discernible stages and turning moments within them.

Identifiable Phases and Turning Points

Amidst the turbulent landscape of mental health crises, careful examination of narratives unveils discernible patterns of identifiable phases (Savenije et al., 2022). These phases, marked by escalating distress, encapsulate individuals' intricate journey during moments of profound vulnerability. Important moments in this story's progression represent a crossroads in which interventions may help heal or worsen the situation.

There is a clear progression in the stories of those who have dealt with mental health crises. A systematic review shows a regular progression with distinct phases, where each stage represents a different kind of suffering and ways of coping. The sequential nature of these stages helps bring some structure to the otherwise disorderly world of mental health crises. The crisis's trajectory may be changed at key junctures throughout these stages, known as turning moments. At certain points in time, interventions (therapeutic, social, or self-initiated) may either help a person go back on the road to recovery or make things far worse. Examining these stories helps to clarify the complex relationship between when treatments occur and how they affect a person's mental health trajectory. Mental health providers and lawmakers benefit greatly from a better understanding of these discernible stages and pivotal junctures. It acknowledges the ever-changing character of these situations and offers a framework that goes beyond a one-size-fits-all crisis response method. Mental health caregivers can better meet the varied needs of individuals at different phases of crisis if they are familiar with these stages. Policymakers may use this acknowledgment as a starting point for crafting mental health policies that are both effective and tailored to certain populations. By recognizing distinct stages and important turning points, lawmakers may fight for solutions that are both timely and tailored to the changing needs of those experiencing mental health crises. This part sets the stage for the next segment, which delves into how the acceptance of mental illness is influenced by life events by stressing the significance of precise interventions.

Life Events and Acceptance of Mental Illness

Within the intricate narratives of mental health crises, a compelling revelation emerges individuals frequently tether their experiences to life events, even in the face of accepting a mental illness diagnosis (Stanghellini, 2023). This interconnection suggests a complex interplay between personal experiences and the acceptance of mental health conditions, challenging conventional understandings and emphasizing the need for holistic approaches in mental health care. The intimate exploration of personal narratives within mental health crises illuminates a recurrent theme—the profound influence of life events. Individuals, even when confronted with a mental illness diagnosis, consistently draw connections between their mental health crises and specific life events. These occurrences cover a wide range, from devastating losses and tragedies to huge life changes and obstacles. These first-person accounts highlight the complex interplay between one's internal mental health and their external environment. The information gathered from these accounts provides credence to the idea that significant life experiences shape the trajectory of mental health crises. In addition, the stories show a complex dynamic where people who have a mental illness nevertheless blame certain moments in their lives for starting or worsening their crises (Scott, 2023).

An important case for more comprehensive approaches to mental health treatment is made when we acknowledge the role that life experiences play in molding an individual's story during a mental health crisis. Mental health providers are encouraged to broaden their attention beyond symptoms and diagnosis when they recognize the relationship between individual experiences and the acceptance of mental health problems. According to this section, effective mental health therapies need to consider more than just a patient's medical history. A holistic approach considers the contextual factors that contribute to mental health crises, offering a more comprehensive foundation for therapeutic strategies. Such an approach aligns with the study's narrative, advocating for a shift towards psychosocial factors, empathetic listening, and community support. As we progress through the chapter, this understanding sets the stage for exploring alternative crisis categories as a diagnostic shift, offering a lens beyond traditional psychiatric classifications.

Alternative Categories as a Diagnostic Shift

In redefining our understanding of mental health crises, a pivotal stride is taken with the proposal of alternative crisis categories. Sourced directly from narratives, these categories challenge the confines of traditional diagnostic labels, offering a pathway to a more nuanced comprehension of diverse crisis experiences that transcend conventional psychiatric classifications. The narratives of individuals navigating mental health crises stand as potent evidence challenging the limitations imposed by traditional diagnostic labels. The proposal of alternative crisis categories arises organically from the richness of these narratives, reflecting the intricate tapestry of experiences that elude simplistic categorization. This data shows that mental health crises may take many forms and that people's experiences with them do not fit neatly into preexisting mental categories (O'Sullivan et al., 2021). The research recognizes and appreciates the diversity of ways people express and overcome their crises by proposing different crisis categories (Lotta et al., 2021). An urgent plea for a paradigm shifts in mental health diagnosis has been made with the suggestion of new crisis classifications.

By rejecting rigid categorizations and focusing attention on the living realities of those impacted, mental health professionals, according to this section, may adopt a more comprehensive perspective on mental health crises. Mental health providers should avoid oversimplifying their patients' experiences by adopting alternative categories that avoid reductionism. This change creates a new way of thinking in which we acknowledge that every crisis is different and is affected by many things beyond what is often considered when making a diagnosis. The point is not to do away with diagnostic frameworks altogether; rather, it is to advocate for a more tailored strategy that considers the variety of people affected by mental health crises. The need for equitable mental health treatments and support is underscored as we go through the chapter, and this diagnostic shift provides the framework for comprehending how socioeconomic class affects crisis care and its aftermath.

Impact of Social Class on Crisis Care and Aftermath

The impact of socioeconomic status on crisis care access becomes apparent within the context of mental health emergencies. While studies show widespread discontent with care after the fact, they also highlight the substantial impact of socioeconomic status on the immediate care situation (Balfour et al., 2022). This provides strong evidence in support of campaigns to promote access to affordable mental health care and to address systemic issues that have persisted long after the crisis has passed.

Research findings consistently indicate that social class exerts a notable influence on access to crisis care during the acute phase of mental health crises (Da Silva et al., 2020). Individuals from different social classes encounter varying degrees of accessibility to timely and quality care, emphasizing systemic disparities that impact immediate outcomes. However, a nuanced shift occurs in the aftermath, where dissatisfaction with care becomes a common thread cutting across social classes. Despite potential differences in the nature and quality of crisis care received, individuals from diverse social backgrounds commonly express discontent with post-crisis support and its enduring impact on their lives.

The evidence presented in this section forms the basis for a crucial argument: advocacy for improved crisis services must extend beyond immediate care accessibility to address systemic disparities and dissatisfaction in the aftermath. Social class, while influencing the initial crisis care experience, diminishes in significance when evaluating overall satisfaction with post-crisis support. This argument underscores the need for mental health advocacy efforts to adopt a holistic perspective. Improving crisis services involves addressing immediate access issues and acknowledging the broader social determinants that persist beyond the crisis. Advocacy initiatives should strive for equitable mental health services that transcend socioeconomic boundaries and deliver consistent, satisfactory support throughout the entirety of an individual's mental health journey. The significance of community involvement and assistance in navigating the intricacies of mental health crises is emphasized as we go forward in the chapter, and this acknowledgment lays the groundwork for investigating coping mechanisms and community resilience.

Coping Strategies and Community Resilience

The complex accounts of these events show a deep investigation of methods of dealing with mental health crises. When people talk about their experiences dealing with mental health issues, it is like seeing a mosaic of resilience. In the face of mental health crises, these stories show how activism, pleasurable pastimes, and community involvement are powerful weapons. People dealing with mental health crises use a diverse array of coping mechanisms, as seen in this study's narratives (Sameer et al., 2020). The National Services Framework encouraged the creation of alternatives to hospitals for individuals in crisis, and acute care and home treatment have grown in popularity in the last several years.

As part of their round-the-clock support, psychiatric nurses, psychiatrists, social workers, and other specialists are on hand to provide in-home care. User happiness and reduced hospital admissions indicate that the service is effective. People who are deemed "psychotic" are not sent there; therefore, it does not assist with the most serious issues. More cost-effectiveness, less loss to follow-up, less family strain, and more acceptance for patients and families were observed in home-based crisis therapy, according to a systematic analysis by Moncrieff et al. (2020). Compared to hospital-based care, home therapy is more cost-effective, produces comparable or better results, and increases client or patient satisfaction (Curioni et al., 2023). It is unknown what kind of assistance would be most helpful and widely accepted or if non-medical crisis housing or home care are appropriate for all persons experiencing a crisis. The optimal course of action for all individuals experiencing a crisis requires more investigation.

In their narratives, individuals consistently showcase resilience in the face of mental health challenges. Community engagement emerges as a source of support and solidarity, offering individuals spaces to share experiences and draw strength from shared narratives. Enjoyable activities become therapeutic outlets, providing solace and moments of reprieve amid crises. Additionally, activism and advocacy serve as tools for personal empowerment and mechanisms for driving systemic change. The evidence of diverse coping strategies presented in this section forms the basis for a compelling argument: Mental health interventions must extend beyond clinical settings to incorporate and amplify the resilience exhibited by individuals in their coping mechanisms (Huey & Palaganas, 2020). It is critical to include community support, as it recognizes the power of community ties in promoting strength and healing. The theory argues that mental health therapies should not function in a vacuum but should instead include and capitalize on the strengths of a variety of coping mechanisms.

Mental health providers may foster a more holistic and flexible approach to crisis treatment by equipping patients with various coping methods. This chapter has community resilience and coping mechanisms to make the case for a radical change in mental health care. At the chapter's end, the authors argue that mental health treatment should be more community-oriented, psychosocially focused, and empathic, emphasizing prevention and all-encompassing crisis care.

Call for Paradigm Shift

Navigating the complex landscape of mental health crises has led to a strong need for a new approach to mental health care (Dalgleish et al., 2020). Together, the stories and analysis highlight the need for a new way of thinking that prioritizes mental health, speaking out for oneself, listening with empathy, and having strong community backing. A persuasive body of evidence is formed when narratives, interwoven with the many threads of human experiences, merge with analytical insights.

The research presented here strongly suggests that conventional approaches to mental health care must give way. Taken as a whole, the stages, turning points, and coping mechanisms that have been found indicate a void in the current discussion, which is mostly based on psychopathology. The realization that mental health crises are not discrete occurrences controlled only by clinical diagnosis has led to the need for a paradigm shift. Instead, they are deeply entwined with the psychosocial fabric of individuals' lives, necessitating an empathetic and comprehensive approach. The evidence advocates for a model that fosters self-advocacy, encourages empathetic listening, and recognizes the pivotal role of community support in mental health care (Kumar & Nayar, 2021). This rallying cry is based on the conviction that better crisis treatment and preventative services may be achieved via a comprehensive strategy that includes psychological elements, self-advocacy, sympathetic listening, and community support. The argument asserts that mental health services, traditionally rooted in the discourse of psychopathology, must evolve to align with the dynamic and complex nature of mental health crises. By prioritizing psychosocial factors, mental health professionals can better understand and address the root causes of crises, moving beyond symptom management to foster lasting resilience. The emphasis on self-advocacy empowers individuals to actively participate in their recovery journeys, while empathetic listening acknowledges the importance of subjective experiences. Lastly, robust community support becomes a linchpin, recognizing the strength and resources embedded within communal networks.

As this chapter culminates, the call for a paradigm shift serves as a compass guiding the way forward. It positions mental health care on a trajectory that transcends conventional boundaries, fostering a system that not only responds to crises but actively works towards prevention, resilience, and improved outcomes for individuals facing mental health challenges. The exploration of mental health crises through the lenses of psychosocial complexity, identifiable phases, life events, alternative categories, social class impact, coping strategies, and a call for a paradigm shift reveals a multifaceted landscape. The evidence gleaned from personal narratives and meticulous analyses coalesces into a call for transformative change in mental health services (Gruber., 2021). This chapter has explored the intricacies of mental health crises, highlighting their psychosocial underpinnings and the identifiable phases individuals traverse. It emphasized the interplay between life events and the acceptance of mental illness, challenging traditional diagnostic labels with the proposal of alternative crisis categories. The social class's influence on crisis cares access and dissatisfaction in the aftermath underscored systemic disparities. Coping strategies, rooted in community resilience, showcased diverse pathways to recovery. The cumulative evidence fervently supports a call for a paradigm shift in mental health services.

SOLUTIONS AND RECOMMENDATIONS

To effectively address the identified structural discrepancies, it is imperative to establish policies that promote equitable access to crisis care. Ensuring that individuals across all income levels can access mental health care requires a concerted effort to eliminate barriers associated with social class. Moreover, there is a need to critically assess and reinforce post-crisis support programs. By scrutinizing and strengthening these programs, we can actively work towards bridging existing gaps and ultimately foster more satisfactory outcomes for individuals from diverse backgrounds.

FUTURE RESEARCH DIRECTIONS

It is crucial to delve further into understanding the role of social support networks and the effectiveness of community-based treatments in addressing mental health crises. Additionally, conducting thorough investigations into the nuanced influence of cultural factors on crisis experiences is essential for the development of culturally sensitive mental health services. Furthermore, the implementation of longitudinal studies can contribute valuable insights into the extended trajectories of individuals when adopting a paradigm-shifted approach to mental health care. This research can provide a comprehensive understanding of sustained recovery and resilience over the long term.

CONCLUSION

In conclusion, our exploration of mental health crises reveals a complex tapestry of experiences, urging a profound reevaluation of mental health services. To translate these insights into actionable change, we propose comprehensive, real-world solutions. Healthcare policies should prioritize equitable access, dismantle social class barriers, and ensure that post-crisis support is universally robust. Intervention strategies must embrace a holistic paradigm, integrating psychosocial factors, fostering self-advocacy, and emphasizing empathetic community support. Therapeutic approaches should evolve to honor diverse coping strategies, recognizing the resilience embedded in community engagement and activism. This holistic transformation, grounded in the realities of lived experiences, charts a course toward a more compassionate and effective mental health care system. The narratives and analyses highlight a profound truth: Mental health crises navigate recognizable phases with crucial turning points. The interplay between life events and the acceptance of mental illness challenges traditional diagnostic frameworks. The proposal of alternative crisis categories reflects the diversity of experiences, prompting a diagnostic shift. The social class's impact on crisis cares illuminates systemic disparities while coping strategies and community resilience advocate for holistic approaches. In the end, there is a strong need for a change in thinking that places more importance on psychosocial variables, self-advocacy, listening with empathy, and community support.

REFERENCES

Baker, J. A., Canvin, K., & Berzins, K. (2019). The relationship between workforce characteristics and perception of quality of care in mental health: A qualitative study. *International Journal of Nursing Studies*, *100*, 103412. doi:10.1016/j.ijnurstu.2019.103412 PMID:31629212

Balfour, M. E., Hahn Stephenson, A., Delany-Brumsey, A., Winsky, J., & Goldman, M. L. (2022). Cops, clinicians, or both? Collaborative approaches to responding to behavioral health emergencies. *Psychiatric Services (Washington, D.C.)*, *73*(6), 658–669. doi:10.1176/appi.ps.202000721 PMID:34666512

Barkataki, I., & Ross, L. (2019). Psychological treatment on the acute ward. *Oxford Textbook of Inpatient Psychiatry*, *245*, 245–252. Advance online publication. doi:10.1093/med/9780198794257.003.0028

Barrett, L. F. (2022). Context reconsidered: Complex signal ensembles, relational meaning, and population thinking in psychological science. *The American Psychologist*, *77*(8), 894–920. doi:10.1037/amp0001054 PMID:36409120

Baumgardt, J., & Weinmann, S. (2022). Using Crisis Theory in Dealing with Severe Mental Illness-A Step Toward Normalization? *Frontiers in Sociology*, *7*, 805604. doi:10.3389/fsoc.2022.805604 PMID:35755483

Bernstein, K. S., & Kaplan, R. (2022). *Psychiatric Mental Health Assessment and Diagnosis of Adults for Advanced Practice Mental Health Nurses*. Taylor & Francis., doi:10.4324/9781003137597

Bowden-Jones, O., & Abdulrahim, D. (2020). *Club Drugs and Novel Psychoactive Substances: The Clinician's Handbook*. Cambridge University Press., doi:10.1017/9781911623106

Cappelletty, G. (2022). *Into the Maelstrom: Toward a Theory of Chaos and Crisis*. Austin Macauley Publishers.

Chan, E. A., Tsang, P. L., Ching, S. S. Y., Wong, F. Y., & Lam, W. (2019). Nurses' perspectives on their communication with patients in busy oncology wards: A qualitative study. *PLoS One*, *14*(10), e0224178. doi:10.1371/journal.pone.0224178 PMID:31648272

Chuang, Y. T., Zargoush, M., Ghazalbash, S., Samiedaluie, S., Kuluski, K., & Guilcher, S. (2023). From prediction to decision: Optimizing long-term care placements among older delayed discharge patients. *Production and Operations Management*, *32*(4), 1041–1058. doi:10.1111/poms.13910

Da Silva, A. G., Baldaçara, L., Cavalcante, D. A., Fasanella, N. A., & Palha, A. P. (2020). The impact of mental illness stigma on psychiatric emergencies. *Frontiers in Psychiatry*, *11*, 573. doi:10.3389/fpsyt.2020.00573 PMID:32636773

Dalgleish, T., Black, M., Johnston, D., & Bevan, A. (2020). Transdiagnostic approaches to mental health problems: Current status and future directions. *Journal of Consulting and Clinical Psychology*, *88*(3), 179–195. doi:10.1037/ccp0000482 PMID:32068421

Dalton-Locke, C., Johnson, S., Harju-Seppänen, J., Lyons, N., Sheridan Rains, L., Stuart, R., Campbell, A., Clark, J., Clifford, A., Courtney, L., Dare, C., Kelly, K., Lynch, C., McCrone, P., Nairi, S., Newbigging, K., Nyikavaranda, P., Osborn, D., Persaud, K., ... Lloyd-Evans, B. (2021). Emerging models and trends in mental health crisis care in England: A national investigation of crisis care systems. *BMC Health Services Research*, *21*(1), 1–12. doi:10.1186/s12913-021-07181-x PMID:34711222

Duggan, M., Harris, B., Chislett, W. K., & Calder, R. (2020). *Nowhere else to go: Why Australia's health system results in people with mental illness getting 'stuck' in emergency departments.*

Edwards, D., Carrier, J., Csontos, J., Evans, N., Elliott, M., Gillen, E., & Williams, L. (2023). Crisis responses for children and young people-a systematic review of effectiveness, experiences and service organisation (CAMH-Crisis). *Child and Adolescent Mental Health.* Advance online publication. doi:10.1111/camh.12639 PMID:36785997

Erchul, W. P., & Schulte, A. C. (2019). Gerald Caplan's contributions to professional psychology: Conceptual underpinnings. In *Consultation in community, school, and organizational practice* (pp. 3–40). Taylor & Francis., doi:10.4324/9781315787077-1

Evans, N., Edwards, D., Carrier, J., Elliott, M., Gillen, E., Hannigan, B., & Williams, L. (2023). Organisation of crisis services. In *Mental health crisis care for children and young people aged 5 to 25 years: the CAMH-Crisis evidence synthesis.* National Institute for Health and Care Research., doi:10.3310/BPPT3407

Gruber, J., Prinstein, M. J., Clark, L. A., Rottenberg, J., Abramowitz, J. S., Albano, A. M., Aldao, A., Borelli, J. L., Chung, T., Davila, J., Forbes, E. E., Gee, D. G., Hall, G. C. N., Hallion, L. S., Hinshaw, S. P., Hofmann, S. G., Hollon, S. D., Joormann, J., Kazdin, A. E., ... Weinstock, L. M. (2021). Mental health and clinical psychological science in the time of COVID-19: Challenges, opportunities, and a call to action. *The American Psychologist*, *76*(3), 409–426. doi:10.1037/amp0000707 PMID:32772538

Guy, A., Brown, M., Lewis, S., & Horowitz, M. (2020). The 'patient voice': Patients who experience antidepressant withdrawal symptoms are often dismissed, or misdiagnosed with relapse, or a new medical condition. *Therapeutic Advances in Psychopharmacology*, *10*, 2045125320967183. doi:10.1177/2045125320967183 PMID:33224468

Harris, J., Clarke, I., & Riches, S. (2023). Developing'Comprehend, Cope and Connect'Training for Acute and Crisis Mental Health Services: Staff, Patient and Carer Perspectives. *Journal of Psychiatric Intensive Care*, *19*(1), 33–50. doi:10.20299/jpi.2023.004

Health, T. L. G. The Lancet Global Health. (2020). Mental health matters. *The Lancet. Global Health*, *8*(11), e1352. doi:10.1016/S2214-109X(20)30432-0 PMID:33069297

Holmes, E. A., O'Connor, R. C., Perry, V. H., Tracey, I., Wessely, S., Arseneault, L., Ballard, C., Christensen, H., Cohen Silver, R., Everall, I., Ford, T., John, A., Kabir, T., King, K., Madan, I., Michie, S., Przybylski, A. K., Shafran, R., Sweeney, A., ... Bullmore, E. (2020). Multidisciplinary research priorities for the COVID-19 pandemic: A call for action for mental health science. *The Lancet. Psychiatry*, *7*(6), 547–560. doi:10.1016/S2215-0366(20)30168-1 PMID:32304649

Huey, C. W. T., & Palaganas, J. C. (2020). What are the factors affecting resilience in health professionals? A synthesis of systematic reviews. *Medical Teacher*, *42*(5), 550–560. doi:10.1080/0142159X.2020.1714020 PMID:31984844

Kelly, B. (2022). *In search of madness: A psychiatrist's travels through the history of mental illness*. Gill & Macmillan Ltd.

Kumar, A., & Nayar, K. R. (2021). COVID 19 and its mental health consequences. *Journal of Mental Health (Abingdon, England)*, *30*(1), 1–2. doi:10.1080/09638237.2020.1757052 PMID:32339041

Lawrance, E. L., Thompson, R., Newberry Le Vay, J., Page, L., & Jennings, N. (2022). The impact of climate change on mental health and emotional wellbeing: A narrative review of current evidence, and its implications. *International Review of Psychiatry (Abingdon, England)*, *34*(5), 443–498. doi:10.1080/09540261.2022.2128725 PMID:36165756

Lindholm, S. K., & Wickström, A. (2020). 'Looping effects' related to young people's mental health: How young people transform the meaning of psychiatric concepts. *Global Studies of Childhood*, *10*(1), 26–38. doi:10.1177/2043610619890058

Lotta, G., Fernandez, M., & Corrêa, M. (2021). The vulnerabilities of the Brazilian health workforce during health emergencies: Analysing personal feelings, access to resources and work dynamics during the COVID-19 pandemic. *The International Journal of Health Planning and Management*, *36*(S1), 42–57. doi:10.1002/hpm.3117 PMID:33502795

Maconick, L., Ikhtabi, S., Broeckelmann, E., Pitman, A., Barnicot, K., Billings, J., Osborn, D., & Johnson, S. (2023). Crisis and acute mental health care for people who have been given a diagnosis of a 'personality disorder': A systematic review. *BMC Psychiatry*, *23*(1), 720. doi:10.1186/s12888-023-05119-7 PMID:37798701

McGorry, P. D., Mei, C., Chanen, A., Hodges, C., Alvarez-Jimenez, M., & Killackey, E. (2022). Designing and scaling up integrated youth mental health care. *World Psychiatry; Official Journal of the World Psychiatric Association (WPA)*, *21*(1), 61–76. doi:10.1002/wps.20938 PMID:35015367

Mitchell, J. T. (2021). Continuum of care for disasters and catastrophes. *International Review of Psychiatry (Abingdon, England)*, *33*(8), 728–739. doi:10.1080/09540261.2022.2030678 PMID:35412427

Moncrieff, J., Gupta, S., & Horowitz, M. A. (2020). Barriers to stopping neuroleptic (antipsychotic) treatment in people with schizophrenia, psychosis or bipolar disorder. *Therapeutic Advances in Psychopharmacology*, *10*, 2045125320937910. doi:10.1177/2045125320937910 PMID:32670542

Montenegro, C., Dominguez, M. I., Moller, J. G., Thomas, F., & Ortiz, J. U. (2023). Moving psychiatric deinstitutionalization forward: A scoping review of barriers and facilitators. Cambridge Prisms. *Global Mental Health (Cambridge, England)*, *10*, e29. doi:10.1017/gmh.2023.18 PMID:37808271

Morant, N., Davidson, M., Wackett, J., Lamb, D., Pinfold, V., Smith, D., Johnson, S., Lloyd-Evans, B., & Osborn, D. P. (2021). Acute day units for mental health crises: A qualitative study of service user and staff views and experiences. *BMC Psychiatry*, *21*(1), 1–12. doi:10.1186/s12888-021-03140-2 PMID:33691668

Morganstein, J. C., & Ursano, R. J. (2020). Ecological disasters and mental health: Causes, consequences, and interventions. *Frontiers in Psychiatry*, *11*, 1. doi:10.3389/fpsyt.2020.00001 PMID:32116830

Naushad, V. A., Bierens, J. J., Nishan, K. P., Firjeeth, C. P., Mohammad, O. H., Maliyakkal, A. M., ChaliHadan, S., & Schreiber, M. D. (2019). A systematic review of the impact of disaster on the mental health of medical responders. *Prehospital and Disaster Medicine*, *34*(6), 632–643. doi:10.1017/S1049023X19004874 PMID:31625487

Newton-Howes, G., & Gordon, S. (2022). The need for a rights-based approach to acute models of care. *World Psychiatry; Official Journal of the World Psychiatric Association (WPA)*, *21*(2), 240–241. doi:10.1002/wps.20965 PMID:35524606

O'Sullivan, K., Clark, S., McGrane, A., Rock, N., Burke, L., Boyle, N., Joksimovic, N., & Marshall, K. (2021). A qualitative study of child and adolescent mental health during the COVID-19 pandemic in Ireland. *International Journal of Environmental Research and Public Health*, *18*(3), 1062. doi:10.3390/ijerph18031062 PMID:33504101

Pavli, A., Theodoridou, M., & Maltezou, H. C. (2021). Post-COVID syndrome: Incidence, clinical spectrum, and challenges for primary healthcare professionals. *Archives of Medical Research*, *52*(6), 575–581. doi:10.1016/j.arcmed.2021.03.010 PMID:33962805

Pilav, S., Easter, A., Silverio, S. A., De Backer, K., Sundaresh, S., Roberts, S., & Howard, L. M. (2022). Experiences of perinatal mental health care among minority ethnic women during the COVID-19 pandemic in London: A qualitative study. *International Journal of Environmental Research and Public Health*, *19*(4), 1975. doi:10.3390/ijerph19041975 PMID:35206163

Pop-Jordanova, N. (2021). Grief: Aetiology, symptoms and management. *prilozi*, 42(2), 9-18. doi:10.2478/prilozi-2021-0014

Radez, J., Reardon, T., Creswell, C., Lawrence, P. J., Evdoka-Burton, G., & Waite, P. (2021). Why do children and adolescents (not) seek and access professional help for their mental health problems? A systematic review of quantitative and qualitative studies. *European Child & Adolescent Psychiatry*, *30*(2), 183–211. doi:10.1007/s00787-019-01469-4 PMID:31965309

Reyes-Mota, A. R., Cerda-Molina, A. L., Mayagoitia-Novales, L., Viveros-Sandoval, M. E., & Borráz-León, J. I. (2021). Reduced cortisol response to traumatic images, self-esteem and stress levels in emergency medical technicians from the Red Cross. *Personality and Individual Differences*, *179*, 110929. doi:10.1016/j.paid.2021.110929

Robin, M., Bellone, L., Belbèze, J., Kazemian, K., Radjack, R., & Corcos, M. (2023). Three-level containment model of hospitalized adolescents with borderline pathology: A holistic therapeutic perspective. *Frontiers in Psychiatry*, *14*, 1110788. doi:10.3389/fpsyt.2023.1110788 PMID:37608992

Sameer, A. S., Khan, M. A., Nissar, S., & Banday, M. Z. (2020). Assessment of mental health and various coping strategies among general population living under imposed COVID-lockdown across world: A cross-sectional study. *Ethics, Medicine, and Public Health, 15*, 100571. doi:10.1016/j.jemep.2020.100571 PMID:32838000

Sampaio, M. L., & Bispo Júnior, J. P. (2021). Towards comprehensive mental health care: Experiences and challenges of psychosocial care in Brazil. *BMC Public Health, 21*(1), 1–12. doi:10.1186/s12889-021-11397-1 PMID:34238266

Savalescu, J., Davies, L. W., Roache, R., Davies, W., & Loebel, J. P. (Eds.). (2020). Psychiatry reborn: Biopsychosocial psychiatry in modern medicine. International Perspectives in. doi:10.1093/med/9780198789697.001.0001

Savenije, A., van Lawick, J., & Reijmers, E. (2022). *Systemic Perspectives in Mental Health, Social Work and Youth Care: A Relational Compass*. Taylor & Francis., doi:10.4324/9781003272038

Scott, E. (2023). *The One Thing We've Never Spoken about: Exposing Our Untold Mental Health Crisis*. Pantera Press.

Sharma, S., & Thapa, R. (2023). Socioeconomic Factors and Their Interaction with Environmental Education and Biodiversity Conservation: Effects on Mental Health and Community Empowerment. *AI. IoT and the Fourth Industrial Revolution Review, 13*(7), 75–90.

Stanghellini, G. (2023). Logics of Discovery II: Lessons from Poetry-Parataxis as a Method That Can Complement the Narrative Compulsion in Vogue in Contemporary Mental Health Care. *Brain Sciences, 13*(10), 1368. doi:10.3390/brainsci13101368 PMID:37891737

Stuijfzand, S., Deforges, C., Sandoz, V., Sajin, C. T., Jaques, C., Elmers, J., & Horsch, A. (2020). Psychological impact of an epidemic/pandemic on the mental health of healthcare professionals: A rapid review. *BMC Public Health, 20*(1), 1–18. doi:10.1186/s12889-020-09322-z PMID:32787815

Thomsen, D. K., Holm, T., Jensen, R., Lind, M., & Pedersen, A. M. (2023). *Storying mental illness and personal recovery*. Cambridge University Press., doi:10.1017/9781108907606

Williams, R., Ntontis, E., Alfadhli, K., Drury, J., & Amlôt, R. (2021). A social model of secondary stressors in relation to disasters, major incidents and conflict: Implications for practice. *International Journal of Disaster Risk Reduction, 63*, 102436. doi:10.1016/j.ijdrr.2021.102436

World Health Organization. (2022). *World mental health report: transforming mental health for all.*

ADDITIONAL READINGS

Komalasari, R. (2022). A Social Ecological Model (SEM) to Manage Methadone Programmes in Prisons. In Handbook of Research on Mathematical Modeling for Smart Healthcare Systems (pp. 374-382). IGI Global. doi:10.4018/978-1-6684-4580-8.ch020

Komalasari, R. (2023). The Relationship Between Cybersecurity and Public Health. In *Handbook of Research on Current Trends in Cybersecurity and Educational Technology* (pp. 78–91). IGI Global., doi:10.4018/978-1-6684-6092-4.ch005

Komalasari, R. (2023). Postnatal Mental Distress: Exploring the Experiences of Mothers Navigating the Healthcare System. In Perspectives and Considerations on Navigating the Mental Healthcare System (pp. 159-181). IGI Global. doi:10.4018/978-1-6684-5049-9.ch007

Komalasari, R. (2023). Designing Health Systems for Better, Faster, and Less Expensive Treatment. In *Exploring the Convergence of Computer and Medical Science Through Cloud Healthcare* (pp. 1–13). IGI Global., doi:10.4018/978-1-6684-5260-8.ch001

Komalasari, R. (2023). The Ethical Consideration of Using Artificial Intelligence (AI) in Medicine. In Advanced Bioinspiration Methods for Healthcare Standards, Policies, and Reform (pp. 1-16). IGI Global. doi:10.4018/978-1-6684-5656-9.ch001

Komalasari, R. (2023). Healthcare for the Elderly With Digital Twins. In Digital Twins and Healthcare: Trends, Techniques, and Challenges (pp. 145-156). IGI Global. doi:10.4018/978-1-6684-5925-6.ch010

Komalasari, R. (2023). Cloud Computing's Usage in Healthcare. In Recent Advancements in Smart Remote Patient Monitoring, Wearable Devices, and Diagnostics Systems (pp. 183-194). IGI Global. doi:10.4018/978-1-6684-6434-2.ch009

Komalasari, R. (2023). History and Legislative Changes Governing Medical Cannabis in Indonesia. In Medical Cannabis and the Effects of Cannabinoids on Fighting Cancer, Multiple Sclerosis, Epilepsy, Parkinson's, and Other Neurodegenerative Diseases (pp. 274-284). IGI Global. doi:10.4018/978-1-6684-5652-1.ch012

Komalasari, R. (2023). Ambient Assisted Living (AAL) Systems to Help Older People. In Exploring Future Opportunities of Brain-Inspired Artificial Intelligence (pp. 84-99). IGI Global. doi:10.4018/978-1-6684-6980-4.ch006

Komalasari, R. (2023). Telemedicine in Pandemic Times in Indonesia: Healthcare Professional's Perspective. In Health Informatics and Patient Safety in Times of Crisis (pp. 138-153). IGI Global. doi:10.4018/978-1-6684-5499-2.ch008

Komalasari, R. (2023). Cloud Computing's Usage in Healthcare. In Recent Advancements in Smart Remote Patient Monitoring, Wearable Devices, and Diagnostics Systems (pp. 183-194). IGI Global. doi:10.4018/978-1-6684-6434-2.ch009

Komalasari, R. (2023). The Relationship Between Cybersecurity and Public Health. In *Handbook of Research on Current Trends in Cybersecurity and Educational Technology* (pp. 78–91). IGI Global., doi:10.4018/978-1-6684-6092-4.ch005

Komalasari, R. (2023). Treatment of Menstrual Discomfort in Young Women and a Cognitive Behavior Therapy (CBT) Program. In Perspectives on Coping Strategies for Menstrual and Premenstrual Distress (pp. 194-211). IGI Global. doi:10.4018/978-1-6684-5088-8.ch011

Komalasari, R. (2023). Healthcare for the Elderly With Digital Twins. In Digital Twins and Healthcare: Trends, Techniques, and Challenges (pp. 145-156). IGI Global. doi:10.4018/978-1-6684-5925-6.ch010

Komalasari, R. (2023). Telemedicine in Pandemic Times in Indonesia: Healthcare Professional's Perspective. In Health Informatics and Patient Safety in Times of Crisis (pp. 138-153). IGI Global. doi:10.4018/978-1-6684-5499-2.ch008

Komalasari, R. (2023). Regulatory Shift Healthcare Applications in Industry 5.0. In Advanced Research and Real-World Applications of Industry 5.0 (pp. 149-165). IGI Global. doi:10.4018/978-1-7998-8805-5.ch008

Komalasari, R. (2023). Exploring Pedagogies of Affect In Secondary School Physical Education For Enhanced Emotional Well-Being. *Pedagogik: Jurnal Pendidikan Guru Sekolah Dasar*, *11*(2), 117–127. doi:10.33558/pedagogik.v11i2.7374

Komalasari, R. (2023). Integrating sport education model and the athletics challenges approach for transformative physical education in Indonesian Middle Schools. *Motion: Jurnal Riset Physical Education*, *13*(2), 118–135. doi:10.33558/motion.v13i2.7372

Komalasari, R. (2023). Efek Ganja Medis pada Pasien Parkinson: A Literature Review of Clinical Evidence. *Journal of Islamic Pharmacy*, *8*(1), 44–48. doi:10.18860/jip.v8i1.17832

Komalasari, R. (2023). Rancangan Program Bagi Keberhasilan Gerakan Mencuci Tangan Yang Sehat Bagi Para Ibu Dan Anak. *Sulolipu: Media Komunikasi Sivitas Akademika dan Masyarakat*, 23(1), 55-60. doi:10.32382/sulolipu.v23i1.3103

Komalasari, R. (2024). Unravelling the Veil: Exploring the Nexus of Insecure Attachment and Functional Somatic Disorders in Adults. In *Discourses, Inquiries, and Case Studies in Healthcare, Social Sciences, and Technology*. IGI Global.

Komalasari, R. (2024). Advancing Healthcare: Economic Implications of Immediate MRI in Suspected Scaphoid Fractures - A Comprehensive Exploration. In *Future of AI in Medical Imaging*. IGI Global.

Komalasari, R. (2024). Women's perceptions of midlife mothering during perimenopause: the impact on health and well-being through life's transitions. In *Utilizing AI Techniques for the Perimenopause to Menopause Transition*. IGI Global.

Komalasari, R. (2024). Machine Learning in Health Information Security: Unraveling Patterns, Concealing Secrets, and Mitigating Vulnerabilities. In *Enhancing Steganography Through Deep Learning Approaches*. IGI Global.

Komalasari, R. (2024). Navigating Complexity: Unraveling the IVHM Requirements Puzzle in Unmanned Aerial Systems Through Innovative IVHM-RD Methodology and Rigorous Data Analysis. In *Ubiquitous Computing and Technological Innovation for Universal Healthcare*. IGI Global.

Komalasari, R. (2024). Trust Dynamics in Remote Patient-Expert Communication: Unraveling the Role of ICT in Indonesia's Private Healthcare Sector. In *Improving Security, Privacy, and Connectivity Among Telemedicine Platforms*. IGI Global.

Komalasari, R. (2024). Cyberbullying in the Health Care Workplace: How to Find Your Way Through the Digital Maze. In *Workplace Cyberbullying and Behavior in Health Professions*. IGI Global. doi:10.4018/979-8-3693-1139-4.ch004

Komalasari, R. (2024). Harmonizing Minds and Machines: A Transformative AI-Based Mental Health Care Framework in Medical Tourism. In *Impact of AI and Robotics on the Medical Tourism Industry*. IGI Global.

Komalasari, R. (2024). Navigating the Future of Healthcare: A User-Centric Approach to Designing Lucrative Business Models for the IoMT. In *Lightweight Digital Trust Architectures in the Internet of Medical Things (IoMT)*. IGI Global.

Komalasari, R. (2024). Biospheric Reverie: Unraveling Indoor Air Quality through Bio-Inspired Textiles, Awareness, and Decision-Making. In *Intelligent Decision Making Through Bio-Inspired Optimization*. IGI Global.

Komalasari, R. (2024). An Integrated Approach to Next-Generation Telemedicine and Health Advice Systems through AI Applications in Disease Diagnosis. In *AI-Driven Innovations in Digital Healthcare: Emerging Trends, Challenges, and Applications*. IGI Global.

Komalasari, R. (2024). Transformative Insights: Harnessing Artificial Intelligence for Enhanced Ovarian Cancer Prediction and Prognosis. In *Biomedical Research Developments for Improved Healthcare*. IGI Global.

Komalasari, R. (2024). Bridging the Gap: Theory of Change Guided Digital Health Implementation in Indonesian Primary Care. In *Analyzing Current Digital Healthcare Trends Using Social Networks*. IGI Global.

Komalasari, R. (2024). Navigating the Digital Frontier: A Socio-Technical Review of Indonesia's NHS E-Health Strategy and the Path to Seamless Healthcare Transformation. In *Inclusivity and Accessibility in Digital Health*. IGI Global.

Komalasari, R. (2024). *Pursuit of Excellence: A Comprehensive Framework for Ensuring Quality in Digital Health Apps. In Multi-Sector Analysis of the Digital Healthcare Industry*. IGI Global.

Komalasari, R. (2024). Fostering Transparency in AI for Disease Detection: Exploring Meaningful Explanations and Interactive Modalities in Healthcare. In *Federated Learning and Privacy-Preserving in Healthcare AI*. IGI Global.

Komalasari, R. (2024). Predictive Pioneers: Bridging the Mental Health Gap in Older Adults through Advanced Digital Technologies. In *Using Machine Learning to Detect Emotions and Predict Human Psychology*. IGI Global.

Komalasari, R. (2024). Unravelling the Veil: Exploring the Nexus of Insecure Attachment and Functional Somatic Disorders in Adults. In *Discourses, Inquiries, and Case Studies in Healthcare, Social Sciences, and Technology*. IGI Global.

Komalasari, R. (2024). Cyberbullying in the Health Care Workplace: How to Find Your Way Through the Digital Maze. In *Workplace Cyberbullying and Behavior in Health Professions*. IGI Global. doi:10.4018/979-8-3693-1139-4.ch004

Komalasari, R. (2024). Navigating Mental Health Crises: Understanding Pivotal Phases, Health Campaigns, and Community Resilience for Recovery and Reform. In *The Role of Health Literacy in Major Healthcare Crises*. IGI Global.

Komalasari, R. (2024). Decoding the Genomic and Proteomic Landscape: Dissemination and Mechanisms of Antibiotic Resistance in Environmental Staphylococci. In *Contemporary Approaches to Mitigating Antibacterial Drug Resistance*. IGI Global.

Komalasari, R. (2024). Unveiling the Future: Blockchain-Powered Digital Twins for Personalized Privacy Preservation in Metaverse Healthcare Data Management. In *Examining the Metaverse in Healthcare: Opportunities, Challenges, and Future Directions*. IGI Global. doi:10.4018/979-8-3693-1906-2.ch017

Komalasari, R. (2024). Safeguarding the Future: Cutting-Edge Time-Stamping Services and Blockchain Technologies for Maintaining EHR Data Integrity Over the Long Term. In *Blockchain and IoT Approaches for Secure Electronic Health Records (EHR)*. IGI Global.

Komalasari, R. (2024). Empowering Informed Healthcare Choices in Rural Areas: SIKDA - A Novel Model for Enhancing Patient Access to Reliable Consumer Health Information in Indonesia. In *Emerging Technologies for Health Literacy and Medical Practice*. IGI Global.

Komalasari, R. (2024). Advancing Trauma Care: Contemporary Cranio-Maxillo-Facial Surgery in Indonesia and Beyond. In *Contemporary Cranio-Maxillo-Facial Surgery: From Trauma to Reconstruction*. IGI Global.

Komalasari, R. (2024). Innovations in Neurodegenerative Disease Diagnosis: Unraveling the Transformative Potential of Deep Learning and MRI Integration. In *Deep Learning Approaches for Early Diagnosis of Neurodegenerative Diseases*. IGI Global.

Komalasari, R. (2024). Secure and privacy-preserving federated learning with explainable artificial intelligence for smart healthcare systems. In *Federated Learning and AI for Healthcare 5.0*. IGI Global.

Komalasari, R. (2024) Optimizing Prostate Cancer Radiotherapy: Advanced Machine Learning in Virtual Patient-Specific Plan Verification. *Indonesian Journal of Cancer.*

Komalasari, R. (2024). Bridging Uncertainties: Exploring the Lived Experiences of Pediatric Long-COVID-19 Through ME/CFS Caregiver Narratives. In G. Rao & S. Dhamdhere-Rao (Eds.), *Clinical Practice and Post-Infection Care for COVID-19 Patients* (pp. 207–227). IGI Global., doi:10.4018/978-1-6684-6855-5.ch009

Komalasari, R., & Mustafa, C. (2023). Combating International Cyber Conflict: A Healthy Just War and International Law Analysis of NATO and Indonesian Policies. Jurnal Pertahanan: Media Informasi tentang Kajian & Strategi Pertahanan yang Mengedepankan Identity. *Nasionalism & Integrity*, *9*(3), 559–570. doi:10.33172/jp.v9i2.16794

Komalasari, R., & Mustafa, C. (2023). Analysis Of The Propulsion And Maneuvering Characteristics Of Autonomous Underwater Vehicles And Their Strategic Defense. *Propeller Jurnal Permesinan*, 1(2).

Komalasari, R., & Mustafa, C. (2023). Amphibious Forces in the Total War Age: Exploring Indonesia's Multifaceted Contributions to Statecraft in the Asia-Pacific Region. *Jurnal Strategi Pertahanan Laut*, *9*(2), 62–77. doi:10.33172/spl.v9i2.12606

Komalasari, R., & Mustafa, C. (2023). The Evolution and Institutionalization of the Naval Partnership between Indonesia and ASEAN. *Jurnal Strategi Pertahanan Laut*, *9*(2), 1–18. doi:10.33172/spl.v9i2.12576

Komalasari, R., & Mustafa, C. (2023). A Healthy Game-Theoretic Evaluation of NATO and Indonesia's Policies in the Context of International Law. *Jurnal Pertahanan: Media Informasi tentang Kajian & Strategi Pertahanan yang Mengedepankan Identity. Nasionalism & Integrity*, *9*(2), 333–349. doi:10.33172/jp.v9i2.16794

Komalasari, R., Nurhayati, N., & Mustafa, C. (2022). Enhancing the Online Learning Environment for Medical Education: Lessons From COVID-19. In Policies and procedures for the implementation of safe and healthy educational environments: Post-COVID-19 perspectives (pp. 138-154). IGI Global. doi:10.4018/978-1-7998-9297-7.ch009

Komalasari, R., Nurhayati, N., & Mustafa, C. (2022). Insider/outsider issues: Reflections on qualitative research. *The Qualitative Report*, *27*(3), 744–751. doi:10.46743/2160-3715/2022.5259

Komalasari, R., Nurhayati, N., & Mustafa, C. (2022). Professional Education and Training in Indonesia. In *Public Affairs Education and Training in the 21st Century* (pp. 125–138). IGI Global., doi:10.4018/978-1-7998-8243-5.ch008

Komalasari, R., Nurhayati, N., & Mustafa, C. (2022). Professional Education and Training in Indonesia. In *Public Affairs Education and Training in the 21st Century* (pp. 125–138). IGI Global., doi:10.4018/978-1-7998-8243-5.ch008

Komalasari, R., Wilson, S., & Haw, S. (2021). A systematic review of qualitative evidence on barriers to and facilitators of the implementation of opioid agonist treatment (OAT) programmes in prisons. *The International Journal on Drug Policy, 87*, 102978. doi:10.1016/j.drugpo.2020.102978 PMID:33129135

Komalasari, R., Wilson, S., & Haw, S. (2021). A social ecological model (SEM) to exploring barriers of and facilitators to the implementation of opioid agonist treatment (OAT) programmes in prisons. *International Journal of Prisoner Health, 17*(4), 477–496. doi:10.1108/IJPH-04-2020-0020

Komalasari, R., Wilson, S., Nasir, S., & Haw, S. (2020). Multiple burdens of stigma for prisoners participating in Opioid Antagonist Treatment (OAT) programmes in Indonesian prisons: A qualitative study. *International Journal of Prisoner Health, 17*(2), 156–170. doi:10.1108/IJPH-03-2020-0018

Mustafa, C. (2020). The influence of sunni islamic values on rehabilitation as judicial decision for minor drug users in Indonesian court. *Ijtihad: Jurnal Wacana Hukum Islam dan Kemanusiaan*, 20(1), 79-96. doi:10.18326/ijtihad.v20i1.79-96

Mustafa, C. (2021). Qualitative Method Used in Researching the Judiciary: Quality Assurance Steps to Enhance the Validity and Reliability of the Findings. *The Qualitative Report, 26*(1), 176–185. doi:10.46743/2160-3715/2021.4319

Mustafa, C. (2021). Key Finding: Result of a Qualitative Study of Judicial Perspectives on the Sentencing of Minor Drug Offenders in Indonesia: Structural Inequality. *The Qualitative Report, 26*(5), 1678–1692. doi:10.46743/2160-3715/2021.4436

Mustafa, C. (2021). The view of judicial activism and public legitimacy. *Crime, Law, and Social Change, 76*(1), 23–34. doi:10.1007/s10611-021-09955-0

Mustafa, C. (2021). The News Media Representation of Acts of Mass Violence in Indonesia. In *Mitigating Mass Violence and Managing Threats in Contemporary Society* (pp. 127–140). IGI Global., doi:10.4018/978-1-7998-4957-5.ch008

Mustafa, C. (2021). The Challenges to Improving Public Services and Judicial Operations: A unique balance between pursuing justice and public service in Indonesia. In Handbook of research on global challenges for improving public services and government operations (pp. 117-132). IGI Global. doi:10.4018/978-1-7998-4978-0.ch007

Mustafa, C., Malloch, M., & Hamilton Smith, N. (2020). Judicial perspectives on the sentencing of minor drug offenders in Indonesia: Discretionary practice and compassionate approaches. *Crime, Law, and Social Change, 74*(3), 297–313. doi:10.1007/s10611-020-09896-0

Suhariyanto, B. (2023). Contradiction Over the Application of Corporate Liability in Corruption Court Decisions in Indonesia. *Indonesia Law Review*, *13*(1), 8.

Suhariyanto, B., Mustafa, C., & Santoso, T. (2021). Liability incorporate between transnational corruption cases Indonesia and the United States of America. *J. Legal Ethical & Regul. Isses*, *24*, 1.

KEY TERMS AND DEFINITIONS

Crisis: A critical turning point or situation marked by intense difficulty or instability, often associated with mental health challenges.

Mental Health: The state of psychological well-being, encompassing emotional, social, and cognitive aspects, is often impacted by various factors, including mental health disorders.

Narratives: personal stories or accounts detailing individual experiences, providing a qualitative understanding of events, emotions, and perspectives.

Psychosocial Factors: Interactions between psychological and social elements influencing mental well-being, including relationships, societal dynamics, and individual coping mechanisms.

Recovery: Regaining health and well-being after a setback, particularly in mental health, encompassing personal growth and adaptation.

Chapter 9
Knowledge, Attitude, and Practices Towards the Use of Psychobiotics for Maternal Health and Well-Being

Suyesha Singh
Manipal University Jaipur, India

Geeta Khanwani
Manipal University Jaipur, India

Manali Datta
https://orcid.org/0000-0002-5335-3446
Amity University, Jaipur, India

ABSTRACT

Health management and sustained mental comfort requires a multidisciplinary approach, with a holistic strategy for maintenance of overall wellbeing. Therapeutic interventions for maternal health need to be designed in such a way that it permits mitigation and prevention of the adverse influences on the health of mother and child both. Good gut health has a significant impact on motivation, and higher cognitive functions involving the neuro-immuno-endocrine mediators. The study aimed to understand the knowledge, attitude and practices of expectant mothers during their pregnancy towards the use of probiotics from different cities of Rajasthan, India. Results of the survey study suggested that a considerable number of mothers were unaware about the health benefits of probiotics consumption during and post-pregnancy and due to partial and ambiguous knowledge towards probiotics, maternal subjects also showed characteristics of disbelief on probiotics consumption during and post-pregnancy, which further contributed towards the decreased consumption of probiotics during and post-pregnancy.

DOI: 10.4018/978-1-7998-9652-4.ch009

INTRODUCTION

Maternal morbidity is one of the major global health concerns wherein about two-third of the complications are well-documented which can be prevented and treated. One of the agenda of 'Sustainable Development Goals' 2030 (SDG-30) aims to reduce maternal mortality rate (MMR). Its objective is to 'Ensure healthy lives and promote wellbeing for all at all ages.' To ensure decline in MMR, in year 2015 World Health Organisation (WHO) published 'Strategies towards ending preventable maternal morbidity' especially maternal health morbidity due to economic disparity as low-middle income countries reported higher maternal morbidity rates as compared to higher income nations (Maternal Health Task Force, 2018; WHO, 2019; WHO, 2015; United Nations Statistics Division, 2016; Geller et al, 2018). In India, MMR declined from 130/100,000 live births to 113/ 100,000 live births between the years 2016-2018, but it needs more attention and efforts to achieve the SDG-2030 target. Although just like global organizations, the Government of India has been constantly forging maternal health-care services among the population yet there is need to address and overcome the massive challenges such as, economic disparities, lack of education, policies and resources, which widens-up the gap between service providers/policy makers and the expectant mothers and their neonates (UNICEF, n.d.). To fight the challenge of increasing maternal morbidity rate, Indian government have adopted antenatal care services as an initiative to safeguard maternal and new-born child health and wellbeing.

Previous studies conducted on preventive and sustainable maternal and child health have reported that pregnancy period triggers metabolic and inflammatory alterations in mother's body which can be prevented from predisposing towards complications by adopting appropriate health-related interventions. The 'Gut Microbiome' based intervention is one of the finest approaches to intervene altered metabolic and inflammatory response of the mother during or after pregnancy as maternal gut microbiome and gut-brain axis gets more sensitize during the peri-natal and post-natal period which can significantly contributes towards the pregnancy outcomes and wellbeing of both mother and child. Imbalance of gut-brain axial may enhance the maternal complications and foetus developmental suppressions especially neurological development depressions, while on the contrary, maintaining maternal health-care, nutrient rich diet and gut-eubiosis by incorporating prebiotics, probiotics, dietary fibres and fermented foods which can be a source of probiotics, can significantly reduce the maternal and foetal health complications during or post-pregnancy. Additionally, it has been reported that lifestyle and dietary modifications can significantly channelise gut-brain axis and therefore, contribute towards boosting maternal gut-microbiome by promoting gut-eubiosis especially during peri and post-natal period (Wang et al, 2017; Dawe et al, 2020; Edwards et al, 2017; Mayer et al, 2014; Borre et al, 2014).

Pregnancy is a period of metabolic fluctuations, hormonal changes, increased dietary demands and elevated risk of inflammation and infections along with the incorporation of prescribed medications and additional supplements during or post-pregnancy acquires the potential to affect maternal and foetal gut-microbiome. Thus, incorporation of probiotics in maternal nutritional intake became a striking area for health-care professionals and researchers especially during or post-pregnancy which can significantly be adopted to overcome from the maternal and foetal complications during the peripartum period.

Probiotics or Psychobiotics

Live microorganisms adequately incorporated in the dietary sources to confer the individual's health benefits by restoring or promoting gut-microbiome are referred as 'probiotics' (Genuis & Genuis, 2016; Chen et al, 2020; Mirghafourvand et al, 2016; He et al, 2020). Probiotics work on the ***'gut-brain axis'*** mechanism (as represented in Figure 1) wherein vital systems of central nervous system such as, enteric nervous system (ENS), autonomic nervous system (ANS) and hypothalamic-pituitary-adrenal (HPA) axis and body's immune system work systematically bidirectionally to circuit route between gut and brain of an individual. It has been reported that if any disturbance or damage takes place in the gut-brain axial routing leads to deterioration of the health and wellbeing of the host. "Psychobiotics" explain the effect of gut-microbiome on gut-brain axis especially focusing on various domains such as emotional, cognitive, physiological, etc. ***"Psychobiotics"*** refers to the live microorganisms previously recognised as probiotics or support to gut-bacteria i.e., prebiotics which when incorporated in an adequate amount can confer health benefits to the host by significantly supporting the gut-brain axis or bacteria-brain axis. (Edwards et al, 2017; Sarkar et al, 2016). With the increasing awareness about the nutrition science and its relevance in individual's health and wellbeing. Consumers are actively adopting food products which claims to be healthy and ensuring wellbeing. Therefore, probiotics and prebiotics containing food products are also widely available in the global food markets in the various forms such as, probiotics or bacterial yoghurt, probiotics milk, other milk confectionaries, fermented foods, etc, under the board label of 'functional or superfoods' category, dietary supplements such as, probiotics powders, capsules, tablets, etc, and in infant formula milk. Due to digitalisation, it has also been quite feasible to circulate any health-related information among the masses quickly, due to which consumers are also consuming the functional or superfoods without any formal prescriptions from the concerning health-care professionals or evidence-based knowledge. Henceforth, it is important to shed more light over the health benefits of psychobiotics/probiotics and consumers behaviour traits such as their knowledge, attitude and practice towards the probiotics especially as a maternal nutrition wherein probiotics products have been considered as one of the preventive therapies from several health complications during or post-pregnancy (Sharma et al, 2019; Cevik Guner & Kissal, 2021; Rutten et al, 2015).

Figure 1. Diagrammatic representation of Gut-Brain Axis

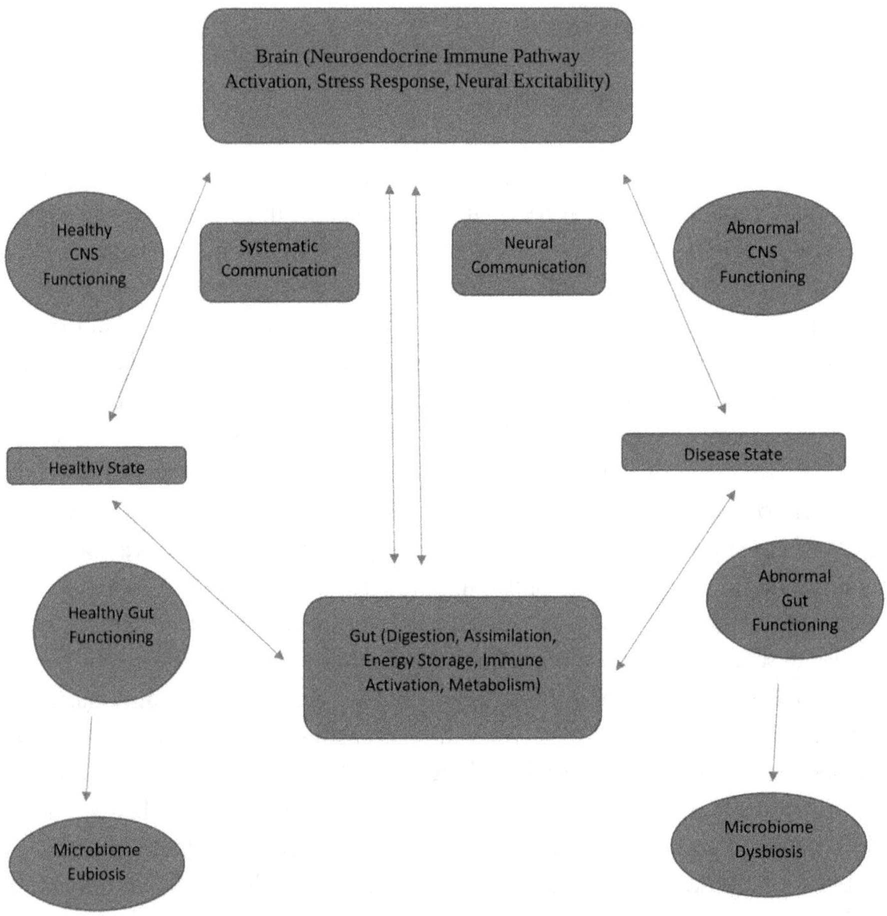

Maternal Gut: Microbiota and Pregnancy Outcomes

Maternal health and wellbeing throughout the perinatal and postnatal period have a significant role in the pregnancy outcomes i.e., maternal health throughout the gestation period and neonate health during and after the pregnancy. There are several factors which have been reported as contributors towards the positive pregnancy outcomes, out of which maternal lifestyle factors have been significantly highlighted as the factors with the efficacy to alter the pregnancy outcomes such as, maternal diet, physical activity, consumption of anti-nutrient products like alcohol, tobacco, etc. It has been indicated that maternal lifestyle factors play a vital role in the alteration of maternal gut-microbiota which also have a relevance on maternal and infant's health and wellbeing. For instance, incorporation of dietary fibres, probiotics and prebiotics food products in the maternal diet influence the production of several nutritionally beneficial components out of which one major component is short chain fatty acids (SCFAs) which has the potential to cross maternal gut mucosal lining and travel to the foetus circulatory system via placenta. SCFAs significantly contributes towards the foetus overall development especially neurodevelopment and set the ground for foetal gut microflora. Thus, maintaining healthy maternal lifestyle by incorporating maternal and child dietary support via adequate dietary fibre, probiotics, prebiotics and all other nutrients, promoting adequate physical activity engagement and avoidance of anti-nutrients in the maternal regimen can significantly contribute towards the positive pregnancy outcomes (Ratsika et al, 2021; McDonald & McCoy, 2019; Spencer et al, 2017; Chu et al, 2016).

Figure 2. Diagrammatic representation of Maternal gut-microbiome and pregnancy outcomes

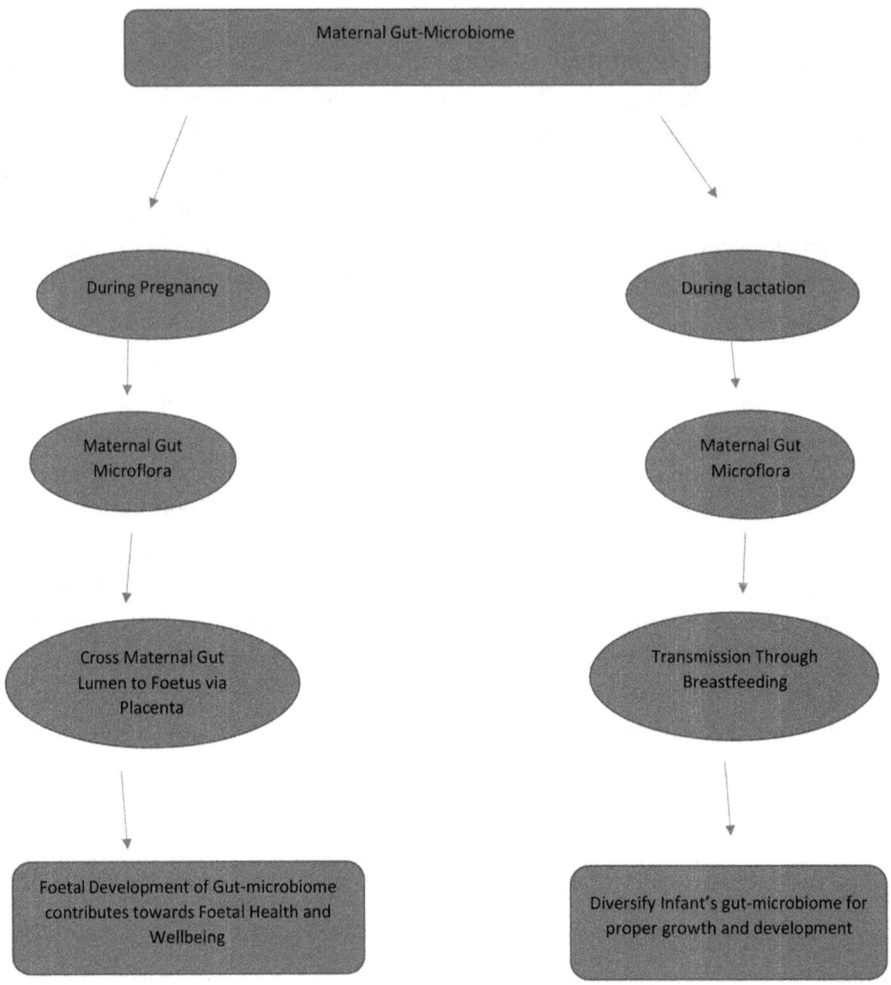

Studies conducted on neonates implied that gut-microflora has a dense distribution of microflora immediately after birth of the baby. Additionally, more diversifying effect has been seen in child's gut-microflora as majority of neonates began with the breastfeeding for the nourishment (Samanta et al, 2011; Hajela et al, 2014; Balamurugan et al, 2008; Kabeerdoss et al, 2013).

Consumer Beliefs and Attitude Towards Probiotics Products

The current Indian market representation showed that about less than 1% contribution has been present from India towards the global market with regard to probiotics products. Presently, markets are equipped with common probiotics products such as, yoghurt/curd, fermented beverages, probiotics beverages, etc. However, with the expansion of gut-microbiome domain, circulation of other probiotics products such as, dietary supplements, infant supplementary formulas, probiotics bar, etc, are gaining popularity among health-conscious population. Majorly, urban population has adopted the inclusion of probiotics formula in their day's diet while it's almost negligible probiotics products acceptance in the rural band of India except the traditional probiotics-based food products. Probiotics products has been distributed in the markets in two major forms i.e., probiotics food products (to enhance gut microbial of the host's body) and probiotics as a medicinal therapy (to treat and prevent specific health conditions or disease). Probiotics products circulated in the Indian market are bound under the guidelines published by Indian Council of Medical Research (ICMR) and Food Safety and Standards Authority of India (FSSAI) (Raghuwanshi et al, 2015; Hajela et al, 2014; ICMR, 2011).

THEORETICAL FRAMEWORK

Knowledge, Attitude and Practice (KAP) Model

The knowledge, attitude and practice model has been a widely adopted model used for the conduction of cross-sectional surveys and formulating structured interviews or survey questionnaire. It demonstrates what is known, believed and practiced by the target population with regard to the specific area of research. This model has also been widely applied to explain individual's health-related behaviours. The model demonstrates health-related behaviours based on three major domains. Firstly, knowledge which refers to an individual's understanding or information regarding a particular health-related behaviours, such as, in the present study, maternal knowledge and understanding with regard to probiotics use especially during or post-pregnancy and how well they are applying their knowledge about the probiotics during or post-pregnancy, in brief, how well they receive the probiotics information, how well they have retained it and how well they are applying it during their gestational period. Secondly, attitude refers to the individual's feelings or opinion about a particular health-related behaviour, i.e., in the present study, maternal attitude or feelings towards the probiotic's consumption during or post-pregnancy which can contribute towards the acceptance or denial of the probiotics-use during their gestational period. Lastly, practices refer to individual's engagement with a certain health-related behaviour followed by their knowledge and attitude towards the same, i.e., in the present study maternal practices or adoption of probiotics products during or post-pregnancy will determine their incorporation or engagement with the probiotics products which can also be influenced by their knowledge and attitude towards probiotics (Siltrakool, 2017; Bano et al, 2013).

Figure 3. Knowledge, Attitude and Practice (KAP) model adopted for the present survey study

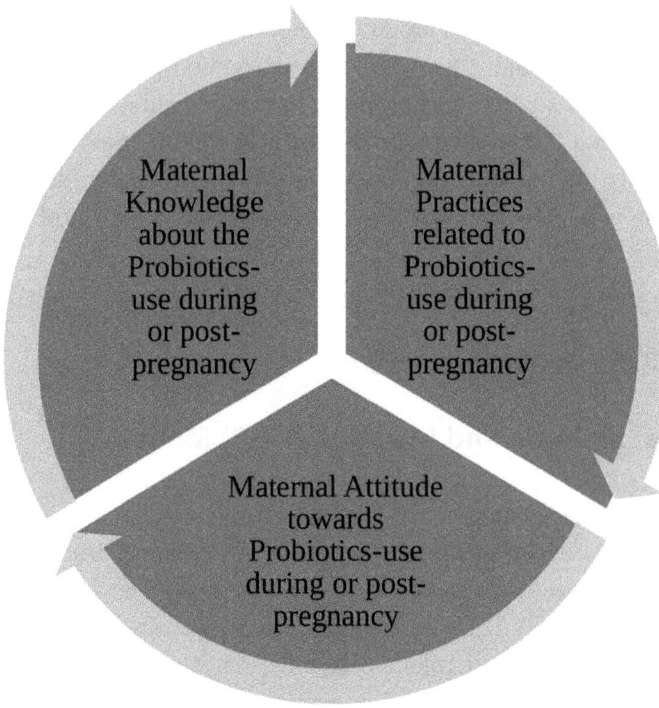

LITERATURE REVIEW

Several health-related research studies have adopted KAP model to demonstrate the knowledge, attitude and practice of target population with regards to explain a specific health-related behaviour. Similarly, several studies have been conducted on probiotics use and its understanding, beliefs and consumption in different population groups, such as, a study was conducted on Indian health-care professionals with aim to access their knowledge, attitude and practice with regards to probiotics-use. The findings of the study highlighted that about 93.25% health-care professionals were correctly aware about the term 'probiotics', while only approximately 54.68% and 66.66% were confident about the efficacy and correct mechanism of probiotics on the human body respectively. Additionally, there was a significant difference found among different health-care professionals out of which medical students and nutrition students showed higher scores to have better knowledge about the probiotics and its health benefits. Therefore, it was concluded that probiotics awareness programmes need to be designed for health-care professionals which will help to revise their knowledge about the probiotics and hence, contribute towards developing attitude and practice regarding probiotics use among the population. Another relative study conducted on health-care professionals in Nigeria also showed relative findings (Otuto Amarauche, 2015; Soni et al, 2018).

Additionally, several studies have highlighted the effectiveness of probiotics/ psychobiotics on maternal and child health. Previous studies suggested that neurogenerative diseases and mental health has been linked with consumption of psychobiotics as a part of maternal nutrition during or post-pregnancy. Psychobiotics/ Probiotics effectively contribute towards routing of gut-brain axis and blood-brain barrier. Henceforth, they significantly contribute towards reduction of maternal and child's various health domains (such as, physical, mental, emotional, cognitive and social) complications, enriching maternal and child's gut-microflora, reduction of autoimmune or genetical disorders in infants, etc, during or post-pregnancy (Cheng et al, 2019; Dawe et al, 2020; Browne et al, 2021; Rutten et al, 2015; Chen et al, 2019; Liang et al, 2020).

Previous studies have indicated towards the relevance of probiotics as a nutritional intervention during and after the pregnancy for both mother and her child. Additionally, several studies have been also conducted to analyse the knowledge, attitude and practice about the probiotics among the various health-care professionals. But it is also important to understand the knowledge, attitude and practice among the expectant and lactating mothers about the probiotics consumption, wherein, quite a limited number of studies have been conducted till date such as, a survey study was conducted on 519 Turkey women with neonates between 6 months to 2 years with an aim to analyse the knowledge, attitude and practice of the mothers regarding probiotics consumption during their pregnancy period and for their infants. The results of the study indicated that about 20.2% mothers knew about probiotics, about 33.1% correctly mentioned about probiotics specific products and lastly, about 49.7% knew that breastmilk contains probiotics. In summary, it was highlighted under the study that there was a statistically significant difference found based on various socio-demographic factors such as, mother's education, age, employment, income, family structure, etc, and variables under the study i.e., maternal knowledge about probiotics, their knowledge about specific probiotics products and knowledge about breast-milk as a source of probiotics (Cevik Guner & Kissal, 2021).

Although several studies have highlighted the role of human gut-microbiome under gut-brain axis route which can contribute towards host's prominent health and wellbeing. Studies have also highlighted the effectiveness of gut-microbiome during the human developmental period especially linking with the maternal nutrition during or post-pregnancy. Ensuring adequate gut-microbiome enrichment during or post-pregnancy among mothers and their neonates, several studies also highlighted the effectiveness of probiotics/psychobiotics on maternal and child health during or post-pregnancy. However, the real challenge is population's understanding, beliefs and acceptance of probiotics products as a source of health benefits. It has been also highlighted in few previous studies that health-care professionals play a moderating role towards building awareness and routing relevant information among the population with regard to probiotics and its effectiveness towards one's health. Therefore, several studies were conducted to understand the knowledge, attitude and practice of probiotics use among various health-care professionals. Although quite a limited number of studies have been conducted to understand the status of knowledge, attitude and practice of probiotics-use among expectant and lactating mothers. Henceforth, it is crucial to understand the knowledge, opinion and acceptance of mothers towards probiotics consumptions during or post-pregnancy period which can contribute towards building prominent maternal nutrition interventions and policies so as to overcome from the one of the most challenging global health concerns i.e., 'Severe MMR'. Therefore, the present study aims to investigate the level of awareness, knowledge, attitude and practices being followed towards the use of probiotics/psychobiotics by Indian expectant and lactating mothers.

METHODOLOGY

The current study was conducted using a mixed method approach. A cross-sectional survey was conducted using a self-report questionnaire based on KAP model which was designed for the purpose of the study. The survey aimed at understanding the prevalent knowledge, attitude and practices among Indian expectant and lactating mothers with respect to probiotics consumption during or after pregnancy and its long-term implications on health. The survey comprised of statements and questions to gather information about the level of awareness and knowledge about probiotics, the behaviours and practices being followed and an attitude towards including probiotics-based food products to enhance the health and well-being of both the mother and the child.

Sample

The sample of the study comprised of 100 Indian expectant and lactating mothers. The data was collected using the convenience sampling method. The inclusion criteria for the sample were: (i) respondents were Indian residents (ii) aged from 18-35 years (iii) Literate and (iv) had access to smartphone/laptop and internet to participate in the survey (v) Indian expectant or lactating women.

Procedure

The survey data was collected in the month of September and October 2021 from the state of Rajasthan, India. Respondents were informed about the purpose of the study, voluntary nature of participation and option for discontinuing at any point of time. Also, participants informed consent was taken and they were assured that all their responses will be kept anonymous, confidential.

Measures

Data was collected with the help of probiotics (KAP) survey questionnaire which was pre-tested by obtaining responses of twenty pregnant and lactating mothers and was later revised and finalized as per their understanding of each statement. The pilot survey schedule comprised of 20 statements and questions for each of the three domains i.e., KAP. The survey questionnaire was then reviewed by the three experts from the relevant fields. After the rankings were obtained from the experts' relevant statements were retained from the original pool of statements for knowledge, attitudes, and practices domains respectively and other statements were discarded.

Knowledge, Attitude and Practices Survey Form

The form consisted of questions regarding subject's age, education, employment status, phase of motherhood (pregnancy/lactation), complications during pregnancy, mode of delivery and breastfeeding status (Figure 4).

The survey questionnaire was divided into three major sections. The first section comprised of 11 questions for assessing mothers' knowledge and awareness about probiotics. The statements intended to understand the subject's understanding about probiotics, sources from where they get relevant information, its use, and benefits during pregnancy (Figure 6, Figure 7 & Figure 12). The second section comprised of 6 statements designed to understand the subject's attitudes, opinions, and beliefs towards probiotics (Figure 9). Lastly, practices related to the use of probiotics during pregnancy were assessed with the help of 9 statements. They were structured to assess the various practices followed by mothers and their frequency of consumption of probiotics products (Figure 10 and Figure 11).

RESULTS AND DISCUSSION

The survey responses were analysed to understand maternal knowledge, attitudes, and practices towards probiotics-use during and after pregnancy.

Figure 4. Maternal status (pregnancy/ lactation), complication related with the pregnancy, mode of delivery of a child (Vaginal or caesarean delivery), type of delivery (pre-term or full-term) and actively breastfeeding status

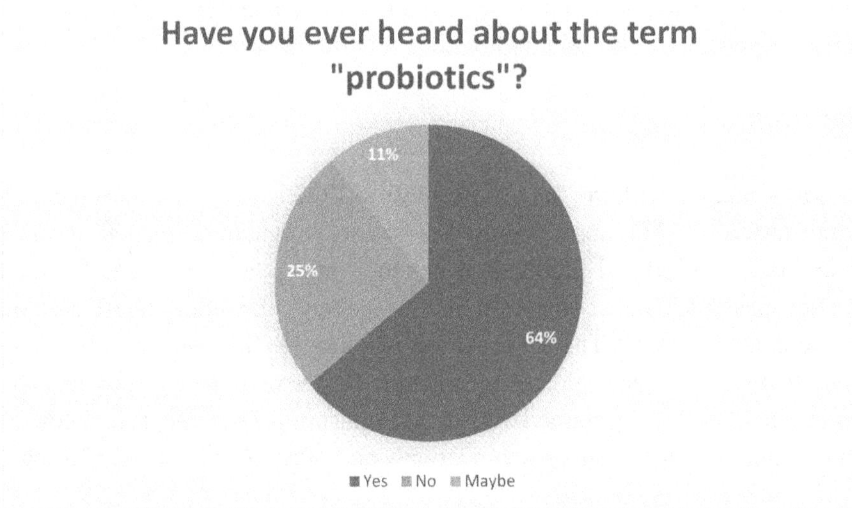

Mothers Knowledge Towards Probiotics-Use During and Post-Pregnancy

The findings of the survey report highlighted that 64% of the total maternal sample was aware about the term 'Probiotics' (Figure 5). Additionally 25% of the total sample was unaware about the term and concept of probiotics and its inclusion in diet and a scanty number of participants i.e., 11% of the total sample was unsure about probiotics term.

Figure 5. Maternal awareness about the term 'Probiotics'

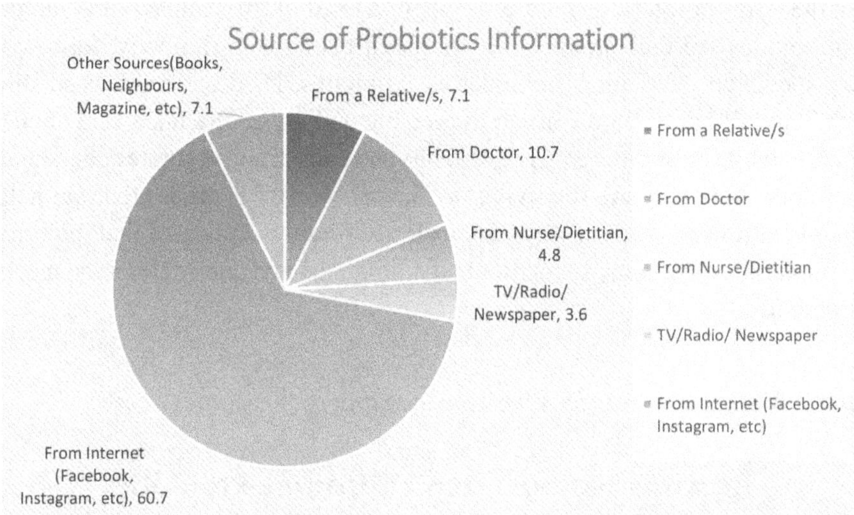

Furthermore, subjects were asked about sources from where they received information about 'probiotics' (Figure 6), wherein majority (60.7%) reported internet as a source of information followed by doctor (10.7%), relatives and other sources such as books, neighbours, etc (7.1%), friend/s (6%), from nurse/ dietitian (4.8%) and TV/Radio/Newspaper (3.6%). Findings indicated internet being a major source of fetching information among the sample while TV, Radio, Newspaper were the least consulted sources of obtaining information about probiotics among the sample.

Figure 6. Source of getting probiotics related information

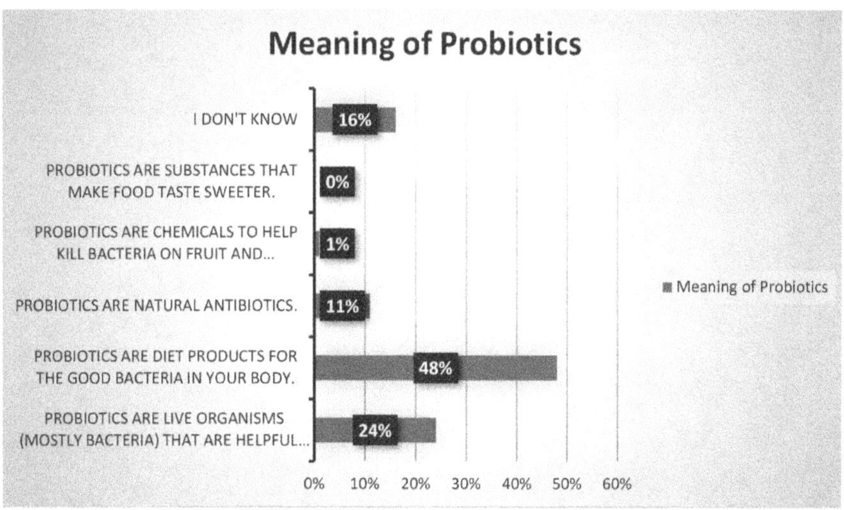

Additionally, subjects were asked about their knowledge and understanding about the term 'Probiotics' (Figure 7), wherein most of the sample (48%) indicated that probiotics are diet products for the good bacteria in the body, followed by 11% respondents describing probiotics as antibiotics, 1% described it as chemicals which help kill bacteria on fruit and vegetable and 16% were not aware about the probiotics while only about 24% respondents had correct and accurate understanding of probiotics i.e., they are the living organisms (mostly bacteria) that are helpful to your health when you eat them. Henceforth, findings indicated that majority of the sample was quite unaware and/or had ambiguous awareness about the meaning of probiotics.

Figure 7. Mothers' knowledge about the meaning of 'probiotics'

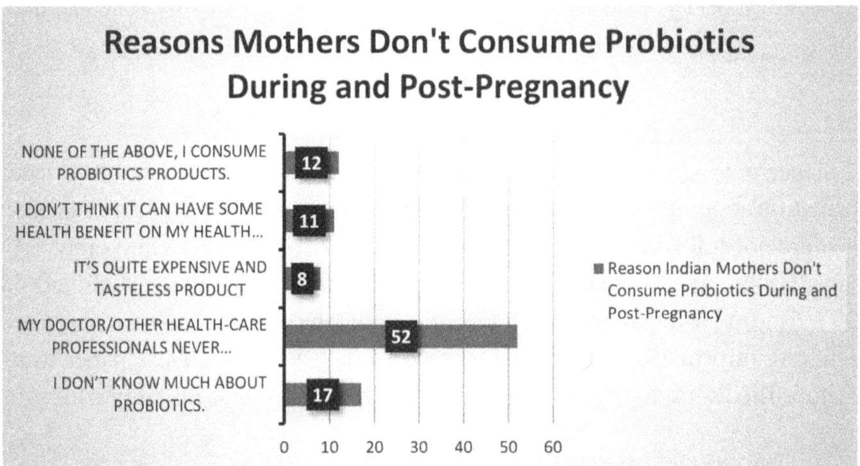

Figure 8. Table representing the knowledge about usage of probiotics during and post-pregnancy

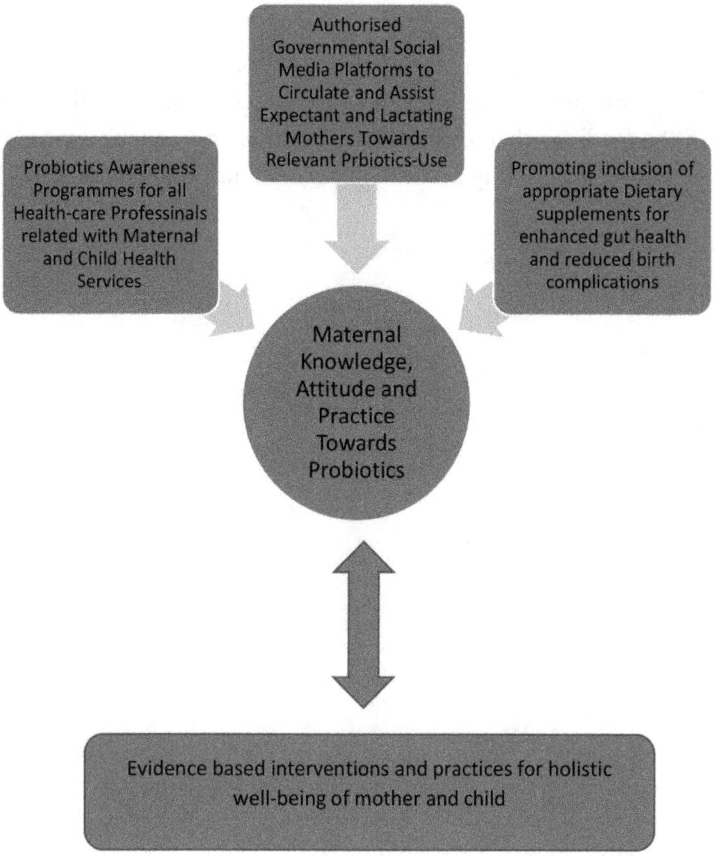

The findings of the study indicated that majority of the mothers (64%) reported no health benefits during or post-pregnancy while only 36% reported that probiotics have health benefits during and post-pregnancy. In addition, there was a slight difference among mothers who were aware about the natural probiotic food items i.e., 43% and who were unaware i.e., 57%. Similarly, there was a slight difference among the mothers who had the understanding that probiotics available in the form of dietary supplements can only work effectively i.e., 48% while 52% reported that probiotics which are available in the form of supplements are not the only effective sources of probiotics. In addition, majority of mothers lacked having sufficient and evidence-based information from credible sources about probiotics which has been indicated in the findings of the present study i.e., 67% of mothers were unaware that probiotics strengthen-up the mother and child's immune system during and post-pregnancy. Similarly, 73% of the mothers were unaware about the fact that probiotics have the ability to support the healthy outcomes of the pregnancy, 69% of the mothers were also unaware about the probiotics serving psychobiotic functions i.e., to support mental health and wellbeing of both mother and her child and 70% mothers were also unaware about the presence of probiotics in the breast milk which can effectively contribute towards child's gut microbiome. Lastly, it was clearly indicated in the findings that 78% mothers were keen to acquire more knowledge about the benefits of including probiotics during and post-pregnancy.

Mothers' Attitude Towards Probiotics-Use During and Post-Pregnancy

Figure 9. Table showing mothers' attitude towards the use of probiotics during and post-pregnancy

(n=100)	
Current Maternal Status:	
Lactation/Breastfeeding	26%
1st Trimester of Pregnancy	8%
2nd Trimester of Pregnancy	27%
3rd Trimester of Pregnancy	39%
Complications Related with Pregnancy	
Yes	21%
No	80%
Mode of Delivery	
Caesarean Delivery	84.6%
Vaginal Delivery	15.4%
Type of Delivery	
Pre-Term	15.4%
Full-Term	84.6%
Breast-feeding Mothers	
Yes	92.3%
No	7.7%

The findings of the study indicated that majority of the mothers i.e., 34% (disagree) and 32% (strongly disagree) with the fact that probiotics are good for maternal and child' health respectively while just about 9% (agree) and 4% (strongly agree) of the sample reported that probiotics provide health benefits to both mother and her child. In contrast, there was a slight difference among mothers who believed that probiotics can be dangerous for maternal and child's health i.e., 28% while about 29% mothers of the total sample disagree with the statement. In addition, 42% of the mothers believed that probiotics do not serve as an alternative for bringing relief for maternal digestive complaints during and post-pregnancy. Similarly, 67% mothers believed that probiotics are not safer than prescribed medicines. Additionally, 57% mothers believed that health claims on probiotics products are not good for the health. Lastly, 64% mothers believed that probiotics cannot make them feel better during and post-pregnancy.

Practices Towards Probiotics-Use During and Post-Pregnancy

Figure 10. Table showing the consumption of probiotics by mothers during and post-pregnancy

Questions for assessing knowledge	Yes	No
	N=100	
Consumption of probiotics can provide benefits to your health and your child health during or post-pregnancy?	36%	64%
Probiotics are also present in natural/traditional food items (such as, curd, fermented foods,etc) which can also be consumed during or post-pregnancy?	43%	57%
Only probiotics in tablets, powder, or capsules that can work effectively in the body during or post-pregnancy?	48%	52%
Probiotics can strengthen-up the mother and child's immune system during or post-pregnancy?	33%	67%
Probiotic can be useful to consume during or post pregnancy for healthy pregnancy outcomes?	27%	73%
Probiotics are good for mental stress and health during or post-pregnancy?	31%	69%
Breast-milk is a good source of probiotics for the new-born baby?	30%	70%
I want to acquire more knowledge about the probiotics?	78%	22%

Findings of the survey study indicated that majority (58%) of the mothers reported that they have never consumed probiotics products during and post-pregnancy.

Additionally, majority i.e., 43% and 38% reported that they have never or rarely searched about probiotics related information during and post-pregnancy respectively. Similarly, majority (64%) of the mothers have never suggested any other mother to consume probiotics products during and post-pregnancy. Additionally, majority i.e., 49% and 32% mothers reported that they have either never or rarely consumed probiotics products to treat digestive complaints during and post-pregnancy respectively. Similarly, majority i.e., 62% mothers reported that their doctors/ health-care professionals never asked them to consume probiotics products to treat digestive complaints during and post-pregnancy. 56% mothers reported they have never consumed probiotics products to enhance their immunity during and post-pregnancy. In contrast, it was reported by 49% of the total sample that they often consume natural products i.e., curd, fermented food, etc, with probiotics/prebiotics nutritional qualities. Lastly, it was also found that 44% mothers reported that they will often consume probiotics if they will be advised to consume probiotics products by their health-care professionals during and post-pregnancy.

Figure 11. represents the reasons behind the limited probiotics consumption among mothers during and post-pregnancy

Statements for assessing attitude	Strongly Disagree	Disagree	Neutral	Agree	Strongly Agree
	N=100				
Probiotics are good for your health and your child's health during or post-pregnancy.	32%	34%	21%	9%	4%
Probiotics can be dangerous for your health and your child's health during or post-pregnancy.	19%	29%	22%	28%	2%
Probiotics may be an alternative option to treat complaints of the maternal digestive system due to pathogenic infections during or post-pregnancy.	20%	42%	26%	9%	3%
Probiotics are safer than prescribed drugs.	7%	67%	13%	10%	3%
Health claims on the Probiotics drugs are good for health.	17%	57%	13%	9%	4%
Probiotics can or make me feel better during or post-pregnancy.	5%	64%	15%	14%	2%

The findings indicated that 52% mothers don't consume probiotics products during and post-pregnancy because their doctors/other health-care professionals never guided them about probiotics followed by 17% respondents who were unclear about probiotics, 11% were having a belief that probiotics doesn't have any health benefits and 8% were of the opinion that probiotics products are expensive and tasteless products while only 12% showed a strong belief towards probiotics consumption.

Findings of the study indicated the status of mothers' understanding and awareness about the probiotic's consumption during and post-pregnancy. Results indicated that majority (64%) of mothers were aware about the term 'probiotics' but only 24% knew the correct meaning of probiotics. Additionally, internet (60.7%) sources showed majority contribution as a source of information about probiotics among the maternal sample of the current study. In addition, results also indicate that 64% subjects were unaware about the probiotics health benefits, 57% subjects were unaware about the presence of probiotics in the natural products, 52% subjects were aware that probiotics are not only present in dietary supplementary sources, 67% subjects lacked awareness towards probiotics efficiency to support body's immunity, 73% subjects were unawareness about the contribution of probiotics in healthy pregnancy outcomes, 69% subjects were not aware about the contribution of probiotics towards the mental health benefits and 70% subjects were also unaware about the fact that breastmilk is a source of probiotics for the child. Lastly, it was also indicated that majority i.e., 78% subjects were keen to acquire more knowledge about the probiotics.

Previous studies conducted among different groups of population such as, students, health-care professionals, general population, clinical population, etc also highlighted that there is quite a limited knowledge and awareness among the population towards probiotics and its health benefits even though many have heard about the term 'probiotics' they were not clear about the actual meaning of probiotics and its health benefits. It has also been reported that source of information towards probiotics has been other sources such as, TV, radio, internet, social groups, etc, rather than the health-care professionals. Studies conducted on health-care professionals also revealed mixed results i.e., on one side health-care professionals were aware about the probiotics and its effectivity while on the other side, there was a significant difference found among the various health-care professional's knowledge and awareness towards probiotics and its health benefits (Sharma et al, 2019; Otuto Amarauche, 2015; Fijan et al, 2019; Arora et al, 2020; Yilmaz-Ersan et al, 2020).

Mothers Attitude Towards Probiotics-Use During and Post-Pregnancy

Findings of the study indicated the extent of understanding and awareness about the probiotic consumption during and post-pregnancy among mothers. Results indicated that majority of mothers in the selected sample believed that there are no health benefits of probiotics consumption during and post-pregnancy (34%), 28% subjects believed that probiotics can be dangerous for health while 29% believed that probiotics are not dangerous for health during and post-pregnancy, 42% subjects believed that probiotics are not the alternative for digestive complaints, 67% subjects believed that probiotics are not safer than prescribed medicines, 57% subjects reported to believe that health claims on probiotics products are not good for health and lastly, 64% subjects believed that probiotics cannot makes feel better during and post pregnancy.

Previous studies showed the relationship between the awareness about probiotics with the attitude towards the probiotics products, studies conducted on different target population showed that group awareness and knowledge about probiotics were more likely to adopt positive attitude towards probiotics consumption while limited understanding towards probiotics leads to disbelief towards the probiotics consumption and its health benefits (Khalesi et al, 2020; Carvalho et al, 2014; Allah & S, 2019; Arshad et al, 2021).

Practices Towards Probiotics-Use During and Post-Pregnancy

58% subjects reported that they have never consumed probiotics products during and post-pregnancy, 43% subjects never searched about probiotics related information, 64% subjects never suggested probiotics consumption to their social groups, 49% subjects never consumed probiotics to treat digestive complaints, 62% subjects reported that they have never been told about probiotics from their health-care professionals, 56% subjects reported that they have never consumed probiotics to enhance their immune system while 49% subjects reported that they have often consumed the traditional food products with probiotics nutritional quality. Additionally, it has been also highlighted that 44% subjects reported that they will consume probiotics if their health-care professional advised them during and post-pregnancy. Lastly, it was also indicated that Indian mothers (52%) don't consume or support probiotics consumption as their health-care professionals never mentioned about the probiotics during and post-pregnancy.

Previous studies have highlighted the relevance of knowledge and attitude towards probiotics consumption or practice. Henceforth, it was highlighted that limited knowledge about probiotics and disbeliefs leads to limited acceptance and incorporation of probiotics products in diet. It is an irony, that people are consuming probiotics in their diet, but they are unaware about the sources, benefits, efficacy, right quantity of probiotics intake due to limited knowledge. Health-care professionals can play a pivotal role in disseminating probiotics-related information and help in fostering favourable attitudes and practices among the clinical and non-clinical population towards probiotics (Pettoello-Mantovani et al, 2019; Barqawi et al, 2021; Sanders et al, 2016; Rutten et al, 2016).

More research needs to be conducted on understanding the efficacy of psychobiotics on maternal and foetal health. This will help the health-care professionals to develop and implement adjunct psychobiotics-based intervention treatment plans during and after the gestation period. However, it has been suggested that incorporation of probiotics in maternal diet during the third trimester i.e., 3-4 weeks before delivery and continuing it for 6 months as a post-natal care, reduces the risk of foetal developmental disorders, maternal pregnancy-related complications and pre-term delivery. It has been observed that beta diversity during the third trimester increases as compared to the first trimester of pregnancy, therefore direct supplementation or dietary inclusion of probiotics can contribute towards the healthy pregnancy outcomes. Studies have suggested continued incorporation of probiotics for 6 months after delivery either in the maternal dietary sources (100 grams twice a day) or direct feeding ($1x10^6$ Cfu/day) to the neonates for the enrichment of beneficial microbiota which can reduce the risk of infant's infections/ diseases (Baldassarre et al, 2018; Swartwout & Luo, 2018; Astbury et al, 2015; Hantoushzadeh et al, 2011).

CONCLUSION

The current study aimed to explore the knowledge level, attitudes and practices of expectant and lactating mothers towards probiotics consumption. The findings of the study revealed that majority (64%) of the mothers were not having relevant information about the probiotics use during and after the pregnancy as they have never been told about the probiotics from their health-care professionals (62%). Although 78% subjects were keen to acquire more knowledge about the probiotics use and 44% reported that they will consume probiotics if their health-care professionals advised then during and after pregnancy. It can be concluded that, a considerable percentage of Indian mothers were unaware about the probiotics efficiency during and post-pregnancy and due to partial or unclear knowledge towards probiotics, maternal subjects also showed characteristics of disbelief on probiotics consumption during and post-pregnancy, which further contributed towards the practice or consumption of probiotics during and post-pregnancy. Interestingly, findings also revealed that probiotics food products were already incorporated in the Indian diet, but the knowledge was quite limited among the sample. Thus, the findings of the present study can contribute to understand that there is limited awareness about the probiotics among the Indian expectant and lactating mothers even when there is an inclusion of probiotics food products in their daily diet which means unconsciously they are practising consumption of probiotics but are not aware or partially aware about it and due to lack of complete understanding about probiotics and its health benefits which can be a foundation stone to develop a better attitudes and beliefs towards probiotics use. The findings of the study intend to pave the way for formulating holistic intervention strategies and polices for maternal and child healthcare.

Figure 12. A suggestive maternal and child health-care model for fostering maternal knowledge, attitudes, and practices

Questions for assessing practices	Never	Rarely	Sometimes	Always	Often
	N=100				
How often you are/have consumed probiotic products during or post-pregnancy?	58%	15%	18%	6%	3%
How often you are/ have searched for additional information regarding probiotics from various sources during or post-pregnancy?	43%	38%	14%	3%	2%
How often you are/have recommended any pregnant or lactating woman to consume probiotics considering the health benefits of the probiotics for mother and child?	64%	19%	13%	2%	2%
How often you are/have consumed any probiotic products to prevent digestive system complaints due to pathogenic infections during or post-pregnancy?	49%	32%	11%	5%	3%
How often your doctor/ health-care professional asked you to consume probiotic products to treat digestive system complaints due to pathogenic infections during or post-pregnancy?	62%	21%	7%	6%	4%
How often you are/have consumed probiotic products to enhance your immune system during or post-pregnancy?	56%	22%	13%	5%	4%
How frequently you are/have consumed natural products such as home-made yogurt, cheese, butter, cow's milk, fermented foods, etc, during or post-pregnancy?	8%	21%	18%	4%	49%
How frequently you will consume probiotics if your doctor/dietitian provides you proper reference about probiotics use during your pregnancy or post-pregnancy?	16%	21%	10%	9%	44%

For fostering relevant information about the efficacy of probiotics use during and after pregnancy, public health agencies need to be actively driven for promoting dietary intervention programmes for the expectant and lactating mothers. Active participation of health-care professionals in circulating the relevant information about the probiotics use during and after the pregnancy needs to be encouraged. Proper training and practice regarding the potential role of dietary intervention therapy needs to be incorporated in the academic curriculum of the health-care professionals dealing with the maternal and foetal health-care unit. Use of mass-media platforms for circulating relevant information about the probiotics use for enhancement of maternal and foetal health by the governing bodies and health-care professionals needs to be encouraged. Standardised assessment and analysis to understand the efficacy of dietary intervention plans needs to be conducted using periodic health surveys by the governing bodies or public health agencies.

Limitations of the Study

A shortcoming of the present survey study is electronic mode of data collection due to which participants with internet- accessibility could only participate in the study which limits the data generation from large population. Another limitation is inclusion of only literate mothers, those who could read the survey questionnaire. This limits the generalizability of the findings to some extent.

Longitudinal study on a large diverse population of expectant and lactating mothers needs to be conducted using methods like face-to-face interview method to address individual biases and limitations of the present study. Additionally, to understand precisely about the potential risks and benefits of psychobiotics during the pre-natal and post-natal period, health-care professionals can significantly contribute towards the relevant data-collection, assessing adequate changes due to dietary modifications and strengthening the present scientific literature.

Research Implications and Future Directions

The present study supports the relevant existing literature and also provides a board realm of understanding on maternal knowledge, attitudes and practices towards probiotics consumption during or after pregnancy which can further contribute to formulate better maternal and child health-related policies and relevant interventions.

For the future investigations, it is recommended a longitudinal or cross-sectional study can be conducted among general population or other specific group of population with regards to their knowledge, attitude and practice towards probiotics which can contribute to an in-depth understanding of individual or community perspective towards probiotics consumption which can help policy-makers and organizations to formulate a better maternal and child health intervention plan and to conquer severe (MMR). In addition, it is also recommended to explore the effectiveness of probiotics consumption among maternal population and formulating a better understanding of interventions for better mother and child health outcomes.

REFERENCES

Allah, H. A., & S, P. M. (2019). The knowledge and perceptions regarding probiotics among the people of al-qassim region, Saudi Arabia. *Journal of Health and Medical Sciences*, *2*(3). Advance online publication. doi:10.31014/aior.1994.02.03.56

Arora, S., Prabha, K., Sharanagat, V. S., & Mishra, V. (2020). Consumer awareness and willingness to purchase probiotic food and beverage products: A study of Sonipat district, Haryana. *British Food Journal*, *123*(8), 2805–2817. doi:10.1108/BFJ-06-2020-0469

Arshad, M. S., Saqlain, M., Majeed, A., Imran, I., Saeed, H., Saleem, M. U., Abrar, M. A., Islam, M., Hashmi, F., Akbar, M., Chaudhry, M. O., Ramzan, B., & Rasool, M. F. (2021). Cross-sectional study to assess the healthcare professionals' knowledge, attitude and practices about probiotics use in Pakistan. *BMJ Open*, *11*(7), e047494. doi:10.1136/bmjopen-2020-047494 PMID:34321300

Astbury, S., Mostyn, A., Symonds, M. E., & Bell, R. C. (2015). Nutrient availability, the microbiome, and intestinal transport during pregnancy. *Applied Physiology, Nutrition, and Metabolism*, *40*(11), 1100–1106. doi:10.1139/apnm-2015-0117 PMID:26499849

Balamurugan, R., Janardhan, H. P., George, S., Chittaranjan, S. P., & Ramakrishna, B. S. (2008). Bacterial succession in the colon during childhood and adolescence: Molecular studies in a southern Indian village. *The American Journal of Clinical Nutrition*, *88*(6), 1643–1647. doi:10.3945/ajcn.2008.26511 PMID:19064526

Baldassarre, M., Palladino, V., Amoruso, A., Pindinelli, S., Mastromarino, P., Fanelli, M., Di Mauro, A., & Laforgia, N. (2018). Rationale of probiotic supplementation during pregnancy and neonatal period. *Nutrients*, *10*(11), 1693. doi:10.3390/nu10111693 PMID:30404227

Bano, R., AlShammari, E., Fatima, S. B., & Al-Shammari, N. A. (2013). A comparative study of Knowledge, Attitude, Practice of nutrition and non-nutrition student towards a balanced diet in Hail University. *IOSR Journal of Nursing and Health Science*, *2*(3), 29–36. https://www.iosrjournals.org/iosr-jnhs/papers/vol2-issue3/E0232936.pdf?id=8220

Barqawi, H. J., Adra, S. F., Ramzi, H. R., Abouaggour, M. A., & Almehairi, S. K. (2021). Evaluating the knowledge, attitudes and practices of the UAE community on microbiota composition and the main factors affecting it: A cross-sectional study. *BMJ Open*, *11*(8), e047869. doi:10.1136/bmjopen-2020-047869 PMID:34404705

Borre, Y. E., O'Keeffe, G. W., Clarke, G., Stanton, C., Dinan, T. G., & Cryan, J. F. (2014). Microbiota and neurodevelopmental Windows: Implications for brain disorders. *Trends in Molecular Medicine*, *20*(9), 509–518. doi:10.1016/j.molmed.2014.05.002 PMID:24956966

Browne, P. D., Bolte, A. C., Besseling-van der Vaart, I., Claassen, E., & De Weerth, C. (2021). Probiotics as a treatment for prenatal maternal anxiety and depression: A double-blind randomized pilot trial. *Scientific Reports*, *11*(1), 3051. Advance online publication. doi:10.1038/s41598-021-81204-9 PMID:33542275

Carvalho, N. B., Costa, T. D., Ferreira, M. A., Simiqueli, A. A., & Minim, V. P. (2014). Consumer attitude regarding products containing probiotics. *Ciência Rural*, *44*(7), 1319–1326. doi:10.1590/0103-8478cr20131178

Cevik Guner, U., & Kissal, A. (2021). Mothers' knowledge, attitudes and practices regarding probiotic use during pregnancy and for their infants in Turkey. *Public Health Nutrition*, *24*(13), 4297–4304. doi:10.1017/S1368980021000951 PMID:33663639

Chen, X., Jiang, X., Huang, X., He, H., & Zheng, J. (2020). Association between probiotic yogurt intake and gestational diabetes mellitus: A case-control study. *Iranian Journal of Public Health*. Advance online publication. doi:10.18502/ijph.v48i7.2946 PMID:31497545

Chen, Y., Li, Z., Tye, K. D., Luo, H., Tang, X., Liao, Y., Wang, D., Zhou, J., Yang, P., Li, Y., Su, Y., & Xiao, X. (2019). Probiotic supplementation during human pregnancy affects the gut microbiota and immune status. *Frontiers in Cellular and Infection Microbiology*, *9*, 254. Advance online publication. doi:10.3389/fcimb.2019.00254 PMID:31380297

Cheng, L., Liu, Y., Wu, C., Wang, S., & Tsai, Y. (2019). Psychobiotics in mental health, neurodegenerative and neurodevelopmental disorders. *Yao Wu Shi Pin Fen Xi*, *27*(3), 632–648. doi:10.1016/j.jfda.2019.01.002 PMID:31324280

Chu, D. M., Antony, K. M., Ma, J., Prince, A. L., Showalter, L., Moller, M., & Aagaard, K. M. (2016). The early infant gut microbiome varies in association with a maternal high-fat diet. *Genome Medicine*, *8*(1), 77. Advance online publication. doi:10.1186/s13073-016-0330-z PMID:27503374

Dawe, J. P., McCowan, L. M., Wilson, J., Okesene-Gafa, K. A., & Serlachius, A. S. (2020). Probiotics and maternal mental health: A randomised controlled trial among pregnant women with obesity. *Scientific Reports*, *10*(1), 1291. Advance online publication. doi:10.1038/s41598-020-58129-w PMID:31992802

Edwards, S. M., Cunningham, S. A., Dunlop, A. L., & Corwin, E. J. (2017). The maternal gut microbiome during pregnancy. *MCN. The American Journal of Maternal Child Nursing*, *42*(6), 310–317. doi:10.1097/NMC.0000000000000372 PMID:28787280

Fijan, S., Frauwallner, A., Varga, L., Langerholc, T., Rogelj, I., Lorber, M., Lewis, P., & Povalej Bržan, P. (2019). Health professionals' knowledge of probiotics: An international survey. *International Journal of Environmental Research and Public Health*, *16*(17), 3128. doi:10.3390/ijerph16173128 PMID:31466273

Geller, S. E., Koch, A. R., Garland, C. E., MacDonald, E. J., Storey, F., & Lawton, B. (2018). A global view of severe maternal morbidity: Moving beyond maternal mortality. *Reproductive Health*, *15*(S1), 98. Advance online publication. doi:10.1186/s12978-018-0527-2 PMID:29945657

Genuis, S. J., & Genuis, R. A. (2016). Preconception care: A new standard of care within maternal health services. *BioMed Research International*, *2016*, 1–30. doi:10.1155/2016/6150976 PMID:27314031

Hajela, N., Balakrish Nair, G., Ramakrishna, B. S., & Ganguly, N. K. (2014). Probiotic foods: Can their increasing use in India ameliorate the burden of chronic lifestyle disorders? *The Indian Journal of Medical Research*, *139*(1). https://www.ncbi.nlm.nih.gov/pmc/articles/PMC3994739/ PMID:24604038

Hantoushzadeh, S., Golshahi, F., Javadian, P., Khazardoost, S., Aram, S., Hashemi, S., Mirarmandehi, B., & Borna, S. (2011). Comparative efficacy of probiotic yoghurt and clindamycin in treatment of bacterial vaginosis in pregnant women: A randomized clinical trial. *The Journal of Maternal-Fetal & Neonatal Medicine*, *25*(7), 1021–1024. doi:10.3109/14767058.2011.614654 PMID:21854132

He, A., Chin, J., & Lomiguen, C. M. (2020). Benefits of probiotic yogurt consumption on maternal health and pregnancy outcomes: A systematic review. *Cureus*. Advance online publication. doi:10.7759/cureus.9408 PMID:32864237

ICMR. (2011). ICMR-DBT guidelines for evaluation of probiotics in food. *The Indian Journal of Medical Research*, *134*(1). https://pubmed.ncbi.nlm.nih.gov/21808130/ PMID:21808130

Kabeerdoss, J., Ferdous, S., Balamurugan, R., Mechenro, J., Vidya, R., Santhanam, S., Jana, A. K., & Ramakrishna, B. S. (2013). Development of the gut microbiota in southern Indian infants from birth to 6 months: A molecular analysis. *Journal of Nutritional Science*, *3*, e2. Advance online publication. doi:10.1017/jns.2013.6 PMID:25191566

Khalesi, S., Vandelanotte, C., Thwaite, T., Russell, A. M., Dawson, D., & Williams, S. L. (2020). Awareness and attitudes of gut health, probiotics and prebiotics in Australian adults. *Journal of Dietary Supplements*, *18*(4), 418–432. doi:10.1080/19390211.2020.1783420 PMID:32588677

Liang, X., Li, Z., Tye, K. D., Chen, Y., Luo, H., & Xiao, X. (2020). The effect of probiotic supplementation during pregnancy on the interaction network of vaginal microbiome. *Journal of Obstetrics and Gynaecology Research*, *47*(1), 103–113. doi:10.1111/jog.14434 PMID:32885568

Maternal Health Task Force. (2018, June 27). *The sustainable development goals and maternal mortality*. https://www.mhtf.org/topics/the-sustainable-development-goals-and-maternal-mortality/

Mayer, E. A., Knight, R., Mazmanian, S. K., Cryan, J. F., & Tillisch, K. (2014). Gut microbes and the brain: Paradigm shift in neuroscience. *The Journal of Neuroscience : The Official Journal of the Society for Neuroscience*, *34*(46), 15490–15496. doi:10.1523/JNEUROSCI.3299-14.2014 PMID:25392516

McDonald, B., & McCoy, K. D. (2019). Maternal microbiota in pregnancy and early life. *Science*, *365*(6457), 984–985. doi:10.1126/science.aay0618 PMID:31488675

Mirghafourvand, M., Homayouni Rad, A., Mohammad Alizadeh Charandabi, S., Fardiazar, Z., & Shokri, K. (2016). The effect of probiotic yogurt on constipation in pregnant women: A randomized controlled clinical trial. *Iranian Red Crescent Medical Journal*, *18*(11). Advance online publication. doi:10.5812/ircmj.39870 PMID:28203450

Otuto Amarauche, C. (2015). Assessing the awareness and knowledge on the use of probiotics by healthcare professionals in Nigeria. *Journal of Young Pharmacists : JYP*, *8*(1), 53–55. doi:10.5530/jyp.2016.1.12

Pettoello-Mantovani, M., Çullu Çokuğraş, F., Vural, M., Mestrovic, J., Nigri, L., Piazzolla, R., Giardino, I., Conoscitore, M., & Namazova-Baranova, L. (2019). Pilot study for the understanding and use of probiotics by different paediatric healthcare professionals working in different European countries. *Italian Journal of Pediatrics*, *45*(1), 57. Advance online publication. doi:10.1186/s13052-019-0648-4 PMID:31053146

Raghuwanshi, S., Misra, S., Sharma, R., & Bisen, P. S. (2015). Indian perspective for probiotics: A review. *Indian Journal of Dairy Science*, *68*(3). https://www.researchgate.net/publication/280704426_Indian_perspective_for_probiotics_A_review

Ratsika, A., Codagnone, M. C., O'Mahony, S., Stanton, C., & Cryan, J. F. (2021). Priming for life: Early life nutrition and the microbiota-gut-Brain Axis. *Nutrients, 13*(2), 423. doi:10.3390/nu13020423 PMID:33525617

Rutten, N., Van der Gugten, A., Uiterwaal, C., Vlieger, A., Rijkers, G., & Van der Ent, K. (2015). Maternal use of probiotics during pregnancy and effects on their offspring's health in an unselected population. *European Journal of Pediatrics, 175*(2), 229–235. doi:10.1007/s00431-015-2618-1 PMID:26319129

Samanta, A. K., Kolte, A. P., Senani, S., Sridhar, M., & Jayapal, N. (2011). Prebiotics in ancient Indian diets. *Current Science, 101*(1).

Sanders, M. E., Merenstein, D. J., Ouwehand, A. C., Reid, G., Salminen, S., Cabana, M. D., Paraskevakos, G., & Leyer, G. (2016). Probiotic use in at-risk populations. *Journal of the American Pharmacists Association, 56*(6), 680–686. doi:10.1016/j.japh.2016.07.001 PMID:27836128

Sarkar, A., Lehto, S. M., Harty, S., Dinan, T. G., Cryan, J. F., & Burnet, P. W. (2016). Psychobiotics and the manipulation of bacteria–gut–Brain signals. *Trends in Neurosciences, 39*(11), 763–781. doi:10.1016/j.tins.2016.09.002 PMID:27793434

Sharma, R., Gupta, S., Gupta, D., & Kushwaha, P. K. (2019). Awareness and knowledge about probiotics among college students. *Journal of Pure & Applied Microbiology, 13*(4), 2201–2208. doi:10.22207/JPAM.13.4.33

Siltrakool, B. (2017). *Assessment of Community Pharmacists' Knowledge, Attitude and Practice Regarding Non-Prescription Antimicrobial Use and Resistance in Thailand* [Master's thesis]. https://www.researchgate.net/publication/322675323_Assessment_of_Community_Pharmacists%27_Knowledge_Attitude_and_Practice_Regarding_Non-Prescription_Antimicrobial_Use_and_Resistance_in_Thailand

Soni, R., Tank, K., & Jain, N. (2018). Knowledge, attitude and practice of health professionals about probiotic use in Ahmedabad, India. *Nutrition & Food Science, 48*(1), 125–135. doi:10.1108/NFS-02-2017-0032

Spencer, S. J., Korosi, A., Layé, S., Shukitt-Hale, B., & Barrientos, R. M. (2017). Food for thought: How nutrition impacts cognition and emotion. *npj Science of Food, 1*(1). doi:10.1038/s41538-017-0008-y

Swartwout, B., & Luo, X. M. (2018). Implications of probiotics on the maternal-neonatal interface: Gut microbiota, Immunomodulation, and autoimmunity. *Frontiers in Immunology, 9*, 2840. Advance online publication. doi:10.3389/fimmu.2018.02840 PMID:30559747

UNICEF. (n.d.). *Maternal health*. https://www.unicef.org/india/what-we-do/maternal-health

United Nations Statistics Division. (2016). —*SDG indicators*. https://unstats.un.org/sdgs/report/2016/

WangQ.Santos FerreiraD. L.NelsonS. M.SattarN.Ala-KorpelaM.LawlorD. A. (2017). Metabolic characterization of menopause: Cross-sectional and longitudinal evidence. doi:10.1101/195909

WHO. (2015). *Strategies toward ending preventable maternal mortality (EPMM)*. World Health Organization. https://www.who.int/reproductivehealth/topics/maternal_perinatal/epmm/en/

WHO. (2019, September 19). *Maternal mortality*. https://www.who.int/news-room/fact-sheets/detail/maternal-mortality

Yilmaz-Ersan, L., Ozcan, T., & Akpinar-Bayizit, A. (2020). Assessment of socio-demographic factors, health status and the knowledge on probiotic dairy products. *Food Science and Human Wellness*, *9*(3), 272–279. doi:10.1016/j.fshw.2020.05.004

Chapter 10
Analysis of Teenage Pregnancy and Contraception Methods on National Family Health Survey (NFHS-5) Data

D. Lakshmi
https://orcid.org/0000-0003-4018-1208
VIT Bhopal University, India

Shreya Santosh Shetye
VIT Bhopal University, India

Karishni Mehta
Dwarkadas J. College of Engineering, India

Vaishnavi Patil
K.J. Somaiya College of Engineering, India

ABSTRACT

To understand the causes and consequences of the rising rates of teenage pregnancy, we utilized the National Family Health Survey (NFHS-5) dataset to explore various factors, including contraception methods employed across India. Employing Python programming, we conducted a cluster analysis to examine data patterns and similarities. Our investigation aimed to establish a potential causal link between adolescent pregnancy and variables such as age, educational attainment, and internet usage. The findings suggest that higher literacy levels are associated with a reduction in teenage pregnancies. Additionally, teenage pregnancies contribute to an increased risk of anemia among pregnant women aged 15-19. Over the past two decades, the prevalence of anemia among Indian women of reproductive age has been 20% higher than the global average. In India, one in every two women is anemic, exceeding the global ratio of one in every three women. Among pregnant women, the incidence of anemia varies from 33% to 89%, with adolescent girls experiencing a rate exceeding 60%.

DOI: 10.4018/978-1-7998-9652-4.ch010

1. INTRODUCTION

Globally, investigations into teenage pregnancy employ both quantitative and qualitative surveys and questionnaires. Many countries prioritize efforts to prevent adolescent pregnancies and enhance newborn health. As indicated by Tripp and Viner (2005), teen pregnancy is more prevalent among those facing financial challenges, with a 60% higher rate of infant mortality and low birth weight compared to infants born to older mothers. Factors contributing to adolescent pregnancy include low literacy, early marriage, unwanted sexual activity due to partner pressure, economic hardship, sexual abuse, insufficient knowledge about contraception methods, hesitancy to use available methods, and fear of acquiring contraceptives, as highlighted by Gipson et al. (2008) and As-Sanie et al. (2004). Conducting thorough research will yield evidence-based insights for health promotion, aiding government agencies in developing targeted initiatives, training programs, and health camps.

Contraception serves as a preventive measure against both pregnancy and Sexually Transmitted Diseases. Adolescents must receive education on contraception to enable informed and health-conscious choices. Curtis et al. (2016) outline various contraceptive options for both women and men, taking into account individual medical conditions and characteristics.

The recent release of the initial data batch from the National Family Health Survey 5 conducted in 2019-20, four years after the previous survey in 2015-16, provides one of the most comprehensive sets of large-scale statistical information on health, family welfare, and emerging issues in this domain. A thorough examination of data from all states reveals a decline in the nutritional status of children under five, with continuous female sterilization being the predominant modern contraception method. There is also a higher prevalence of anemia among women compared to men and an uptick in adolescent pregnancies. Evidence-based reviews derived from this data aid in identifying effective interventions, ensuring optimal resource utilization. It's important to note that these review results are meant for those involved in the development and administration of programs; they do not guide health practitioners on program implementation.

The chapter is organized as follows. Section 2- Materials and Methods include data description, cleaning, and analysis; Section 3- Inferences and Discussions; Section 4- Conclusion.

2. MATERIAL AND METHODS

2.1 Data Description

The NFHS survey is a comprehensive, multi-round examination of households in India. Its main objectives are twofold: firstly, to provide crucial information on health and family welfare for the Ministry of Health and Family Welfare and other government agencies to inform policy and program development; and secondly, to gather data on emerging health and family welfare issues. The statistics utilized in this research for analysis and conclusions primarily originate from the NFHS-5, which surveyed 6.1 lakh households in the year 2019-20. The dataset was acquired through an email request to the official website (Open database, 2022).

In this study, the following features are considered in the analysis:

- Fertility
- Infant and child mortality
- The practice of family planning
- Maternal and child health
- Reproductive health
- Nutrition
- Anemia
- Utilization and quality of health and family planning services

The NFHS-5 gathered information on the percentage of women and men who accessed the Internet for the first time in 2019. The dataset comprises 36 rows, each representing states and union territories of India, with an additional row providing an overview of the entire country. Each of these rows contains 131 features. In this study, 23 specific features are of interest, including data on 'Women aged 15-19 years who were already mothers or pregnant at the time of the survey (%)', 'The adolescent fertility rate for women aged 15-19 years', 'Female sterilization (%)', and others. Tables 1 and 2 display a sample dataset.

Table 1. Features

	Indicators in the NFHS-5 dataset
F1	**Female population age 6 years and above who ever attended school (%)**
F2	Population below age 15 years (%)
F3	Sex ratio of the total population (females per 1,000 males)
F4	Sex ratio at birth for children born in the last five years (females per 1,000 males)
F5	Children under the age of 5 years whose birth was registered with the civil authority (%)
F6	Deaths in the last 3 years registered with the civil authority (%)
F7	Population living in households with electricity (%)
F8	Population living in households with an improved drinking-water source1 (%)
F9	Population living in households that use an improved sanitation facility2 (%)
…	
F129	Men aged 15 years and above who use any kind of tobacco (%)
F130	Women aged 15 years and above who consume alcohol (%)
F131	Men aged 15 years and above who consume alcohol (%)

Table 2. Sample data

	Indicators	F1	F2	F3	F4	F5	F6	F7	F8	F9	….	F129	F130	F131
0	AN	71.8	26.5	1020	929	89.1	70.8	96.8	95.9	70.2	….	38	1.3	18.8
1	AP	83.5	20.8	963	914	97.4	90.9	97.6	96.3	88	….	58.7	5	39.1
2	AR	65.6	22.2	1045	934	92.2	80.2	99.5	96.7	77.3	….	22.6	0.5	23.3
3	AS	71.2	27.1	997	979	87.7	34.5	94.8	93.7	82.9	….	50.3	24.2	52.7
4	BR	78.2	28.3	1012	964	96.3	65.5	92.6	86	68.6	….	51.8	7.3	25.1

Figure 1 depicts the methodology applied to the data analysis. The following steps are carried out: a) data cleansing and data preparation; b) elimination of null values; c) extraction of essential information; d) exploratory analysis; and e) clustering.

Figure 1. Methodology used in data analysis

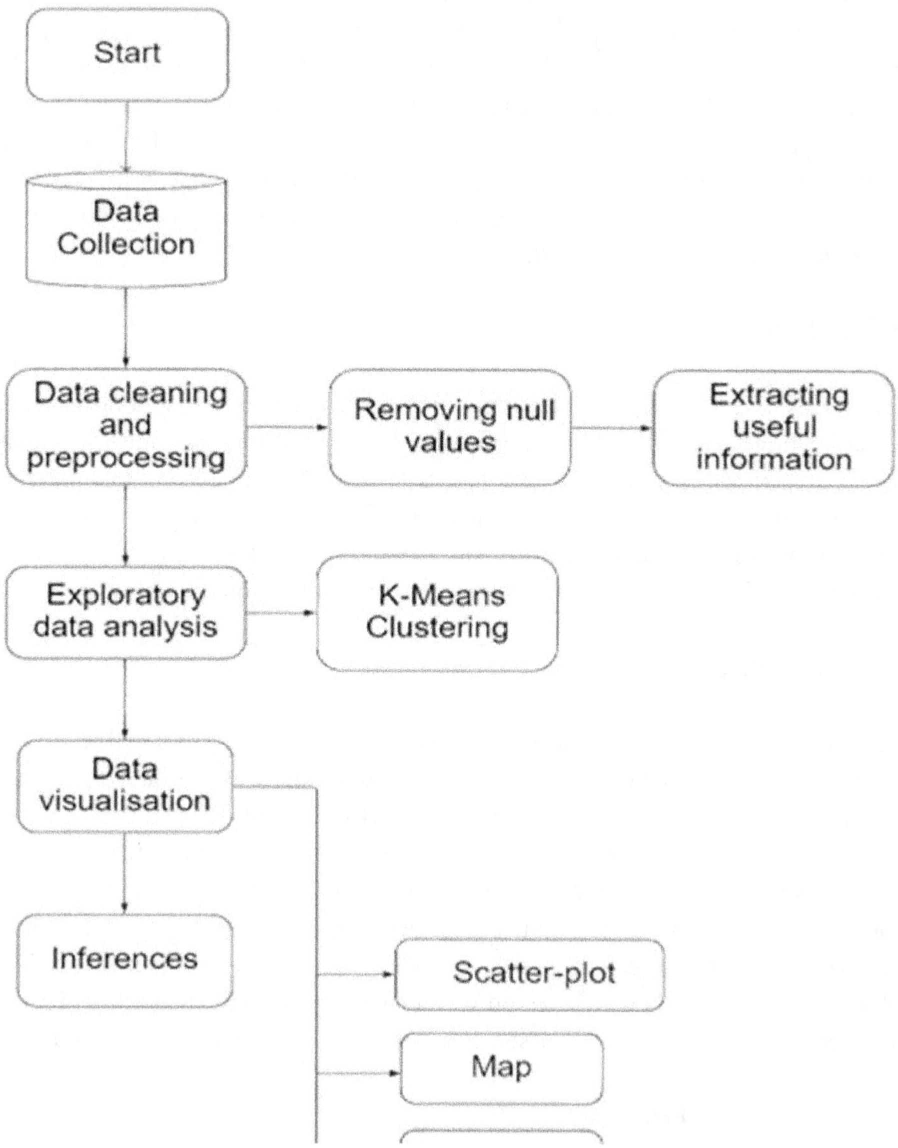

2.2 Data Cleaning

The process of data cleaning encompasses tasks such as eliminating unnecessary rows and columns, handling null values through deletion or replacement, and consolidating well-organized data into a single table or linked tables for analytical purposes. According to Simpson (2015), cleaning and transforming datasets into a machine-learning format contributes to improved performance.

Before training the clustering and correlation models, preprocessing was applied to the NFHS dataset. The clustered data retained specific columns like '% of women with ten or more years of education,' 'percentage of males with ten or more years of education,' 'percentage of women aged 15-19 who were already mothers or pregnant at the time of the survey,' and 'States.' In our study examining the relationship between women's education and teenage pregnancy rates, crucial components have been preserved.

2.3 Data Analysis

Data Analysis is the process of cleaning, converting, and modeling data so that we can identify significant and relevant information for decision-making (Sutton & Austin, 2015). In this paper, the necessary inferences are made for the decision-making on the welfare of the general population of the Indian nation. The goal is to extract usable information from data and make decisions based on that knowledge. The analysis was done on the records of all the states as well as the union territories of India.

2.3.1 Correlation

Correlation relates to two or more variables statistically. These variables may be raw data used to predict our target variable. Correlation measures how one variable affects another. It shows the relationship between two variables (Schober et al., 2018).

This paper evaluates the association between external variables such as 'women married before 18', 'women and men with 10 or more years of schooling, and 'women and men who have used the internet' and teen pregnancy rates in each state using Pearson correlation approach. Teen pregnancy correlates positively with Child Marriage, but adversely with Men and Women with 10+ years of schooling. Teenage pregnancy was also negatively associated with internet access and knowledge.

2.3.2 Data Visualisation

The graphical depiction of information and data is known as data visualization. It enables us to gain insights into massive amounts of data and recognize new patterns and flaws. Making sense of these patterns allows us to focus on regions that raise red flags or signal progress. As a result of this process, it is easier to make good, sound decisions that lead toward decision-making (Midway, 2020).

- Creating bar plots

There are many different ways to display data. A Bar Plot is an important graphic that is used in many applications and presentations. We have plotted a bar graph that shows us the distribution of the number of teenage girls who were already pregnant when the NFHS survey was being conducted.

- Maps

Geospatial maps allow one to create a context using shapes and colors to change the visual focus. We have shown the distribution of teenage pregnancy rates across various states, with dark blue being the states with the highest teenage pregnancy rates and dark red with the lowest.

- Scatterplots

Scatter plots have been used to help visualize the relationship between teenage pregnancy rates in the states of India vs. various external attributes like the level of education of both men and women, child marriage, and access to the internet.

2.4 Clustering

Clustering algorithms were used to analyze NFHS data. Clustering is an unsupervised learning algorithm. It classifies samples or data points into groups so they are comparable to each other and distinct from other groupings (Benabdellah et al., 2019).

We clustered using K-Means. K-Means clusters data by dividing samples into n equal variance groups while lowering the inertia or sum-of-squares criterion. This method requires cluster counts. It can process massive amounts of data and has been used in many sectors (Sinaga & Yang, 2020) and (Jin & Han, 2011).

K-Means Clustering was based on 'the percentage of women with at least 10 years of schooling' and 'the percentage of 15- to 19-year-old moms or pregnant at the time of the survey. Once the number of clusters, k, was calculated, each data point in this two-dimensional space was randomly assigned to one. Then, each data point is reassigned to the cluster centroid that is closest to it. Repeat the two methods until global equilibrium is reached. The programme ends if no data point is reassigned for two iterations.

3. INFERENCES AND DISCUSSIONS

3.1 Identifying teenage pregnancy as an important issue in India

As per the news report (Observer Research Foundation, 2020), 15% of young women globally give birth before the age of 18. Maternal disorders are a leading cause of disability-adjusted life years (DALYs) and death in 15-19-year-old girls globally. 6.8% of 15-19-year-old women were moms or pregnant at the time of the survey, while India's adolescent fertility rate is 43%. Teen pregnancy costs India $7.7 billion annually, according to the UN. The health ministry reports that adolescent pregnancies account for 12% of the nation's GDP expenditure.

Child marriage, teen pregnancies, and adolescent malnutrition haven't improved in India. Given that India will have the world's highest adolescent girl population of 95 million by 2030, it's crucial to reduce child marriages and teenage pregnancies to improve mother and infant mortality rates. Figure 2 shows India's teen birth rate per state.

Figure 2. State-wise representation of adolescent fertility rate
(Dark blue and dark red represent low and high adolescent fertility rates respectively.)

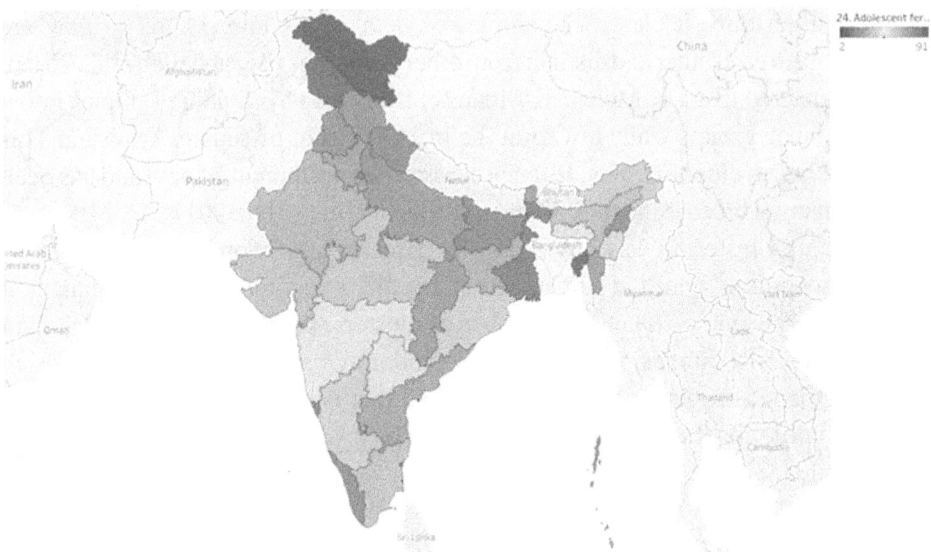

3.2 Analyzing teenage pregnancy across all states in India

Figure 3 illustrates the percentage of teenage girls who were already mothers at the time of the NFHS survey completion in each state.

Figure 3. Bar chart representation of teenage pregnancy across all states

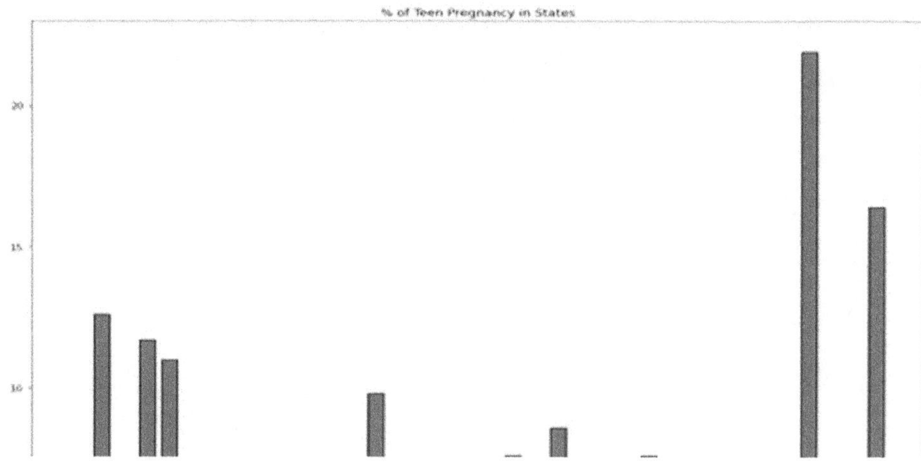

Figure 4 shows the percentage of adolescent moms in each state during the NFHS survey. Tripura, West Bengal, Andhra Pradesh, Assam, and Bihar have the highest teen pregnancy rates; Kerala, Lakshadweep, J&K, Chandigarh, and Ladakh have the lowest. Four of the top five states are in eastern India, while the fifth is in the south. Northern and southern India have low teen pregnancy rates.

Figure 4. Geographical representation of women aged 15-19 who were pregnant or already mothers (Dark blue and dark red represent the least and highest number of women 15-19 who were pregnant or already mothers respectively)

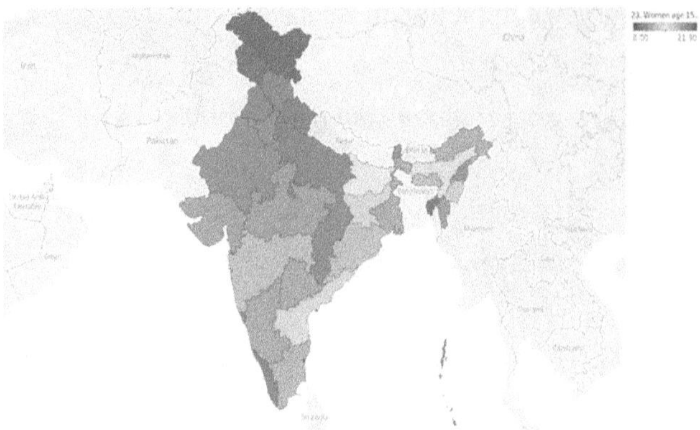

3.3 Correlating external factors with teenage pregnancy

In this section, we aim to identify the factors influencing adolescent pregnancies and those that can help reduce them. Here, we rely on the correlation coefficient between adolescent pregnancies and other variables.

3.3.1 Child marriages

In India, 23.3% of 20-24-year-old women were married before age 18. The 0.84 is the correlation between women married before 18 and adolescent moms. This is disturbing, especially considering Karnataka had the most child marriages during Covid-19. In 2020-2021, 296 child marriages were reported, up 49% from 2019-2020. Karnataka enters the top ten states with the most young mothers due to teen pregnancies.

Despite efforts, underage weddings are rising in several states. Tripura (40.1%, up from 33.1% in 2015-16), Manipur (16.3%, up from 13.7%), and Assam (31.8%, up from 30.8%) have seen increases in child weddings, while West Bengal (41.6%) and Bihar (40.8%) have high rates. Figure 5 depicts the association between early marriage and adolescent fertility in India.

Figure 5. Scatter plot between adolescent fertility rate and women married before 18 years

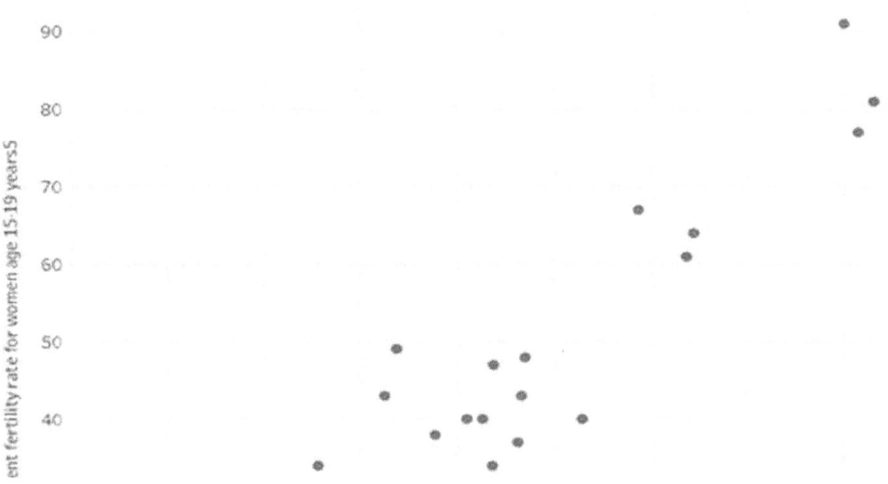

3.3.2 Literacy

The correlation coefficient between adolescent fertility and women with 10 or more years of schooling is -0.61, and that of men with 10 or more years of schooling is -0.67, as shown in Figures 6a and 6b. Literacy and adolescent pregnancy are negatively connected, leading to the conclusion that, despite the mild correlation, raising the literacy rate will significantly aid in reducing the teen pregnancy rate. As shown in Figure 6b, there is also a significant correlation between increasing the education level of men and decreasing teenage pregnancy.

Figure 6. (a) Scatter plot between adolescent fertility and men with 10 or more years of schooling and (b) Scatter plot between adolescent fertility and women with 10 or more years of schooling

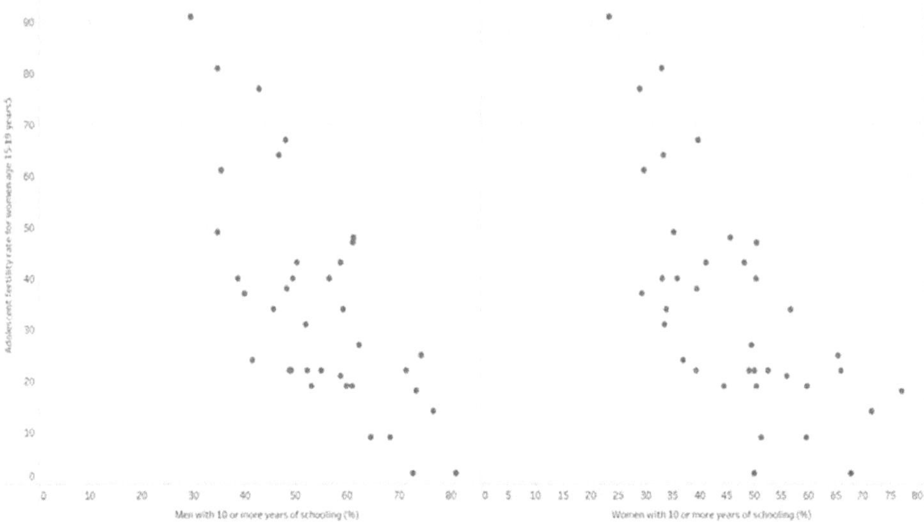

3.3.3 Internet usage

According to Figures 7a and 7b, there is a moderate correlation of -0.6 and -0.65 between teenage pregnancy and women and men who have access to and use the internet. This shows that the usage of the internet, by both men and women, has a positive effect on the population and can help to reduce teenage pregnancy, it being a source of knowledge.

Figure 7. (a) Scatter plot between adolescent fertility rate and women who have used the internet and (b) Scatter plot between adolescent fertility rate and men who have used the internet

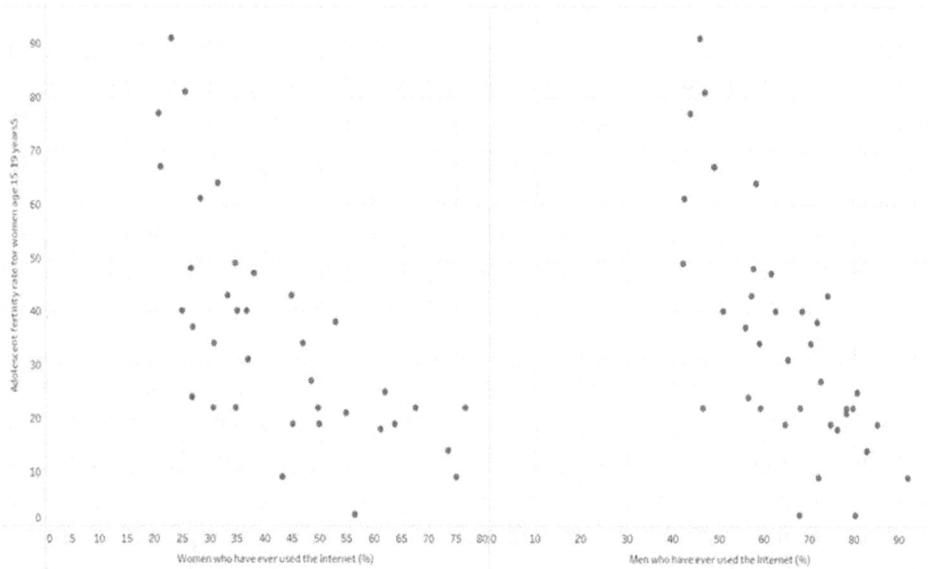

3.4 Causes and Effects of Teenage Pregnancy

3.4.1 Anemia

As per the news report (News Editorials, 2021), among all women in the age group 15-19 years, about 59.1% were anemic. Anemia rates in Indian states have risen among children under five (58.6% to 67%), women (53.1% to 57%), and men (22.7% to 25%), surpassing the 20%-40% moderate incidence range. It can be stated that anemia is seen to be much higher in women as compared to men.

A pregnant woman needs 15 milligrams of iron per day to survive herself and the baby. Iron deficiency raises the risk of maternal mortality. India has low maternal health. India has 80% of all anemia-related maternal deaths, whereas Southeast Asia has 50%.

Despite a considerable rise in IFA tablets (Mithra et al., 2014) used by pregnant women for 180 days or longer, anemia incidences have grown in half the States/UTs during NFHS-4. Teenage mothers had a higher risk of anemia, according to a study. Teenage pregnancies raise anemia risk in 15 to 19-year-olds. Iron supplements reduce neonatal complications. Anemia affects 33% to 89% of pregnant women and 60% of adolescent girls. Figure 8 shows adolescent pregnancy and anemia in India, where we can observe that all states except Kerala have "severe anemia" (39.4%).

Figure 8. The Ratio of Adolescent Pregnancy and Anaemic in States of India
The size of the dot represents the teenage pregnancy rate. Bigger sizes represent higher rates. Dark blue and dark red colors of the dots represent low and high numbers of anemia patients in each state.

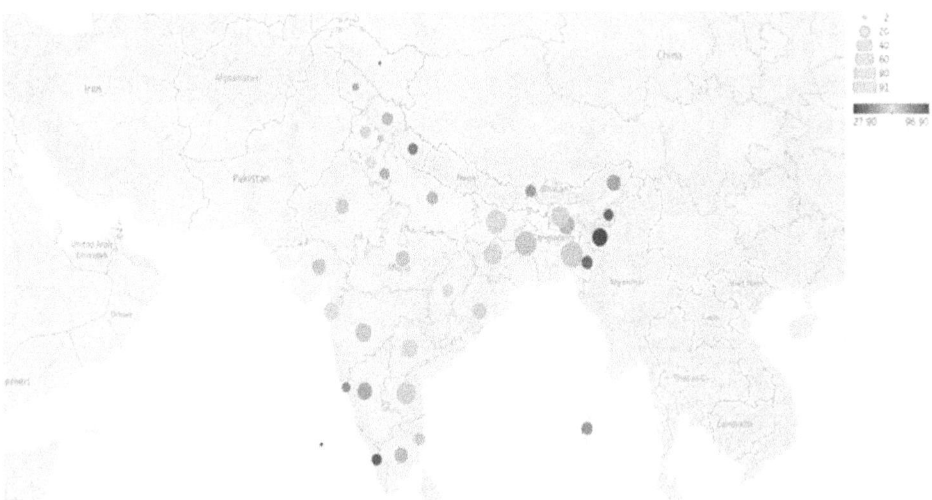

3.4.2 Use of contraception

Female sterilization (Stuart & Ramesh, 2018) was the most common method of contraception in Andhra Pradesh (98%), Telangana (93%), Kerala (88%), Karnataka (84%), Bihar (78%), and Maharashtra (77%). Figure 9 displays India's family planning practices. Female sterilisation was at a maximum of 37.9% of all procedures employed. Condom (9.5%), pill (5.1%), IUD PPIUD (2.1%), injectables (0.6%), and male sterilisation followed (0.3 percent). Only 66.7% of Indians practice family planning, while 56.5% use modern methods. In India, just 23.9% of health workers had ever talked to female non-users about family planning, and no data exists for male non-users.

Figure 9. Pie chart showing the distribution of types of contraceptives used in India

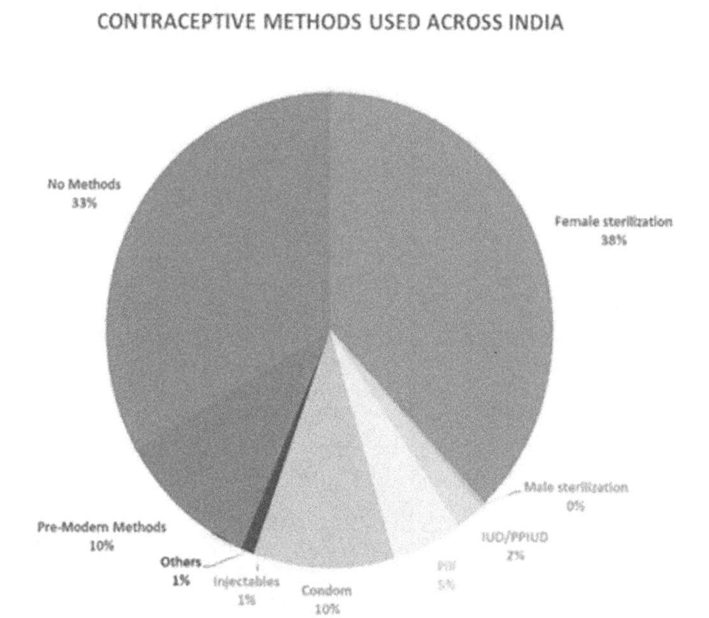

3.5 Clustering

NFHS data were clustered based on the percentage of women with 10 or more years of schooling and the percentage of 15-19-year-old moms or pregnant women at the time of the survey. Three clusters were found. Figure 10 shows states with a larger percentage of women with 10 or more years of schooling and a lower percentage of 15-19-year-old mothers or pregnant women. These were northern and southern Indian states. The purple cluster shows states with a moderate percentage of women with 10 or more years of schooling and 15-19-year-old moms or pregnant women at the time of the survey. These included India's northern, southern, and eastern states. The third teal cluster reflects states with fewer women with 10 or more years of schooling and more 15-19-year-old moms or pregnant women at the time of the survey. These states are in India's central belt. Clustering helped us divide India's states based on women's education and adolescent pregnancy.

Figure 10. Women With 10 Or More Years Of Schooling Versus Teenage Pregnancy

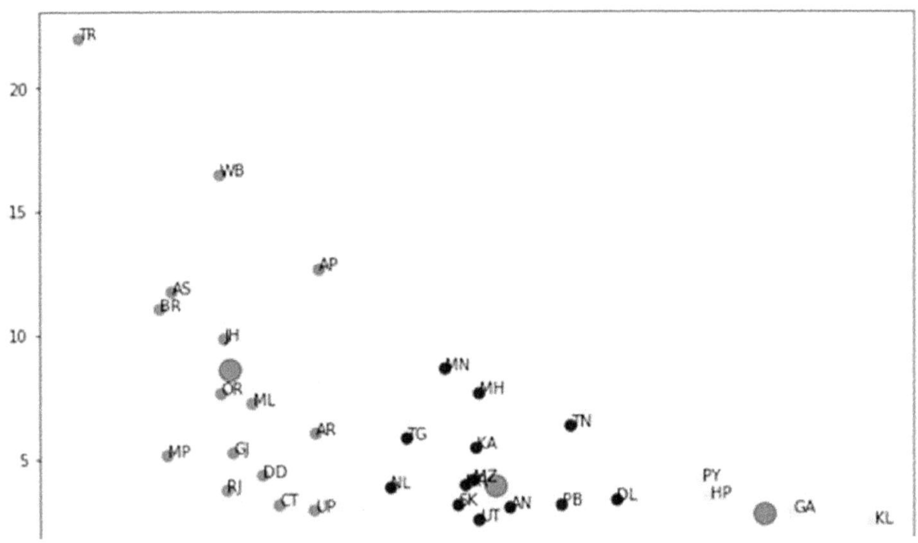

By visualizing the states on a map of India we further realize trends in the distribution of the categories in Figure 11.

Figure 11. Clusters formed during K-means are represented on the Indian Map

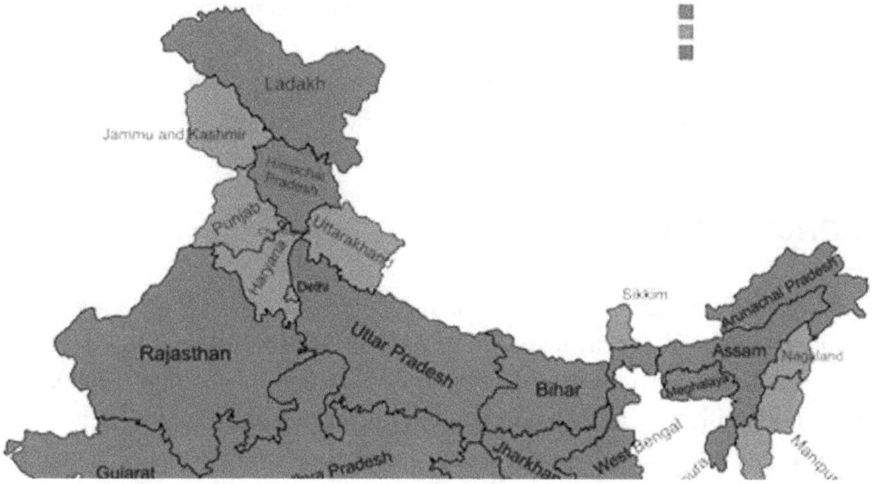

(The blue, pink and red states from figure 11 are represented by the teal, purple and yellow clusters in figure 10 respectively)

Factors Affecting Teenage Pregnancy

1. Early marriage
2. Poor literacy
3. No Internet Access

4. RECOMMENDATIONS

This section contains data-driven advice to help India overcome the aforementioned difficulties. The best solution to this problem is health literacy. Although educating adults is difficult, we can start with the young. We also need to highlight the significance of frequent checkups and encourage women to contact their doctors, especially gynecologists, to discuss contraceptives that are best for them.

In rural areas, men often refrain from opting for sterilization due to entrenched beliefs, such as skepticism toward female doctors. We advocate sending as many male doctors/social workers as possible to explain the male sterilization procedures (Reference Manual for Male Sterilization, 2019) such as promoting condoms, tablets,

IUDs, and injectables as viable family planning methods. We recommend using celebrities to increase awareness.

To discourage young girls from getting married and pregnant, advocate giving incentives to young women and their families to keep them in school; one such incentive could be introducing job training programmes for unmarried and/or pregnant young women, that guarantee a job after the training.

5. CONCLUSION

The research findings indicate that an increase in literacy is associated with a reduction in teenage pregnancies. To address teen pregnancy, it is beneficial to promote education and internet usage in rural India. Family planning methods other than female sterilization are considered safer and less detrimental to a woman's well-being. Despite female sterilization being the most prevalent form of birth control in India at 37%, male sterilization (0.3%), condoms, and pills are seldom utilized. Health or family planning workers play a crucial role in educating users about safer contraceptive methods, potential side effects, and appropriate actions in case of side effects. With only 5.6% of condom users in India, there is a need to emphasize the shared responsibility of family planning between men and women, addressing the significant issue of men's lack of education and accountability. Promoting education and internet use, especially in rural areas of India, can be instrumental in addressing the challenge of teenage pregnancy. It is vital to encourage the adoption of family planning methods that are considerably safer and less harmful to women's health than female sterilization.

REFERENCES

As-Sanie, S., Gantt, A., & Rosenthal, M. S. (2004). Pregnancy prevention in adolescents. *American Family Physician*, *70*(8), 1517–1524. PMID:15526738

Benabdellah, A. C., Benghabrit, A., & Bouhaddou, I. (2019). A survey of clustering algorithms for an industrial context. *Procedia Computer Science*, *148*, 291–302. doi:10.1016/j.procs.2019.01.022

Curtis, K. M., Tepper, N. K., Jatlaoui, T. C., Berry-Bibee, E., Horton, L. G., Zapata, L. B., ... & Whiteman, M. K. (2016). US medical eligibility criteria for contraceptive use, 2016. *Morbidity and Mortality Weekly Report: Recommendations and Reports*, *65*(3), 1-103. DOI: http://dx.doi.org/ icon doi:10.15585/mmwr.rr6503a1external

Gipson, J. D., Koenig, M. A., & Hindin, M. J. (2008). The effects of unintended pregnancy on infant, child, and parental health: A review of the literature. *Studies in Family Planning, 39*(1), 18–38. doi:10.1111/j.1728-4465.2008.00148.x PMID:18540521

Jin, X., & Han, J. (2011). *K*-Means Clustering. In C. Sammut & G. I. Webb (Eds.), *Encyclopedia of Machine Learning*. Springer., doi:10.1007/978-0-387-30164-8_425

Midway, S. R. (2020). Principles of effective data visualization. *Patterns (New York, N.Y.), 1*(9), 100141. Advance online publication. doi:10.1016/j.patter.2020.100141 PMID:33336199

Mithra, P., Unnikrishnan, B., Rekha, T., Nithin, K., Mohan, K., Kulkarni, V., Holla, R., & Agarwal, D. (2014). Compliance with iron-folic acid (IFA) therapy among pregnant women in an urban area of south India. *African Health Sciences, 14*(1), 255–260. doi:10.4314/ahs.v14i1.39 PMID:26060488

News Editorials. India: [updated 2021 Nov 27]. Available from: https://www.drishtiias.com/daily-news-editorials/nfhs-5-a-closer-look

Observer Research Foundation. India: [updated 2020 Jan 14]. Available from: https://www.orfonline.org/research/theres-a-need-to-end-teenage-pregnancies-in-india-its-harming-the-national-economy-60307/

Open database: National Family Health Survey (NFHS5) certified by the Ministry of Health and Family Welfare (MoHFW), India http://rchiips.org/nfhs/data1.shtml

Reference Manual for Male Sterilization. Family Planning Division Ministry of Health and Family Welfare Government of India. [updated October 2019]. Available from: https://nhm.gov.in/images/pdf/programmes/family-planing/guidelines/Reference_Manual_for_Male_Sterilization-NSV-Oct_2013.pdf

Schober, P., Boer, C., & Schwarte, L. A. (2018). Correlation coefficients: Appropriate use and interpretation. *Anesthesia and Analgesia, 126*(5), 1763–1768. doi:10.1213/ANE.0000000000002864 PMID:29481436

Simpson, S. H. (2015). Creating a data analysis plan: What to consider when choosing statistics for a study. *The Canadian Journal of Hospital Pharmacy, 68*(4), 311. doi:10.4212/cjhp.v68i4.1471 PMID:26327705

Sinaga, K. P., & Yang, M. S. (2020). Unsupervised K-means clustering algorithm. *IEEE Access : Practical Innovations, Open Solutions, 8*, 80716–80727. doi:10.1109/ACCESS.2020.2988796

Stuart, G. S., & Ramesh, S. S. (2018). Interval female sterilization. *Obstetrics and Gynecology*, *131*(1), 117–124. doi:10.1097/AOG.0000000000002376 PMID:29215509

Sutton, J., & Austin, Z. (2015). Qualitative research: Data collection, analysis, and management. *The Canadian Journal of Hospital Pharmacy*, *68*(3), 226. doi:10.4212/cjhp.v68i3.1456 PMID:26157184

Tripp, J., & Viner, R. (2005). Sexual health, contraception, and teenage pregnancy. *BMJ (Clinical Research Ed.)*, *330*(7491), 590–593. doi:10.1136/bmj.330.7491.590 PMID:15761001

Chapter 11
The Intersectionality of the Opioid Crisis and Cancer Treatment

Siddhi Surawkar
Polygence Research Academy, USA

ABSTRACT

Since the 1990s, more than 500,000 deaths have been recorded in the U.S. due to opioids, and the opioid crisis has become a leading cause of death. This risk is higher for individuals with cancer as they are prone to becoming addicted but need these drugs to manage chronic pain. In fact, about 75% of cancer patients use opioids but at least 19% of them show signs of misuse. The crisis has cost the U.S. billions of dollars in federal funding. Although the U.S. has increased the accessibility of substance abuse treatments and patient education programs, the stigma of seeking treatment for substance abuse and the necessity of opioids as an analgesic for cancer patients remain. To solve the American opioid crisis's impact on individuals with cancer, an awareness campaign is proposed, allowing for a decrease in stigmatization.

INTRODUCTION

The term "opioid" refers to a wide variety of drugs that can bind to opioid receptors (Krieger, n.d.). Opioids can be naturally derived from poppy plants or manufactured synthetically (Krieger, n.d.), with the latter becoming more popular in recent years due to greater potency (Synthetic opioids, 2020). Both methods of production create an analgesic that binds to opioid receptors, blocking those receptors from receiving

DOI: 10.4018/978-1-7998-9652-4.ch011

pain signals. This creates a numbing feeling which can be essential for those who suffer from severe chronic pain, like in the case of cancer patients (Bruera & Paice, 2015). However, these drugs are not without risk of side effects, including nausea, constipation, sedation, and addiction (Bruera & Paice, 2015). Higher doses have been shown to increase the threat of addiction, as have certain genetic factors (Bugada et al., 2020). However, genetic testing is not widely accessible, and higher doses may be necessary for individuals experiencing particularly severe pain, such as cancer patients (Bennett et al., 2018). Therefore, these issues regarding opioids are especially pertinent to Americans with cancer.

The first wave of the opioid crisis began in 1996 due to an increase in pharmaceutical advertising and an increased focus on patient comfort and quality of life, which led to more opioids being prescribed and about 20,000 opioid-related deaths occurring annually during this period (Understanding the opioid overdose epidemic, 2023; U.S. Congress Congressional Budget Office, 2022). The opioid crisis has continued in waves. The second wave occurred in 2010, with the rise of heroin, accounting for about 25,000 deaths each year. The third wave in 2013, occurring as fentanyl use increased, led to approximately 50,000 deaths per year (Understanding the opioid overdose epidemic, 2023; U.S. Congress Congressional Budget Office, 2022). A fourth wave seems to be imminent as more and more Americans begin mixing manufactured opioids with psycho-stimulants, such as cocaine and methamphetamine (Understanding the opioid overdose epidemic, 2023; U.S. Congress Congressional Budget Office, 2022).

In the last 30 years, more than 500,000 opioid-related deaths have been recorded, making them one of the top 10 leading causes of death in the United States (U.S. Congress Congressional Budget Office, 2022). The U.S. has spent billions of dollars and instituted several bills to attempt to mitigate this crisis by increasing access to substance abuse treatments, educating communities about opioids, and providing services to those affected by substance abuse disorders (U.S. Congress Congressional Budget Office, 2022). However, opioids are a necessary analgesic for many patients with chronic conditions, namely those with cancer, and these bills have not been effective in curbing the crisis in this unique population.

BACKGROUND

Prevalence

According to a 2017 study, more than 40 million people worldwide use opioids (Cheetham et al., 2022). This overuse of a powerful and addictive drug has caused concern in the U.S. as opioid drugs have become one of the top 10 causes of death

(U.S. Congress Congressional Budget Office, 2022). In fact, from 2000 to 2022, there was approximately a 5-fold increase in opioid-related deaths, accounting for 500,000 deaths (Rosoff et al., 2021). About 10,000 people died due to prescription opioids in 2020 alone (U.S. Congress Congressional Budget Office, 2022). This does not mean opioids are inherently dangerous, however; they become dangerous when misused. In fact, 4.3 million Americans aged 12 and older admitted to using prescription opioid analgesics for non-medical reasons (Gasior et al., 2015). This has resulted in more than 16,500 deaths each year which equals about 46 deaths per day (Gasior et al., 2015). These drugs can also lead to long-lasting health issues. In the case of one woman who became addicted to opioids and then began purchasing street drugs to maintain the high, she developed hearing loss, digestive issues, and throat damage (Real Stories, 2020). Similar examples of opioid-users developing chronic health issues when misusing the drug have been widely reported. This issue is further compounded by opioid-users who sell their drugs to others once they no longer need them, as these opioids can land in the hands of Americans who misuse (Real Stories, 2020). In fact, more than 90% of opioid pills that are misused come from surplus prescription medication distributed by friends or family members (Beauchemin & Cogan, 2022).

Although opioids may be utilized as a drug of abuse, many Americans legitimately require opioids to manage pain, particularly patients with cancer. There are currently an estimated 16.9 million individuals with cancer in the U.S., with 1.9 million more individuals being diagnosed each year (Bulls et al., 2021). Approximately 75% of these millions of people use opioids to manage their chronic pain (Bulls et al., 2021; Page & Blanchard, 2019). Of this number, 19% showed signs of opioid misuse (Yennurajalingam et al., 2021), and 17% of cancer patients who received a mastectomy (Farmer, 2022) were found to have misused opioids. Due to the necessity of opioids as analgesics for Americans with cancer, it is important to understand how the opioid crisis affects this vulnerable population.

Community Impact

Opioid addictions detrimentally affect both opioid users and their communities. Opioid users struggle to find and maintain jobs, resulting in financial difficulty and strain on families (Gilbert, 2023; Greene et al., 2018; Sigurdsson et al., 2012). In fact, adults 50 years and older who had misused opioids were 40% less likely to be employed and currently employed older adults who had misused opioids were twice as likely to have experienced unemployment (Costa & Evans, 2022). Compounding this issue, is the evidence that every 1% increase in the unemployment rate is correlated with a 3.6% increase in the rate of opioid-related deaths and a 7% increase in the rate of opioid-related emergency department visits (Bohler et al., 2021). This leads to a vicious cycle of unemployment increasing due to the opioid crisis which in turn rises due to unemployment. As the unemployment rate rises (Overview United States, 2018), less money is put back into local economies and more funding is needed for public welfare programs. In fact, $55.7 billion of the national budget was allocated to reducing the misuse of prescription opioid analgesics in 2007 (Gasior et al., 2015). Between 2017 and 2020, the federal budget to alleviate the opioid crisis tripled from $2.1 billion to $6.1 billion (U.S. Congress Congressional Budget Office, 2022). This burden can be even higher when focusing on cancer patients who have developed an addiction, as they require treatment for not only opioid misuse disorders but also alternative medications, which are often expensive, to continue treating their chronic pain after they are weaned off opioids. Many communities with high rates of opioid use do not have the built-in funds to solve this crisis and thus must resort to redirecting funds from other sectors, such as education and local businesses.

Increased opioid use in communities also increases the likelihood of injury and illness, including an increase in traffic accidents and increased rates of infectious diseases like HIV and hepatitis; the risk for HIV in individuals who use opioids is 1.4% versus 0.3% risk for HIV in individuals who do not use opioids, and a 6.5% risk for hepatitis in individuals who use opioids versus 0.2% risk for hepatitis in individuals who do not use opioids. Furthermore, opioid misuse presents an increased risk for acute bacterial infections (Gasior et al., 2015). These rates may be higher among individuals with cancer due to the immunocompromising nature of cancer treatment. These contagious diseases can quickly spread through a community. Additionally, using opioids for at least 30 days increases an individual's chance of depression by 25% and approximately 30% of individuals with major depressive disorder show signs of opioid misuse (Rosoff et al., 2021). This creates the threat of additional trauma due to the suicide of loved ones and secondary depression cases. This increased rate of disease, injury, and death, both strains resources as well as causes emotional and physical trauma for community members who lose loved ones and must compensate by taking on additional responsibilities. For example, increased opioid use is correlated with a greater number of children in foster care which is a traumatizing experience for the child and the child's relatives, as well as a burden on the community's foster system (Bohler et al., 2021).

In addition, many first responders reported burnout due to the trauma of regularly assisting and attempting to save overdose victims, with 95% of first responders believing the increased rate of opioid use is affecting their job (Pike et al., 2019). In a series of interviews questioning these professionals about this burnout, they cited a lack of gratitude after revival, in addition to physical and mental exhaustion from reviving the same patient multiple times (First-Responder trauma and the opioid crisis, 2020). First responders rarely witness positive outcomes or full recovery for these individuals which can be demoralizing (First-Responder trauma and the opioid crisis, 2020). These effects are especially detrimental in low-income communities that do not have the resources to invest in effective opioid control (Bohler et al., 2021) and are targeted by law enforcement due to high rates of drug use (Kain, 2011). The opioid crisis strains low-income communities' limited and essential human and financial resources.

Relationship Between Cancer and the Opioid Crisis

Evidence shows 53% of cancer patients experience pain during or after treatment, and about 75% of cancer patients use opioids to manage their pain as these analgesics have shown to be largely effective (Bennett et al., 2018). However, as the body builds tolerance, one opioid becomes ineffective and another type must replace it, which can lead to increased tolerance and addiction to multiple types of opioids (Bruera & Paice, 2015; Mercadante, 1999; Real Stories, 2020). Many patients are not warned of the side effects of prolonged opioid use and thus may use them unnecessarily or take more than prescribed (Real Stories, 2020).

However, some individuals may misuse these drugs. Approximately 20% of cancer patients have a higher risk of developing a substance abuse disorder and misuse opioids within 8 weeks of a follow-up care appointment (Arthur & Bruera, 2022). Individuals with cancer also use prescribed opioids to manage the emotional distress (Bruera & Paice, 2015) and high levels of depression, anxiety, and hopelessness reported by cancer survivors (Harsanyi et al., 2023). This is especially pertinent after the COVID-19 pandemic which was especially isolating for those who were immunocompromised (Bohler et al., 2021) and thus could not build or maintain a support system during this time. Specific risk factors for opioid misuse disorders include being young, male, single, having a history of substance abuse, coming from a lower socio-economic background, or possessing a combination of these factors (Bruera & Paice, 2015). These patients are likely to switch to more potent drugs, such as heroin (Synthetic opioids, 2020), once their prescribed opioids run out or if their prescribed drugs stop giving them the same high that allows them to maintain their emotional condition and avoid withdrawal symptoms (Real Stories, 2020).

Individuals who use opioids often face barriers when seeking healthcare. They are frequently seen as unreliable sources of information regarding their health and their opinions are often dismissed (Cheetham et al., 2022). They are more likely to experience lower empathy, lower engagement, lesser encouragement for follow-up appointments, and face a paternalistic rather than collaborative approach to their care. Suspicions of misuse and professional biases result in these patients being labeled as "difficult" or attention-seeking and thus experiencing insufficient or interrupted care (Bulls et al., 2021). They may also be barred from participating in clinical trials due to concerns regarding the validity of their feedback (Cheetham et al., 2022). Americans battling cancer often rely on clinical trials for accessible and effective treatment. Thus, being prohibited from entering trials can be detrimental to their health. This negative patient experience partially occurs because medical staff who prescribe opioids are required to complete additional training which creates the false notion of opioids being an inherently dangerous and unnecessary class of drugs (Cheetham et al., 2022). It is also partially due to doctors who prescribe opioids often being blamed for overdoses and thus, can become burned out and dissatisfied with their job (Bulls et al., 2021). More than 70% of health care providers were concerned about the development of an opioid use disorder among their cancer patients, which made them less likely to prescribe opioid analgesics in order to mitigate this risk (Harsanyi et al., 2023). This has caused the opioid prescribing rate for patients on Medicare to drop by 21% among oncologists and 23% among all doctors between 2013 and 2017 (29). Patients using opioid analgesics may face verbal and non-verbal negative attitudes from the pharmacists who distribute these opioids (Cheetham et al., 2022). They may refuse to sell syringes or other medical equipment based on assumptions made from physical appearance (Cheetham et al., 2022). This bias can be particularly detrimental to individuals with cancer who may show more signs of drug use due to high and constant doses of various medications to manage the side effects of cancer treatment. In fact, 40% of oncological practices reported that their patients had trouble filling their prescriptions (Page & Blanchard, 2019) and globally, approximately 6 million individuals with cancer have inadequate or no access to opioids (Bennett et al., 2018). This has resulted in 32% of cancer patients in developed countries, such as the U.S., being undertreated for their pain (Bennett et al., 2018; Harsanyi et al., 2023). In such cases, stigma and oversight of the opioid prescription process cause cancer patients, who often desperately need opioids to manage their chronic pain, to face barriers in treatment which lessens their quality of life.

Relation to Health Literacy

Low health literacy among cancer survivors makes them more susceptible to opioid misuse. In fact, one in every six cancer survivors reported low health literacy, and about 5% reported they found it difficult to understand medical advice, while 9% reported they found it difficult to understand written or verbal medical instructions (Coughlin et al., 2022). This is consistent with evidence that individuals with chronic pain tend to find it more difficult to find, understand, and apply information regarding pain management options (Rogers et al., 2019). Additionally, evidence shows that most health education materials are written at a level too complex for most average Americans to understand (Rogers et al., 2019). Most guidelines suggest that such information not surpass a recommended 8th-grade reading level to be accessible to all Americans (Prince et al., 2019). However, these guidelines are often not met and more complicated medical jargon is used which affect readability and dissemination of information. Particular risk factors for lower health literacy include not having a high school diploma, having a lower household income, being unemployed, not having health insurance, and being black or Hispanic (Coughlin et al., 2022). This is greatly due to the lack of resources and information these populations have access to because of medical biases and institutionalized barriers to healthcare access. Additionally, patients are not commonly screened for health literacy levels when admitted to the hospital, which makes it difficult for physicians to gauge their level of understanding and speak in terms that the patient can comprehend and retain (Truong & Fenton, 2022). This lack of health literacy leads to less informed decisions being made regarding analgesics to manage chronic pain, which can increase a patient's likelihood of becoming addicted (Rogers et al., 2019). Many Americans, especially older individuals, state that they are confused by prescription instruction and feel that their usage directions need clarification (Improving opioid misuse prevention literacy between older adults and health care providers , 2019). In two public hospitals, 40% of patients could not understand the instructions they were given on their medication intake (Rogers et al., 2019). In fact, about 25% of patients prescribed opioids misuse them due to a lack of understanding of their proper usage (Wagner, 2023). Many patients cite that a lack of explanation regarding opioid prescriptions is particularly common among oncologists, who most commonly interact with cancer patients (Harsanyi et al., 2023).

Additionally, it should be considered that in the case of opioid misuse among cancer patients, it is essential for these Americans to not only understand the medical terminology associated with their care but also the policies that affect their ability to access opioids (Improving opioid misuse prevention literacy between older adults and health care providers , 2019). The governmental regulation of opioids results in strict policies that both prescribers and users must adhere to. This information may be difficult to understand, especially for cancer patients who must also simultaneously absorb medical information related to their treatment plans. This can result in a lack of understanding of the law (Improving opioid misuse prevention literacy between older adults and health care providers , 2019), which then creates fear around seeking out treatment as patients fear penalization and are unsure if they are eligible to receive help. It can also create a sense of shame as patients feel they are doing something wrong as they do not understand what protections these governmental policies provide them.

Current State of the Opioid Crisis

Due to the increased morbidity rates from opioid misuse (Bulls et al., 2021), the federal government created several regulations to counter the opioid crisis in America. In 2016, a series of several healthcare bills were passed, including the Comprehensive Addiction and Recovery Act (CARA), the 21st Century Cures Act, and the Substance Use-Disorder Prevention that Promotes Opioid Recovery and Treatment (SUPPORT) for Patients and Communities Act (U.S. Congress Congressional Budget Office, 2022). Together, these bills limit the supply of opioids; lower barriers to treatment by increasing Medicaid coverage; provide funds to popularize naloxone, methadone, and buprenorphine; and reunite families affected by opioid misuse disorders (U.S. Congress Congressional Budget Office, 2022). In 2021, the U.S. government approved $1.5 billion for preventing substance use disorders and $30 million for increased community support by distributing naloxone and creating syringe disposal sites (U.S. Congress Congressional Budget Office, 2022). These laws were moderately successful in increasing safe access to opioids and increasing community awareness.

However, despite these changes and additional funding, the opioid crisis continues due to institutional bias in the criminal justice system and mismanaged substance abuse treatment programs (Cheetham et al., 2022). Overregulation regarding drug distribution has resulted in opioid abuse treatment programs that contradict best practices due to a lack of accessibility to alternative, more effective methods (Treatment for U.S. opioid addicts often inadequate, researchers say, 2013). Such overregulation also causes alternative medications to be expensive, further complicating the process of weaning individuals off of opioids while still providing them with analgesics, a common goal for cancer patients (Treatment for U.S. opioid addicts often inadequate, researchers say, 2013). This hinders both cancer patients and non-cancer patients alike from accessing substance abuse treatment, and the limits on opioid prescriptions can lead to a lack of access to safe drugs for individuals with cancer.

In the U.S. there continues to be an emphasis on criminalization of drugs rather than an emphasis on rehabilitation (Islam & Mcrae, 2014; Kain, 2011). Therefore, people with opioid addictions often do not seek out the resources made available to them, as they fear being penalized or feel as though these resources do not provide adequate support (Stigma and discrimination, 2022; Treatment for U.S. opioid addicts often inadequate, researchers say, 2013). Stigma remains a major barrier to treatment, with 61% of cancer patients using opioids having faced stigma and 29% displaying stigma-related habits such as taking less medication despite their doctor's instructions (Bulls et al., 2021; Islam & Mcrae, 2014). Many reported feeling the need to reduce their use to prevent criticism from their community, which made them feel embarrassed and isolated (Anson, 2021). This results in many cancer patients refusing opioid medications as they associate opioids with shame (Cheetham et al.,

2022) and death (Bulls et al., 2021). These patients were also more likely to not share pain complaints with their physicians for fear of being judged or considered as liars due to the prevalent stigma towards those who seek out opioid analgesics (Harsanyi et al., 2023). Such concerns may reduce their quality of life as opioids are an important pain-management tool for those with cancer.

Most destigmatization campaigns have been family- or survivor-led and encourage people with substance abuse disorders to seek treatment. However, these programs are often hindered by existing stigma and a lack of national funding and attention. Individuals taking opioids are often seen as dangerous or weak, leading to ostracization (Cheetham et al., 2022) of the user and their loved ones, meaning these destigmatization programs are often ignored by the public. This is partially because, over a period of 15 years, less than 5% of media coverage of the opioid crisis mentioned the need for expanded substance abuse treatment programs, while greater than 60% stated that law enforcement was the solution (Bulls et al., 2021). The media often highlights instances of individuals lying to get opioids, leading to increased stigma for patients of color or of low socioeconomic backgrounds as these particular groups are most often suspected of falsely reporting their need for opioids due to systematic racial and classist biases in American society (Bulls et al., 2021). This leads to oversight that prevents individuals with cancer from getting necessary drugs while also criminalizing those patients who do get addicted. Evidence shows black and Hispanic cancer patients, particularly black men, in end-of-life care received fewer and smaller doses of opioids than white patients with comparable circumstances (Ben-Ari, 2023). They were also more likely to undergo urine drug tests, which further highlights how medical racial biases can create a barrier to access to necessary opioids (Ben-Ari, 2023). This hinders health literacy efforts that could allow patients to better understand and utilize the analgesics they are using because it discourages patients' questions due to the fear of being further stigmatized (McCurry et al., 2022). This fear leads to patients continuing to misuse opioids as they continue believing harmful misconceptions and fear seeking new information or assistance.

Some states have begun training law enforcement officials in the proper use of naloxone (an emergency treatment for opioid overdoses), or have passed Good Samaritan laws which provide immunity for those who call 911 when witnessing an overdose (Wagner et al., 2016). Although these have slightly decreased stigma, they are not widespread and many people of color who are often victimized by law enforcement still distrust this system. In fact, only 63% of overdose witnesses call 911, with 52% of them hesitating for 5 or more minutes due to a fear of being arrested (Wagner et al., 2016).

Current State of Health Literacy

Currently, most health literacy programs are focused on individuals with chronic illnesses, particularly prostate and skin cancer (Truong & Fenton, 2022). Some health literacy interventions make efforts to include researches and other academic sources, health professionals from the community and larger corporations, the patient's loved ones, and the patient themselves when developing the information (Truong & Fenton, 2022). However, this is not a widespread practice and most programs continue to primarily rely on academics and researchers rather than the local community and patients (Truong & Fenton, 2022). This is something that must be changed as most patients reported that they preferred to learn through connecting with others and being involved in their care team (Truong & Fenton, 2022). Improved patient outcomes, such as being more confident in their ability to communicate with medical providers, previously unmet needs being met, and being less likely to be misinformed by other community members, have been reported when patient and public involvement is encouraged (Truong & Fenton, 2022).

In particular, Chronic Disease Self-Management Education (CDSME) programs have been growing in popularity across the country (Improving opioid misuse prevention literacy between older adults and health care providers , 2019). This model of opioid use treatment among patients with chronic illnesses like cancer emphasizes voluntary participation and personal goal-setting (Improving opioid misuse prevention literacy between older adults and health care providers , 2019). It is led by individuals who have personal experience with the condition of the learners and encourage participants to deeply examine varying options for pain management and creating healthcare goals (Improving opioid misuse prevention literacy between older adults and health care providers , 2019). This allows for patients to take control of their treatment plans and advocate for their needs and wants. However, this does not ensure that cancer patients using opioids feel comfortable advocating for themselves to their medical providers. This can be due to a variety of factors, including a lack of comfort and transparency in the patient-physician relationship, a lack of confidence in their own knowledge, and medical biases that may prevent physicians from acknowledging and adapting to patients' needs. Additionally, the additional financial and temporal costs of attending these programs leaves disadvantaged populations, specifically those from a lower socioeconomic background, at risk as they often do not have the resources or the free time to attend such classes. It also affects cancer patients who often have frequent appointments as they also lack the time and sometimes energy to attend such classes due to their treatments. Other health literacy methods have also been shown to be lacking and experts encourage them to be re-evaluated and revamped to fit modern American's needs utilizing the new information we now have on treating opioid use disorders among cancer patients (Rogers et al., 2019).

PROPOSED SOLUTION

Public Campaign

The proposed solution is a national public destigmatization campaign focused on educating communities particularly affected by the opioid crisis, and professionals who regularly interact with individuals using opioids. The campaign would emphasize that Americans fighting cancer need opioids and also need community support to access substance abuse treatment. This campaign should focus on sharing personal stories, perhaps through partnerships with grassroots advocacy groups. It should also emphasize substance abuse treatments and explain the structural barriers to treatment that Americans with addictions may face (including a lack of insurance, medical programs, or alternative sources of necessary drugs) (Cheetham et al., 2022). This will increase knowledge of opioid addiction (Real Stories, 2020) and reduce fear of opioid users and opioids (Bulls et al., 2021; Harsanyi et al., 2023). Raising awareness can allow for more donors and ambassadors to get involved in the mission of ending the opioid crisis, as well as starting conversations (Beck, 2015) which is crucial to disseminating information and solving the root of the issue. Utilizing simple, relatable language and providing visual education has been shown to increase knowledge among cancer patients of their condition, allowing them to make better informed decisions (Housten et al., 2020). Health education has also been shown to enable patients to make a more accurate assessment of the risks of their medical decisions (Housten et al., 2020), allowing them to better understand the consequences of using and abusing opioids. Additionally, patients will be better informed, thus having the information they need to discuss concerns with their physicians and community (Harsanyi et al., 2023; Housten et al., 2020), instead of continuing to operate based on dangerous misconceptions due to a fear of being stigmatized. Reducing stigma will allow more patients to seek treatment, as they may feel less isolated and could become more open to admitting they need help. Reducing stigma among healthcare professionals will also lessen emotional and physical suffering for cancer patients by lessening the likelihood of physicians refusing to sell certain medical equipment, like syringes, due to personal biases (Harsanyi et al., 2023). Overall, this solution will make opioids and substance abuse treatments more accessible for individuals with cancer as they will face fewer societal barriers due to decreased stigmatization of opioids.

Counter Arguments

Some organizations and individual Americans may be critical of the outlined proposals. For one, many grassroots organizations may be resistant to national oversight of such a campaign due to a concern about local voices being silenced (Mikolajczak, 2015). Underprivileged communities are often hesitant to adopt suggestions from national organizations that do not share their background and thus may be less likely to understand their needs (Local is better than national, 2017; Mikolajczak, 2015). However, involving the federal government adds legitimacy and allows for public institutions - such as the justice system - to be reformed and destigmatized on a larger scale. This would aim to promote better treatment systems and a national sharing of financial and labor resources that is not currently present. This sharing of resources is especially important to underprivileged communities as it can reduce the strain on local resources which are often relatively limited. Furthermore, this solution allows the focus to remain on elevating community voices, even on a national level, affording underprivileged populations more representation. Partnerships between larger health corporations and small, local community organizations have had some efficacy (Improving opioid misuse prevention literacy between older adults and health care providers , 2019). Allowing trained experts from national organizations to speak with the local community with the publicized support of neighborhood organizations that the community trusts helps to build a path of open communication (Improving opioid misuse prevention literacy between older adults and health care providers , 2019). This allows the community members to gain knowledge that can enable them to make better informed medical decisions and also provides larger organizations with the information they need to adapt their approach to better aid these communities. Open dialogue should also be emphasized during these events so that patients feel that they have the ability to voice their concerns and experiences (Improving opioid misuse prevention literacy between older adults and health care providers, 2019), and receive information that is helpful and relevant to them.

Another possible point of contention is the idea of destigmatization excusing addiction (Christiano & Neimand, 2017), and it not being the public's responsibility. However, stigma is a huge barrier to treatment and so without a destigmatization campaign, many of these individuals who become addicted to prescription opioids will not be able to reintegrate into their community. This harms both the individual and the community due to higher rates of unemployment, greater social welfare costs, and the high threat of communicable illnesses if people with opioid addictions can not access treatment. These broad community impacts of the opioid crisis make it a public health crisis, and it must be addressed as such.

Many members of the public may believe these solutions are a waste of funding to solve a relatively small issue. However, the U.S. currently spends billions of dollars on mismanaged and ineffective programs (Gasior et al., 2015; U.S. Congress Congressional Budget Office, 2022). These programs have been criticized by many health experts as contradicting currently recommended best practices for treating opioid addictions (Treatment for U.S. opioid addicts often inadequate, researchers say, 2013). These funds could be redirected toward more impactful policies, such as a destigmatization campaign and opioid monitoring program that focuses on cancer patients. Therefore, funding is generally not a concern; however, a significant impact can still be made with limited funds by focusing on a specific subset of patients: those who are found to escalate their opioid dose quickly or frequently, those that often complain of 10/10 pain, and those at risk for chemical coping (Bruera & Paice, 2015).

Other individuals may believe there is no opioid crisis among Americans with cancer as less than 5% of patients with chronic illnesses that are prescribed opioids misuse them (Gasior et al., 2015). However, of the 100 million Americans who face chronic pain - a large number of which are cancer patients - approximately one-third report signs of opioid dependence (Islam & Mcrae, 2014), making the total amount of people affected approximately 33 million. This number becomes even greater when considering that individuals who abuse prescription opioids that have been shared with them by their family members are not counted as part of these statistics (Bruera & Paice, 2015; Real Stories, 2020).

Another group that may show resistance to these policies is law enforcement and judicial officials, due to America's focus on drug criminalization (Islam & Mcrae, 2014; Kain, 2011). However, decreased criminalization would be beneficial, as being incarcerated increases the likelihood of an overdose by 40 times (Bohler et al., 2021; Wagner et al., 2016), decreases tax revenue as funds are redirected to incarceration programs from community welfare programs, and makes the public unlikely to call 911 (Wagner et al., 2016) due to a poor view of law enforcement. Law enforcement officials who received training on overdose treatment rather than pressing criminal charges formed better relationships with their community (Wagner et al., 2016), which improved trust between parties and boosted job satisfaction. Law enforcement professionals can also help issue drug treatment referrals (Wagner et al., 2016) under the aforementioned policy, which will help shift the narrative from punitive to sympathetic. This allows populations who medically need opioids, namely cancer patients, to access them without fear of unnecessary prosecution and empowers them to freely seek help if they are struggling with addiction.

Other individuals advocate for the use of new biomedical technologies in battling the crisis, namely drug recipe modification and individualized medicine. However, these are currently not FDA-approved, have not been widely studied, and are not feasible to be produced on a large-scale basis due to their immense financial costs (Bruera & Paice, 2015). Another popular theoretical solution is individualized medicine as it can result in 24% more effective pain medication, reduce hospital readmission by 54%, and decrease mortality by 85% (Bugada et al., 2020). If widely implemented, an average of $4,382 will be saved per patient per two months (Bugada et al., 2020). However, this approach is lengthy and requires comprehensive genetic testing (Bugada et al., 2020), which may not be possible at this time in low-income communities and heightens the threat of insurance discrimination. Therefore, more data must be collected and more public support garnered in order to ensure the success of any further steps.

Future Directions

By implementing a national destigmatization campaign centered around cancer patients using opioids, the stigma surrounding opioids can be lessened and will, in turn, improve current policies, such as law enforcement training, as it will create a culture of understanding and emphasis on recovery. This will improve interactions opioid users have with their community, thus making them more likely to seek out help as needed.

By not only decreasing stigma but also increasing the knowledge of opioid users' communities and physicians, it is hopeful that cancer patients using opioids will feel more comfortable asking questions and bringing up concerns surrounding their use of opioid analgesics. This will allow physicians to better assess the patient's risk of opioid misuse and ideally prevent it. By fostering understanding and open communication, cancer patients should be able to better understand their treatment options and thus make more informed decisions when managing their chronic pain. This should aid in reducing the opioid crisis as pain medication is less likely to be misused by more informed patients (Rogers et al., 2019).

In addition, care must be taken to prevent both oversight and restriction to opioid access (Bulls et al., 2021; Wood, 2018) as this often greatly impacts individuals with cancer in communities that are commonly discriminated against. The destigmatization campaign will encourage greater access to opioids for pain management in individuals with cancer, allowing this vulnerable population to get the treatment they need. However, it should be noted much current research informing the proposed policies is limited and generalized to all Americans using opioids rather than concentrating on cancer patients who use opioids. Therefore, more data is necessary to inform future policies and changes could be considered if collected data supports alternative approaches. Additionally, as new technologies arise rapidly, they could be used in conjunction with the proposed solution to make the destigmatization campaign more efficient and effective.

CONCLUSION

The proposed solution of a national public destigmatization campaign exists to increase community support and assistance with treatment plans. This is especially important for individuals who need opioids to manage cancer pain but may not be advised on or adhere to best practices. This has caused the U.S. to expend its financial, labor, and temporal resources on this crisis through increased access to treatment, community education, and public welfare services for those with opioid addictions. However, opioids remain one of the leading causes of death and thus the U.S. must reevaluate its policies and create more impactful solutions, such as the one proposed in this paper, to ensure cancer patients can safely access these drugs while still managing the risk of addiction.

REFERENCES

Anson, P. (2021, May 25). *How opioid hysteria affects cancer patients*. Pain News Network. Retrieved August 10, 2023, from https://www.painnewsnetwork.org/stories/2021/5/25/how-opioid-hysteria-affects-cancer-patients

Are cancer patients getting the opioids they need to control pain? (2020, September 16). National Cancer Institute at the National Institutes of Health. Retrieved August 10, 2023, from https://www.cancer.gov/news-events/cancer-currents-blog/2020/opioids-cancer-pain-oncologists-decreasing-prescriptions

Arthur, J., & Bruera, E. (2022). Managing cancer pain in patients with opioid use disorder or nonmedical opioid use. *JAMA Oncology*, *8*(8), 1104. doi:10.1001/jamaoncol.2022.2150 PMID:35771548

Beauchemin, M., & Cogan, J. (2022, June 1). *Addressing opioid misuse in cancer pain management* (Interview by M. A. Farmer) [Transcript]. Columbia University. Retrieved February 2, 2024, from https://www.cancer.columbia.edu/news/ addressing-opioid-misuse-cancer-pain-management

Beauchemin, M. P., Raghunathan, R. R., Accordino, M. K., Cogan, J. C., Kahn, J. M., Wright, J. D., & Hershman, D. L. (2022). New persistent opioid use among adolescents and young adults with sarcoma. *Cancer*, *128*(14), 2777–2785. doi:10.1002/cncr.34238 PMID:35599575

Beck, J. (2015, April 21). What Good Is 'Raising Awareness?'. *The Atlantic*. https://www.theatlantic.com/health/archive/2015/04/what-good-is-raising-awareness/391002/

Ben-Ari, E. (2023, February 14). Study finds disparities in access to opioids for cancer pain at end of life. *Cancer currents.* https://www.cancer.gov/ news-events/cancer-currents-blog/2023/disparities-opioids-cancer-pain-end-of-life

Bennett, M., Paice, J. A., & Wallace, M. (2018). Pain and opioids in cancer care: Benefits, risks, and alternatives. *American Society of Clinical Oncology Educational Book, 37*(37), 705–713. doi:10.1200/EDBK_180469 PMID:28561731

Bohler, R., Thomas, C.P., Clark, T.W., & Horgan, C.M. (2021, February). *Addressing the opioid crisis through social determinants of health: What are communities doing?* Opioid Policy Research Collaborative at Brandeis University.

Bruera, E., & Paice, J. A. (2015). Cancer pain management: Safe and effective use of opioids. *American Society of Clinical Oncology Educational Book*, (35), e593–e599. doi:10.14694/EdBook_AM.2015.35.e593 PMID:25993228

Bugada, D., Lorini, L. F., Fumagalli, R., & Allegri, M. (2020). Genetics and opioids: Towards more appropriate prescription in cancer pain. *Cancers (Basel), 12*(7), 1951. doi:10.3390/cancers12071951 PMID:32708424

Bulls, H. W., Chu, E., Goodin, B. R., Liebschutz, J. M., Wozniak, A., Schenker, Y., & Merlin, J. S. (2021). Framework for opioid stigma in cancer pain. *Pain, 163*(2), e182–e189. doi:10.1097/j.pain.0000000000002343 PMID:34010940

Cheetham, A., Picco, L., Barnett, A., Lubman, D. I., & Nielsen, S. (2022). The impact of stigma on people with opioid use disorder, opioid treatment, and policy. *Substance Abuse and Rehabilitation, 13*, 1–12. doi:10.2147/SAR.S304566 PMID:35115860

Christiano, A., & Neimand, A. (2017, Spring). Stop raising awareness already. *Essentials of Social Innovation.* https://ssir.org/articles/entry/stop_raising_awareness_already#

Costa, T., & Evans, L. L., Jr. (2022, February 23). *Older workers: Opioid misuse and employment outcomes* [Letter to Robert P. Casey, Jr. & Susan M. Collins]. https://www.gao.gov/assets/gao-22-104491.pdf

Coughlin, S. S., Datta, B., Vernon, M., Hatzigeorgiou, C., & George, V. (2022). Health literacy among cancer survivors. *Medicine, 101*(9), e29010. doi:10.1097/MD.0000000000029010 PMID:35244079

Farmer, M. A. (2022, June 1). *Addressing opioid misuse in cancer pain management.* Columbia University Herbert Irving Comprehensive Cancer Center. Retrieved July 12, 2023, from https://www.cancer.columbia.edu/news/addressing-opioid-misuse-cancer- pain-management

First-Responder trauma and the opioid crisis. (2020, June). *Catching Up With COSSAP*, 1-3. https://www.cossapresources.org/Content/Documents/Articles/Final_TASC_AHP_First_Responder_Trauma.pdf

Gasior, M., Bond, M., & Malamut, R. (2015). Routes of abuse of prescription opioid analgesics: A review and assessment of the potential impact of abuse-deterrent formulations. *Postgraduate Medicine*, *128*(1), 85–96. doi:10.1080/00325481.2016.1120642 PMID:26566680

Gilbert, A. (2023, July 6). *After the addiction, opioid users struggle to get back to work.* Bloomberg Law. Retrieved February 2, 2024, from https://news.bloomberglaw.com/daily-labor-report/ after-the-addiction-opioid-users-struggle-to-get-back-to-work

Greene, D., & King, N. (Hosts), & Noguchi, Y. (Writer). (2018, April 18). Anguished families shoulder the biggest burdens of opioid addiction [Radio broadcast]. In Morning edition. NPR.

Harsanyi, H., Cuthbert, C., & Schulte, F. (2023). The stigma surrounding opioid use as a barrier to cancer-pain management: An overview of experiences with fear, shame, and poorly controlled pain in the context of advanced cancer. *Current Oncology (Toronto, Ont.)*, *30*(6), 5835–5848. doi:10.3390/curroncol30060437 PMID:37366920

Housten, A. J., Gunn, C. M., Paasche-Orlow, M. K., & Basen-Engquist, K. M. (2020). Health literacy interventions in cancer: A systematic review. *Journal of Cancer Education*, *36*(2), 240–252. doi:10.1007/s13187-020-01915-x PMID:33155097

Improving opioid misuse prevention literacy between older adults and health care providers [Video]. (2019, April 2). YouTube. https://www.youtube.com/watch?v=9m7NYDUlCzc&t=10s

Islam, M. M., & Mcrae, I. S. (2014). An inevitable wave of prescription drug monitoring programs in the context of prescription opioids: Pros, cons and tensions. *BMC Pharmacology & Toxicology*, *15*(1), 46. Advance online publication. doi:10.1186/2050-6511-15-46 PMID:25127880

Kain, E. (2011, June 29). *The war on drugs is a war on minorities and the poor.* Forbes. Retrieved August 5, 2023, from https://www.forbes.com/sites/erikkain/2011/06/28/the-war-on-drugs-is-a-war-on-minorities-and-the-poor/?sh=258062dc624c

Krieger, C. (n.d.). *What are opioids and why are they dangerous?* Mayo Clinic. Retrieved July 13, 2023, from https://www.mayoclinic.org/diseases-conditions/prescription-drug- abuse/expert-answers/what-are-opioids/faq-20381270

Local is better than national. (2017). *A Better Way*. Retrieved August 5, 2023, from https://www.betterway.network/local-is-better-than-national

McCurry, M. K., Avery-Desmarais, S., Schuler, M., Tyo, M., Viveiros, J., & Kauranen, B. (2022). Perceived stigma, barriers, and facilitators experienced by members of the opioid use disorder community when seeking healthcare. *Journal of Nursing Scholarship*, *55*(3), 701–710. doi:10.1111/jnu.12837 PMID:36317787

Mercadante, S. (1999). Opioid rotation for cancer pain. *Cancer*, *86*(9), 1856–1866. doi:10.1002/(SICI)1097-0142(19991101)86:9<1856::AID-CNCR30>3.0.CO;2-G PMID:10547561

Mikolajczak, C. (2015, June 1). Local initiatives or national policies: What's best for our planet? *Cafe Babel*. https://cafebabel.com/en/article/local-initiatives-or-national-policies-whats-best-for-our-planet-5ae00a0ff723b35a145e5d48/

Overview United States (OECD Economic Surveys). (2018, June). OECD.

Page, R., & Blanchard, E. (2019). Opioids and cancer pain: Patients' needs and access challenges. *Journal of Oncology Practice / American Society of Clinical Oncology*, *15*(5), 229–231. doi:10.1200/JOP.19.00081 PMID:31013181

Pike, E., Tillson, M., Webster, J. M., & Staton, M. (2019). A mixed-methods assessment of the impact of the opioid epidemic on first responder burnout. *Drug and Alcohol Dependence*, *205*, 107620. doi:10.1016/j.drugalcdep.2019.107620 PMID:31675545

Prince, L. Y., Mears, S. C., Watson, J. C., & Hadden, K. B. (2019). Health Literacy Evaluation of Opioid Patient Education Materials for Orthopaedic Surgery. *Journal of Surgical Orthopaedic Advances*, *28*(3), 232–236. PMID:31675301

Real Stories. (2020, December 3). Centers for Disease Control and Prevention. Retrieved July 13, 2023, from https://www.cdc.gov/rxawareness/stories/index.html

Rogers, A. H., Bakhshaie, J., Orr, M. F., Ditre, J. W., & Zvolensky, M. J. (2019). Health literacy, opioid misuse, and pain experience among adults with chronic pain. *Pain Medicine*, *21*(4), 670–676. doi:10.1093/pm/pnz062 PMID:30938818

Rosoff, D. B., Smith, G. D., & Lohoff, F. W. (2021). Prescription opioid use and risk for major depressive disorder and anxiety and stress-related disorders. *JAMA Psychiatry*, *78*(2), 151. doi:10.1001/jamapsychiatry.2020.3554 PMID:33175090

Sigurdsson, S. O., Ring, B. M., O'Reilly, K., & Silverman, K. (2012). Barriers to employment among unemployed drug users: Age predicts severity. *The American Journal of Drug and Alcohol Abuse*, *38*(6), 580–587. doi:10.3109/00952990.2011.643976 PMID:22242680

Stigma and discrimination. (2022, June 1). National Institute on Drug Abuse. Retrieved February 2, 2024, from https://nida.nih.gov/research-topics/ stigma-discrimination

Synthetic opioids [Leaflet]. (2020). Department of Justice.

Treatment for U.S. opioid addicts often inadequate, researchers say [TV program]. (2013, August 5). In News hour. PBS.

Truong, M., & Fenton, S. H. (2022). Understanding the Current Landscape of Health Literacy Interventions within Health Systems. *Perspectives in Health Information Management*, *19*(Spring), 1h. PMID:35692852

Understanding the opioid overdose epidemic. (2023, August 8). Centers for Disease Control and Prevention. Retrieved August 17, 2023, from https://www.cdc.gov/opioids/basics/epidemic.html

U.S. Congress Congressional Budget Office. (2022, September). *The opioid crisis and recent federal policy responses*. Government Publishing Office.

Wagner, K. D., Bovet, L. J., Haynes, B., Joshua, A., & Davidson, P. J. (2016). Training law enforcement to respond to opioid overdose with naloxone: Impact on knowledge, attitudes, and interactions with community members. *Drug and Alcohol Dependence*, *165*, 22–28. doi:10.1016/j.drugalcdep.2016.05.008 PMID:27262898

Wagner, T. (2023, March 22). *Opioid overdose: A deadly cross-roads of health literacy and patient safety*. https://www.safercaretexas.org/opioid-overdose-a-deadly-cross-roads-of- health-literacy-and-patient-safety/

Wood, S. P. (2018, June 8). *Prescription monitoring programs: Helpful or harmful?* https://www.health.harvard.edu/blog/prescription-monitoring-programs-helpful-or-harmful-2018060814001#:~:text=Good%20intentions%20aside%2C%20there%20are%20some%20unintended%20and,than%20good%2C%20including%20taking%20away%20much%20needed%20medications

Yennurajalingam, S., Arthur, J., Reddy, S., Edwards, T., Lu, Z., Rozman de Moraes, A., Wilson, S. M., Erdogan, E., Joy, M. P., Ethridge, S. D., Kuriakose, L., Malik, J. S., Najera, J. M., Rashid, S., Qian, Y., Kubiak, M. J., Nguyen, K., PharmD, Wu, J., ... Bruera, E. (2021). Frequency of and factors associated with nonmedical opioid use behavior among patients with cancer receiving opioids for cancer pain. *JAMA Oncology*, *7*(3), 404–411. doi:10.1001/jamaoncol.2020.6789 PMID:33410866

KEY TERMS AND DEFINITIONS

Analgesic: A broad term used to describe a drug meant to lessen or eliminate pain.

Destigmatization: The act of reducing stigma, thus decreasing shame or discrimination for individuals with a certain condition.

Good Samaritan Laws: Laws that allow bystanders to assist a person in need without risk of liability, typically in the case of a medical emergency.

Health Literacy: An individual's ability to gather, comprehend, and apply information regarding their health, treatment options, and available healthcare services.

Naloxone: A medication often used in emergencies to quickly treat an opioid overdose by reversing opioids' effects.

Opioid Misuse Disorder: A condition characterized by the individual not using the opioids strictly as prescribed; this can present with varying symptoms and behaviors and also includes risk behaviors such as prescription sharing.

Opioids: A class of drugs that bind to opioid receptors, typically used to manage pain.

Socioeconomic Status: A person's calculated status in society and the economy based on various factors such as income, education, occupation, residence, and sometimes race or ethnicity.

Chapter 12
Health Literacy for Disabled Students:
A Case Study of Curriculum Development in Japanese Special Schools

Taku Murayama
Tokyo Gakugei University, Japan

ABSTRACT

Health literacy and related practical issues have been the subject of discussion in recent research. During COVID 19 times, the discussion and practice on health literacy are also critical for safe schooling and classroom activities. The purpose of this chapter is to discuss the chief issues on health literacy for the children with the special educational needs, especially focused on the intellectually and developmentally disabled students. In this chapter, the case for the curriculum development and lesson studies in the special educational schools for the intellectually and developmentally disabled are studied. The author of chapter plays a role as a supervisor for the school and have been in the participant observation in lesson study for the practice on the theme of the difference between COVID-19 virus and influenza virus.

1. LOCATION AND PURPOSE OF THE PROBLEM

The purpose of this chapter is to examine the learning issues in children's health literacy education for the intellectually disabled. Health literacy, as a further development from the concept of health promotion, is positioned as a key concept in health education (Nutbeam, 2000). It is considered to be a concept that goes further

DOI: 10.4018/978-1-7998-9652-4.ch012

from a process that allows people to control and improve their own health and to recognize patients and their families as entities that can actively acquire health. Health literacy and related practical issues have been the subject of discussion recent research. In with-COVID 19 times, the discussion and practice on the health literacy are also critical in the schooling, for the safe schooling and classroom activities. The purpose of this chapter is to discuss the chief issues on health literacy for the children with the special educational needs, especially focused on the intellectually and developmentally disabled students.

This chapter will also focus on the recent characteristics of health literacy. The importance of maintaining children's mental and physical health and supporting their recovery from mental and physical illnesses has become increasingly strong. One example is the acquisition of hygiene concepts and the habituation of hygiene behaviors due to the spread of the novel coronavirus infection (COVID-19). The spread of the COVID-19 infection has not only affected the maintenance of one's own health and health care, but also the maintenance of health in relation to close others, such as family members, and the wearing of masks in public spaces. In May 2023, the World Health Organization (WHO) declared the end of the "public health emergency of international concern (PHEIC)" for COVID-19, but the challenges of maintaining and managing health, including the so-called sequelae, continue. Challenges to health maintenance, including the so-called after-effects, continue. This is one of the possibilities of health literacy education, not only for health care of the self but also for concern regarding health in the public sphere at large. This chapter tries the theoretical and case studies in Japanese classes how students with special educational needs learn and acquire the health literacy through the daily lessons, and how health literacy program relate the other learning fields such as natural sciences, physical education, media literacy education, and so on.

In Japan's special education schools and other special-needs education, learning about independent activities is positioned as an essential part of the curriculum. In the self-reliance activities stipulated in the curriculum guidelines for special-needs schools in Japan, six categories and 27 learning contents are presented (Ministry of Education, Culture, Sports, Science and Technology, 2019). For example, in the category of "health maintenance," the content includes matters related to the formation of lifestyle habits, understanding of disease states, and life management (Ibid.). Independent activities are required to be implemented not only in special-needs schools but also in special-needs classes and day classes. The 27 learning contents are expected to be selected, organized, and embodied as appropriate learning tasks in accordance with the actual conditions of individual students. For example, when considering learning issues related to health in the context of education for the intellectually disabled, the emphasis is not only on disease and the maintenance of health, but also on "developing the ability to manage one's own health." This emphasis is not only on the prevention of disease through daily life, but also on the long-term issue of social participation after graduation.

The same can be said not only for independent activities but also for combined instruction in each subject area, for example, in the teaching of daily life and life-unit learning. Furthermore, students need to be able not only to manage their own health but also to choose their own activities and communicate with others on that basis. The ability to be aware of one's physical condition and disease status and to accurately judge what one can do and to what extent one can do it under exiting circumstances is also emphasized.

It is the position of this paper that the characteristics of learning tasks related to health, including independent activities, are deeply related to health literacy. In other words, it is noteworthy that learning content related to improving and overcoming learning and living conditions caused by disabilities and illnesses includes aspects of learning how the individual perceives his/her own disability or illness and how to deal with limitations in life. Through examination of these issues, it is expected that it may be possible to obtain clues for exploring the life issues of children with intellectual disabilities who study at special-needs schools and other schools, and the characteristics of learning for social participation.

2. HEALTH LITERACY AND SOCIAL CONTEXT

2.1 Characteristics of the Health Literacy Concept

Health literacy has reportedly been defined in various ways, but according to Nakayama's (2016) organization, two points are common to the various definitions of health literacy. The first point is that "informed decision making" should be considered a priority. The second point is that "decision-making is an action to solve a problem, and information is what is needed to know the options for solving a problem and to evaluate the advantages and disadvantages of each option.

Based on the theory of health promotion, health literacy is positioned as a type of critical literacy for working with the wider environment to maintain or improve one's own health, the health of immediate others, and the health of community members. In this context, literacy is classified into three types. First is functional literacy, which corresponds to basic reading and writing skills. Second is interactional literacy, which involves using one's own communication and other skills to proactively obtain and extract information. Third is critical literacy, which involves critically examining, analyzing, and integrating information and using that information in response to situations and circumstances. Health literacy emphasizes the critical literacy aspect. This is because it leads to the ability to adjust and change the social and environmental factors of one's illness and health. Nutbeam, a leading theorist of the health literacy concept, follows the same three categories of literacy (Nutbeam, 2000).

Health literacy is considered a concept that utilizes the health belief model in the 1960s to promote behavior change for health (Nakayama, 2016). The health belief model is explained as "a health behavior theory that identifies 'threat perception' and 'balance of benefits and disadvantages' as drivers of health behavior" (Sawada, 2019). The "threat perception" is defined as "feeling that one's life as it is now is likely to lead to illness or complications" or "feeling that if one were to become ill or have complications, the consequences would be serious" (Ibid.). The consequences here are broad, including health, economic, and social isssues. Another facilitating factor is the feeling that the benefits of taking appropriate action in terms of health outweigh the disadvantages.

In with and after COVID-19 society, each individual is required to manage their own health in the positive way and proactively participate in decision-making with respect to the health and medical care that they wish to receive. Of the many definitions of health literacy, the most commonly cited is the definition provided by the World Health Organization (WHO) in "Healthy People 2010". In "Healthy People 2010", health literacy is defined as "the degree to which individuals have the capacity to obtain, process, and understand basic health information and services needed to make appropriate health decisions". Previous studies on health literacy have mainly been conducted in multi-ethnic nations such as the United States that encompass various populations with lower levels of literacy. In such studies, health literacy has been measured in the same way that basic literacy is measured, only in terms of health information, with the main focus being on functional literacy (Murayama, 2016).

2.2 Health Literacy and Social Background

Attempts have already been made to measure and compare health literacy. Data from U.S. adults indicate that as of 2003, only one in nine could clearly understand the meaning of medical terms (Kunter et al. 2006). Japanese health literacy has also been shown to be relatively low. A Japanese version of the HLS-EU (a survey of eight European countries) was developed and a national survey was conducted in 2014 (Nakayama, et al. 2015). According to the survey, the percentage of people with health literacy difficulties in a survey of the general population and patients was about 85%, much higher than in the eight European countries (Nakayama, 2022). National surveys in six Asian countries and regions, including Taiwan, are also said to approximate those in Europe (ibid.). From this, it can be said that the status of health literacy attainment is low in Japan.

Nakayama (2022) cites three reasons for the low level of health literacy in Japan. First is the inadequacy of primary care in Japan. In Europe, primary care physicians are often responsible for the health education of local residents. In contrast, Japanese primary care physicians are not said to be doing this. Second, there is a lack of reliable and easy-to-understand public websites. Nakayama (2022) gives an example regarding cancer treatment, using Ogasawara et al. (2018) as an example. According to Ogasawara et al. (2018), when trying to obtain information about cancer diseases and treatments, the percentage of harmful information is higher than reliable information (Ogasawara et al. 2018). Third, "education from an early age may influence the development of the ability to evaluate information" in Japan. Early education in Japan has not been aimed at developing the ability to make judgments or decisions based on information; the focus has been on understanding information, which may reflect the characteristics of health literacy in Japan, according to the report.

Health literacy also needs to address a wide range of educational levels and to focus on the socioeconomic setting. Wynia, & Osborn (2010) found that limited health literacy is associated with poor health. They then point out that improving the quality of health literacy is effective in maintaining and improving health. This is because matters related to the maintenance and management of health are also directly related to lifestyle and diet. In this respect, health literacy is tied to the new public health. The concept is considered particularly important in health education. In addition, in special needs education, it is strongly connected to the independent activity curriculum and learning activities in dealing with one's own health challenges.

3. LEARNING HEALTH LITERACY IN EDUCATION FOR CHILDREN WITH INTELLECTUAL DISABILITIES

In this chapter, the case for the curriculum development and lesson studies in the special educational schools for the intellectually and developmentally disabled are studied. The author of chapter plays a role as a supervisor for the school and have been in the participant observation in lesson study for the practice on the theme of the difference between COVID-19 virus and influenza virus. Two case studies are discussed to explore the characteristics and possibilities of health literacy education in intellectual disability education. In both cases, the descriptions have been adjusted to protect information about individuals to the extent that the original intent is not compromised.

3.1 Examples of Learning Activities Related to COVID-19 Infection Control

The first case study is a study of the living arrangements related to the COVID-19 infection in an upper secondary school for special needs students with intellectual disabilities.

The lesson, which was put into practice in a small group study, began with students making a list of things they do on a daily basis to prevent the spread of infection. These included frequent hand washing, regular opening of classroom windows for ventilation, and wearing masks. Regarding frequent hand washing, the students shared information about when they wash their hands at certain times in their school life situations. For example, immediately after arriving at school, during recess, when returning to the classroom from the playground, before serving school lunch, and before eating school lunch. In the case of students in the upper grades, this also included situations in which multiple students shared the same teaching materials, depending on the subject. This is one of the typical forms of combined instruction, such as when students share equipment and tools in work study, or when students pass tools and materials to each other.

It was also confirmed that hand washing and wearing masks are useful not only for maintaining the health of individual students, but also for maintaining the health of others close to them, such as family and friends, and that they should take care of each other. Although not directly confirmed in class, the class members also assumed that if a student at this school were to become infected or ill, he or she would likely not be able to stay in the hospital alone due to personal independence and cognitive and emotional limitations.

In the second half of the study, using a tablet device, students proceeded with an activity to research COVID-19 using the Internet. Students summarized their research on a worksheet and then presented it to each other. Students were given individual assistance in entering keywords according to their cognitive and language abilities, but at the same time, the keywords they selected were adjusted individually.

3.2 Examples of Learning Tasks Related to Cooking and Eating Habits

The second case study concerns cooking and eating in the middle school of a special-needs school for the intellectually disabled. Individual learning tasks were set not as subject-specific instruction in home economics, but as instruction combined with independent activities. For the study, learning groups were organized across grade levels, and group work on cooking was developed based on the division of labor and collaboration. The learning group included students with a variety of learning difficulties and needs, including those who had difficulty using scissors, kitchen knives, and other cutting tools, those who had good hand-eye coordination but were not encouraged to use cutting tools due to emotional constraints, and those who had difficulty touching raw foods due to sensory sensitivity. In addition, the class members were expected to activate communicative activities in group work.

In a cross-grade cooking class that was held about once a month, students worked in groups to select menus using the Internet and to assign roles in cooking activities. In setting up the menus, the degree of food categorization was set according to the cognitive development of each student. For example, a simplified food exchange list was used. After the selection of the menu, the roles of the cooking activities were assigned to the groups. For example, tasks such as washing food, cutting food with a knife, etc. were set according to the cooking skills of each student and reflected in the individualized instructional plans for the cooking unit.

In group work in the cooking study, discussion activities are necessary. The upperclassmen led the discussion while consulting with and advising each other. When deciding on menus, students not only listed the menus they wanted to eat or cook, but also selected ingredients that were expected to be effective in managing the physical condition of their families and grandparents, and exchanged opinions with each other about nutritional balance.

3.3 Public and Individual Learning

In recent years, there have been changes in the forms of information gathering about health and nutrition, as well as in the forms and structures of communication that accompany such information. In this regard, health literacy education is characterized not only as patient education but also as education with a preventive aspect. It can be seen as a learning issue where highly personal issues such as health maintenance, health management, and disease prevention, and highly public issues such as being aware of the health management of family members and others close to one, and cooking practice for meals with family members, are interlaced.

As the students with intellectual and developmental disabilities come to learn and use the health literacy as functional literacy, it is critically important that curriculum development and the learning activities for the students with special educational needs. The points of view are as follows. The first is the curriculum development for the students' context of their daily livings. In the view of the author, the special education curriculum has two genealogical roots by the emphasis of learning in the living situation and by the emphasis of learning the topic in the situation and materials along with the students' individuality, cognitive abilities, and so on. Therefore, the topics learned in the schooling are compositive and multi-strata issues as a matter of necessity. The second is the process of curriculum development for health literacy includes the change and arrange of the message by the agents of the public-hygiene and policy makers into teaching contents for the students with the literacy-handicap.

In the U.S. health policy "Healthy People 2020," health communication using information technology was positioned as one of the pillars of the policy (U.S. Department of Health and Human Services, 2012). The Internet has come to play a central role in the collection of information, and "much of the information is provided by national professional organizations" (Nakayama, 2016). The successor "Healthy People 2030" also calls for the promotion of health communication via IT media as "Health IT" (U.S. Department of Health and Human Services, 2021, Services, 2021).

As regards to the literacy acquisition for the public health, the designing the lesson for health literacy are with arrangement of the knowledge and skills of the health into the simple term. This concern is common to the related field such as medicine and another rehabilitation in the view of adaptation for talking with the semi-literate patients, science communication between the professional and novice in the field, and so on. The third are the health literacy are suitable the collaborative learning and investigative activities in the lesson. The topic in this case, COVID-19 are unknown virus, so textbooks and packaged teaching materials are not always useful both to students and teachers. Through the learning process with the inquiry and investigation of these virus, it is expected that students acquires that the media literacy in learning health literacy because they often use the Internet instead of the paper books and textbooks.

4. HEALTH PSYCHOLOGICAL ISSUES FOR INTELLECTUALLY DISABLED CHILDREN

4.1 Psychological Challenges for Children With Intellectual Disabilities

Three psychological challenges children with intellectual disabilities face will be discussed here.

The first concerns physical discomfort brought about directly by physical and mental illness. This is true not only when the child has subjective symptoms or directly feels pain, but also when the child does not have subjective symptoms. In recent years, an increasing number of children have complained of subjective symptoms including those outside the original site of the lesion. It is possible to focus on physical discomfort by including these symptoms as well. Second, there is psychological and emotional anxiety, which is difficult to see when the child is in good health. This includes anxiety about treatment and inability to have a time perspective on his or her future life. Third, the child is unable to verbalize his or her anxiety. Some children show physical symptoms as a result of this. In addition, some children may express their anxiety as rejection of life or aggressive attitudes toward those close to them due to their inability to verbalize their anxiety. The Japanese Courses of Study Commentary for special educational schools indicates that for children who are psychologically unstable, "it is important to achieve psychological stability by allowing them to confide their worries and express their anxious feelings" (Ministry of Education, Culture, Sports, Science and Technology, 2019).

It is necessary to check for restrictions in the child's daily life. Physical and mental discomfort and distress, dietary restrictions, and low self-esteem may be observed. In addition, anxiety about physical condition and prognosis, changes in appearance due to side effects of treatment, anxiety about maintaining friendships, and complexes about physical and psychological aspects of the disease may be considered. In addition, school-aged children may show a decreased sense of belonging to a group, such as a learning group at school.

Children's social skills should also be noted. Children's social skills also vary based on mental and choronogical age, developmental stage, family environment, and support from others. There are four main challenges for school-aged children with intellectual disabilities. First, there is a delay in academic achievement and social skills. Cases of maladjustment to school have also been reported. Second, the impact of friendships and school maladjustment on overall psychological adjustment; friendships and school adjustment are also important predictors of later psychological adjustment. Third is the influence factor of friendships. Friendships are affected by the limitation of treatment activities and changes in appearance due to side effects (Vanneta et al. 1998). Fourth, it is difficult to establish and maintain friendships. It has also been noted that students' changes in appearance can lead to a negative self-image.

Next, an overview of the challenges of adolescence and young adulthood are suggested. First, as in school age, one can point to the side effects of treatment and feelings of inferiority due to having the disease or disabilities. Support for the intellectually disabled child can be said to be a scheme and awareness of self-management of one's own health problems. It has also been noted that family problems affect the psychological adjustment and maladjustment of the child. Self-management and self-care involves dealing with one's own mind and body on a long-term basis. This includes not only so-called treatment, but also diet and medication management.

There are four elements of psychological support for the disabled children. First, it is important to check the child's own understanding of the illness and its treatment, and to gather information. It is important for the intellectually disabled child to be able to identify what he or she knows and does not know about his or her illness and treatment, in accordance with his or her age and ability to understand. Second, cognitive-behavioral therapeutic activity is used to alleviate mental distress. Fourth, the resolution of daily life problems. Fifth, the promotion of positive life experiences. This has been shown to be effective in improving patients' own sense of accomplishment and self-efficacy through the incorporation of creative activities.

4.2 Psychological Support for Children With Intellectual Disabilities

Health literacy is used as a key concept in health education. This is a concept that can be utilized not only for children with diseases, but also for a broad range of healthy individuals. Health literacy is not viewed as literacy in the narrow sense, but rather as functional. Thus, the focus is on the ability to verbalize one's complaints and concerns to one's doctor and medical staff, to understand the doctor's explanations, and to communicate these in one's own words to family members and others. Appropriate behavior in daily living is also an issue, such as the ability to manage medication, lifestyle, and dietary restrictions in accordance with the treatment plan decided with the doctor and medical staff, and the ability to rest when necessary or to request rest on one's own. Health literacy is a common challenge for adults as well, but for children in particular, it has been pointed out that it is important to create a supportive environment for health literacy rather than to rely solely on the child's personal abilities (Nutbeam 2000).

Using Nutbeam's (2000) description of functional literacy as a support, it is important to use one's own communication skills to proactively acquire information about illness and treatment. In addition, the ability to adjust and change social and environmental factors regarding one's illness and health is also important. For example, it is necessary to examine what changes can be expected from mental health literacy education. One example known to the author is a junior high school student's comment, "I realized that mental illnesses and mental disorders are more familiar to me than I thought." In addition, the author has seen an improvement in students' knowledge of mental illness and mental disorders, as well as their motivation to acquire knowledge, such as "If I increase my knowledge, I can protect myself and my friends," and "It is important to learn about mental illness and mental disorders because it may happen to me." Based on a narrow definition of literacy education, it could be limited to knowledge about mental ill health. However, by examining the acquisition and application of knowledge, the perspective of taking literacy in a broader sense can be said to be more emphatic.

5. DISCUSSION AND CONCLUSION

Through the case study, the range and critical role of health literacy have been raised in the context of theoretical and practical research on students' learning about health, virus, and health promotion. It is also expected to clarify the progress and limitations of current research. This chapter will focus on four main aspects of health literacy: the definition of health literacy, assessment of health literacy, translation into health education, and health literacy focus on the virus. Given the contextual background above, much attention has been paid to the concept of "health literacy" as a means for all individuals to be able to promote their own health condition.

The primary goal of school health education is to develop health literacy among school-aged children. That said, in the Japanese context, education for the disabled and culturally disadvantaged is rarely practiced. After reviewing the literature and case studies, the following points of discussion have identified into the following points. First, further theoretical discussion regarding the definition of health literacy and its translation into specific educational theory and practice is needed. Especially for the disabled and disadvantaged. Second, further analysis regarding language and other barriers to understanding and applying health literacy is needed. Third, few, if any, studies have dealt with health literacy among those with health conditions and the disabled. Almost all of the previous research presumes that the students and adults receiving health literacy instruction do not have specific illnesses, impairments, and disabilities. This is one of the limitations of the previous research. One of the practical challenges facing schools is inclusive education, the goal of which is to include students with mild disabilities and health conditions in any types of schools. This is the case in terms of the social lives for the youth and adults. That said, while the educational system is able to teach literacy it is unable to teach health literacy. Health literacy is multifaceted and requires a multi-sectorial approach involving society as a whole. Therefore, it is anticipated that health literacy and its practical application will serve as foundation for building an inclusive society. Finally, the author would like to address three issues for the future. First, the importance of health literacy is widely shared. On the other hand, health literacy education for intellectually disabled children, the topic of this chapter, includes many individual issues. Therefore, it includes points that differ from broadly targeted health literacy education. This has similar characteristics to patient education in health care. It is not simply a dichotomy that can be explained in terms of whether one has good health or is undergoing treatment. In particular, there is a commonality in the fact that the education is condition-specific. In this regard, it is necessary to wade through health literacy programs and consider psychological support for children with cognitive limitations.

Second, the study should examine differences in the developmental stages of health literacy according to the child's intellectual and cognitive disability status, differences by developmental status, and differences in the structure and content of health communication with health care providers and school personnel. This could also be a powerful resource for learning about intellectually disabled children and children with health risks.

REFERENCES

Kunter, M., (2006). The health literacy of America's adults: Result from the 2003 National Assessment of Adult Literacy. *Education*, *6*, 1–59.

Ministry of Education, Culture, Sports, Science and Technology (2019) *The Japanese Courses of Study Commentary for Special Educational Schools*, Kairyudo P ublication. Tokyo. (originally in Japanese).

Murayama, T. (2016). Key Issues of Health Literacy: A Literature Review. *The Journal of East Asian Educational Research*, *2*, 83–91.

Nakayama, K. (2016). What is Health Literacy? Fukuda, H. & Eguchi, Y. (eds.) Health Literacy: New Key Word for Health Education. Taishukan Co. Ltd., 1-22. (originally in Japanese)

Nakayama, K., Osaka, W., Togari, T., Ishikawa, H., Yonekura, Y., Sekido, A., & Matsumoto, M. (2015). Comprehensive health literacy in Japan is lower than in Europe: A validated Japanese-language assessment of health literacy. *BMC Public Health*, *15*(505), 505. doi:10.1186/s12889-015-1835-x PMID:26001385

Nakayama, K. (2022) Health Literacy for Info-pro, *Information Science & Technology, 72(4),* 122-127.(originally in Japanese)

Nutbeam, D. (2000). Health Literacy as a public health goal: A challenge for contemporary health education and communication strategies into the 21st century. *Health Promotion International*, *15*(3), 259–267. doi:10.1093/heapro/15.3.259

Ogasawara, R., Katsumata, N., Toyooka, T., Akaishi, Y., Yokoyama, T., & Kadokura, G. (2018). Reliability of Cancer Treatment Information on the Internet: Observational Study. *JMIR Cancer*, *4*(2), e10031. doi:10.2196/10031 PMID:30559090

Sawada, S. Health Belief Model, https://www.e-healthnet.mhlw.go.jp/information/dictionaries/exercise, (Last Accessed on 9th, October, 2023.) (originally in Japanese)

U.S. Department of Health and Human Services. (2012) Healthy People 2020, https://wayback.archive-it.org/5774/20220413183808/https://www.healthypeople.gov/2020/dat a-search, last accessed on 22nd, May, 2023.

U.S. Department of Health and Human Services, Office of Disease Prevention and Health Promotion. (2021)Healthy People 2030, https://health.gov/healthypeople, last accessed on 24th, May, 2023.

Vannatta, K., Gartstein, M. A., Short, A., & Noll, R. B. (1998). A controlled study of peer relationships of children surviving brain tumors: Teacher, peer, and self ratings. *Journal of Pediatric Psychology*, *23*(5), 279–287. doi:10.1093/jpepsy/23.5.279 PMID:9782676

Wynia, M. K., & Osborn, C. Y. (2010). Health literacy and communication quality in health care organizations. *Journal of health communication*, 15 Suppl 2(Suppl 2), pp.102–115.

Chapter 13
Health Literacy Initiatives in the Donation Landscape:
Educating for Impact

Susmita Chakrabarty
Centurion University of Technology and Management, India

Monali Priyadarsini Mishra
Centurion University of Technology and Management, India

ABSTRACT

Health literacy plays a pivotal role in the landscape of organ and blood donation, influencing individuals' understanding of the process, its benefits, and the critical need for donations. This abstract provides an overview of a comprehensive study that examines health literacy initiatives and their impact on the donation landscape. The research delves into the various strategies employed to enhance health literacy, including educational campaigns, digital platforms, and community engagement. The study aims to shed light on the effectiveness of these initiatives in increasing awareness, dispelling myths, improving comprehension of the donation process, and ultimately driving higher participation in life-saving donations. Additionally, the research explores the challenges faced in promoting health literacy and suggests recommendations to further optimize educational approaches in the context of organ and blood donation.

DOI: 10.4018/978-1-7998-9652-4.ch013

INTRODUCTION

Health literacy is a fundamental skill that encompasses an individual's ability to access, understand, evaluate, and apply health information in ways that promote and maintain good health. It's a multifaceted concept that influences how people interpret and act upon health-related information, navigate the healthcare system, and make informed decisions about their well-being. When applied to the realm of donation—be it blood, organs, or tissue—health literacy plays a pivotal role in empowering potential donors to make informed and confident choices. This chapter explores the profound impact of health literacy on the decision-making process of donors, highlighting how an informed and literate individual can contribute to a more efficient and ethical donation system (Liu, 2020).

In the complex and ever-evolving field of medicine, health literacy plays a pivotal role in ensuring optimal patient outcomes. Defined as the ability to obtain, process, and understand basic health information, health literacy is crucial in empowering patients to make informed decisions about their healthcare. Whether it's deciphering medical jargon, understanding treatment options, or comprehending the potential risks and benefits of a procedure, health literacy equips individuals with the tools they need to actively participate in their own care (Van den Broucke, 2014). Blood transfusion and organ donation are two critical areas in medicine where health literacy proves indispensable. When it comes to blood transfusions, patients need to be well-informed about the procedure itself, the risks involved, and the importance of pre- and post-transfusion care. Understanding the different blood components and their respective indications is essential for patients to grasp the rationale behind a transfusion. Additionally, knowledge of potential complications, such as transfusion reactions or infections, enables patients to promptly report any adverse events to their healthcare providers. With a comprehensive understanding of blood transfusion, patients can actively engage in shared decision-making, ensuring their treatment aligns with their individual goals and preferences. Similarly, health literacy is vital in the realm of organ donation. Organ transplantation offers hope and a new lease on life for countless individuals, but it also comes with its own set of challenges. Successfully navigating the organ transplantation process demands a high level of health literacy. Patients must comprehend the intricacies of organ allocation, waitlist dynamics, and the criteria for listing eligibility. Understanding the benefits and potential risks of transplantation, including the side effects of immunosuppressive medications, empowers patients to make educated decisions about pursuing this life-saving intervention. Moreover, informed patients are better equipped to manage their post-transplant care, including adhering to medication regimens, monitoring for rejection signs, and recognizing potential complications (Coughlin, 2020). Inadequate health literacy not only hampers patients' ability to make informed decisions but also has serious implications for their overall health outcomes. Limited health literacy has been associated with poorer management of chronic conditions, increased emergency room utilization, and higher healthcare costs. Patients with low health literacy often face challenges in understanding medication instructions, interpreting lab results, and following treatment plans, leading to suboptimal health outcomes. This highlights the critical role that health literacy plays in empowering patients to actively participate in their care and make informed decisions that can positively impact their health (McCray, 2005). To address the importance of health literacy in medical settings, healthcare providers must play an active role in facilitating patients' understanding of their healthcare information. This involves utilizing clear and simple language when communicating with patients, providing written materials with appropriate health literacy levels, and incorporating visual aids to enhance comprehension. Additionally, healthcare providers should actively engage patients in discussions about their treatment options, ensuring that patients have the necessary information to make choices aligned with their values and preferences. By fostering a patient-centred approach, healthcare providers can empower individuals with the knowledge they need to actively participate in their own care and improve health outcomes (Cristofori, 2022). Health literacy holds immense significance in the field of medicine. By enabling patients to obtain, process, and understand health information, health literacy empowers individuals to make informed decisions about their healthcare. Within the contexts of blood transfusion and organ donation, health literacy plays a critical role in facilitating patients' understanding of complex procedures, potential risks, and treatment options. Inadequate health literacy hampers patients' ability to actively engage in their care, leading to poorer health outcomes. Healthcare providers have a responsibility to promote health literacy and ensure patients have the necessary tools to make informed decisions. By doing so, we can bridge the gap in health disparities and pave the way for improved patient outcomes.

BACKGROUND

Understanding Health Literacy

Health literacy is often described as the ability to understand and use health information effectively to make appropriate health decisions. It encompasses a range of skills, including reading, listening, analytical thinking, and decision-making. A health-literate individual can interpret health-related information, comprehend the implications of medical conditions, and evaluate the risks and benefits associated with healthcare choices.

Health literacy involves more than just being able to read medical instructions or understand a doctor's advice. It encompasses various dimensions, including:

- Functional Literacy: The ability to read, write, and comprehend basic health information needed to function effectively in the healthcare environment.
- Interactive Literacy: The ability to extract information and derive meaning from different forms of communication, such as verbal instructions from healthcare providers or written materials.
- Critical Literacy: The capacity to evaluate the credibility and accuracy of health information and apply it to make informed decisions about one's health.

The Impact of Health Literacy on Individuals (Ahern, 2006):

1. Informed Decision-Making

Health literacy equips individuals to understand the benefits, risks, and alternatives related to their health decisions. Informed decision-making is crucial in healthcare, ensuring that individuals actively participate in their care plans and choose options aligned with their values and preferences.

2. Preventive Health Practices

Health-literate individuals are more likely to engage in preventive health practices, such as vaccinations, regular screenings, healthy eating, and physical activity. They comprehend the importance of prevention in maintaining good health and reducing the risk of chronic diseases.

3. Medication Management

Understanding medication instructions, dosage, and potential side effects is essential for proper medication management. Health literacy enables individuals to adhere to prescribed regimens, reducing medication errors and improving treatment outcomes.

4. Access to Healthcare Services

Health-literate individuals can navigate the healthcare system effectively, accessing appropriate services, scheduling appointments, and understanding insurance coverage. This ensures timely medical care and the utilization of healthcare resources efficiently.

5. Health Communication

Health literacy enables individuals to communicate effectively with healthcare professionals, ask relevant questions, and seek clarification, leading to improved doctor-patient relationships and a better understanding of diagnoses and treatment options.

Barriers to Health Literacy (Ferguson, 2019):

Several barriers can impede health literacy, including:

- Language and Vocabulary: Complex medical jargon and unfamiliar terminology can be challenging for individuals with limited language proficiency.
- Education Level: Lower levels of education can hinder the understanding of health information, making it difficult to comprehend written materials or follow complex health instructions.
- Cultural Differences: Cultural beliefs, norms, and practices may impact health literacy levels and influence health-seeking behaviours and understanding of health information.
- Healthcare System Complexity: The complexity of the healthcare system, including insurance, forms, and processes, can overwhelm individuals, especially those with low health literacy.

Promoting Health Literacy

To enhance health literacy, efforts should focus on:

- Simplifying Communication: Healthcare providers should use plain language and avoid medical jargon, ensuring that information is easily understood by everyone.
- Education and Awareness: Public health campaigns and educational programs should raise awareness about health literacy's importance and equip individuals with essential health information.
- Patient-Centred Care: Healthcare should be tailored to individual needs and preferences, encouraging active participation and informed decision-making (Baldry, 1986).
- Accessible Health Information: Providing information in multiple formats (written, verbal, visual) and in different languages can enhance accessibility and understanding.
- Empowering Communities: Empowering communities to advocate for their health, ask questions, and seek clarification fosters a culture of health literacy.

Health literacy is essential for individuals to make informed decisions regarding medical procedures such as blood and organ transplantation. Here are key health literacy requirements for these procedures:

Blood Transplantation

Understanding the Procedure: Clear and concise explanation of the process of blood transfusion, its purpose, and potential risks and benefits.

Informed Consent: Thorough understanding of the consent form, including risks, alternatives, and implications of refusing or accepting a blood transfusion.

Blood Types and Compatibility: Education about blood types, compatibility, and potential adverse reactions that may occur due to incompatible blood transfusions.

Safety Measures: Knowledge about safety protocols followed during blood transfusion to prevent infections and ensure safe and appropriate transfusions.

Preparation and Aftercare: Information regarding pre-transfusion preparations, post-transfusion monitoring, and signs of adverse reactions or complications.

Organ Transplantation

Understanding the Procedure: Comprehensive understanding of the organ transplantation process, including pre-transplant assessments, the surgery itself, and post-transplant care.

Informed Consent: Detailed comprehension of the consent form, risks associated with the surgery, potential benefits, alternative treatment options, and the lifelong commitment to follow-up care.

Organ Matching and Waiting Lists: Knowledge about organ matching, organ allocation systems, waiting lists, and the factors affecting priority for organ transplantation.

Immunosuppressive Medications: Education about the necessity of immunosuppressive medications, potential side effects, compliance requirements, and their role in preventing organ rejection.

Post-Transplant Care and Lifestyle Changes: Information about post-transplant care, lifestyle modifications, dietary changes, physical activity, medication adherence, and long-term follow-up care.

Emotional and Psychological Support: Awareness of the emotional and psychological aspects of organ transplantation, including potential stress, coping strategies, and available support services.

Health information on the internet (Berland, 2001)

Health information on the internet can be a valuable resource, providing access to a vast amount of information on various medical conditions, treatments, and general wellness. However, it's important to approach online health information with caution and critical thinking. Here are some tips for navigating health information on the internet:

Verify the Source: Check the credibility of the website or source. Look for information from reputable health organizations, medical institutions, government health agencies, or known experts in the field.

Check the Date: Ensure that the information is current and up-to-date. Medical knowledge evolves, and outdated information may not be accurate or applicable.

Cross-Reference Information: Verify information by cross-referencing it with multiple reliable sources. Consistency across reputable sources increases the likelihood of accuracy.

Consult Healthcare Professionals: If in doubt or if the information is about a specific medical condition, consult healthcare professionals for personalized advice. They can provide guidance based on your individual health needs.

Beware of Biased Information: Be cautious of information that seems overly promotional or biased, especially if it's associated with a particular product or service. Look for a balanced and evidence-based presentation.

Understand the Limitations: Recognize the limitations of online information. Not all health content online is reviewed by experts, and some sources may lack scientific rigor.

Be Sceptical of Miracle Cures: Be wary of claims about miracle cures or treatments that seem too good to be true. Consult with healthcare professionals before trying any new treatments or therapies.

Privacy and Security: Protect your privacy when seeking health information online. Use reputable and secure websites, especially when providing personal information.

Educate Yourself: Improve your health literacy to better understand and evaluate health information. This can help you distinguish between reliable and unreliable sources.

Consider the Context: Understand that not all health information is applicable to everyone. Factors like age, gender, medical history, and lifestyle can influence the relevance of information to an individual.

Enhancing Knowledge for Informed Decisions

One of the primary ways health literacies empowers donors is by providing them with accurate and comprehensive information. Knowledge is the bedrock upon which informed decisions are made. When potential donors have access to clear and detailed information about the donation process, its significance, and potential outcomes, they can assess the situation and decide whether to participate.

For example, a health-literate individual understands the importance of blood donation in emergency situations, surgeries, and treating various medical conditions. They also comprehend the eligibility criteria, potential side effects, and the impact their donation can have on the lives of others. Armed with this knowledge, they can confidently opt to donate blood, knowing the positive impact it can make in the community (Moritsugu, 2013).

Building Confidence in the Decision-Making Process

Health literacy instils confidence in donors, enabling them to engage actively in the decision-making process. When individuals are well-informed, they are more likely to participate willingly and without hesitation. Confidence in the decision to donate arises from a clear understanding of the benefits and risks involved, fostering trust in the healthcare system and the donation process.

For instance, a potential organ donor with adequate health literacy comprehends the transplantation process, the significance of matching, and the potential benefits of saving a life. This understanding instils confidence in their decision to become a donor, knowing they are making a substantial and positive difference in someone else's life.

Fostering Informed Consent and Autonomy

Informed consent is a fundamental principle in healthcare that respects an individual's autonomy and right to make decisions regarding their own body. Health literacy ensures that potential donors can provide informed consent for their donations, understanding the procedures, risks, and potential outcomes involved.

In the case of organ transplantation, an informed consent process involves discussing the procedure, its potential benefits and risks, alternative treatment options, and the post-operative care required. Health-literate donors can engage meaningfully in this process, ensuring their decisions are well-informed and aligned with their personal beliefs and values.

Encouraging Consideration of Ethical and Cultural Factors

Health literacy extends beyond medical facts and embraces ethical considerations and cultural beliefs. Empowered donors, with a strong foundation in health literacy, can weigh the ethical implications of their donation decisions. They can reflect on their actions in the broader context of society and their personal values.

For example, a potential organ donor with a good grasp of health literacy may consider the ethical implications of opting to donate to a family member versus a stranger on a transplant waiting list. They can also consider how their cultural or religious beliefs may influence their decision and how they can align their choices with their ethical and cultural framework.

Facilitating Effective Communication and Advocacy

Health literacy enhances communication between donors, healthcare professionals, and the wider community. A well-informed donor can effectively communicate their decisions, concerns, and expectations regarding the donation process. They can advocate for themselves, ensuring their wishes are respected and their questions are addressed adequately.

In addition, health-literate donors can spread awareness about donation, dispel myths, and encourage others to become donors by sharing accurate information. Their ability to communicate effectively amplifies the impact of their decision, encouraging a culture of donation within their communities.

Overcoming Barriers and Addressing Disparities

Addressing health literacy challenges and disparities is essential in ensuring equitable access to donation opportunities. Many individuals, particularly those from disadvantaged socioeconomic backgrounds or with limited access to education, may face barriers in understanding the importance of donation and the processes involved.

Efforts to improve health literacy, through targeted education and accessible information, can bridge these gaps and empower individuals across diverse communities. By doing so, we can work towards a more inclusive and representative pool of donors, ultimately benefitting those in need of life-saving donations.

Barriers to Health Literacy

Health literacy refers to an individual's ability to obtain, understand, and apply health information to make informed decisions about their well-being. However, several barriers can hinder health literacy, making it challenging for individuals to access and comprehend essential health information. Here are some examples of barriers to health literacy:

Language and Vocabulary

Challenge: Medical terminology can be complex and unfamiliar to many individuals.

Impact: Limited vocabulary may lead to misunderstandings of health instructions, prescriptions, or educational materials.

Limited Literacy Skills

Challenge: Some individuals may struggle with basic reading and writing skills.

Impact: Difficulty in understanding written health information, including medication instructions, appointment schedules, and preventive care guidelines.

Cultural and Diversity Factors

Challenge: Diverse cultural backgrounds may influence health beliefs and practices.

Impact: Misinterpretation of health information or reluctance to seek medical help due to cultural differences.

Limited Access to Information

Challenge: Socioeconomic factors, including lack of internet access or information resources.

Impact: Difficulty in accessing reliable health information, missing out on preventive measures, and being unaware of available healthcare services.

Healthcare Jargon

Challenge: Use of technical and jargon-heavy language in healthcare settings.

Impact: Patients may feel overwhelmed or intimidated, hindering effective communication with healthcare providers.

Digital Divide

Challenge: Unequal access to digital technology and online health resources.

Impact: Limited access to online health information and digital health tools, affecting the ability to engage in telehealth or use health apps.

Limited Time with Healthcare Providers

Challenge: Short appointment durations and limited communication time with healthcare professionals.

Impact: Incomplete understanding of medical conditions, treatment options, and preventive measures.

Healthcare System Complexity

Challenge: Complex healthcare systems with multiple providers, insurance policies, and administrative processes.

Impact: Confusion about navigating the healthcare system, leading to delayed or inadequate care.

Stigma and Discrimination

Challenge: Fear of judgment or discrimination in healthcare settings.

Impact: Reluctance to seek care, disclose health concerns, or follow through with recommended treatments.

Low Health Literacy Awareness

Challenge: Lack of awareness about the importance of health literacy.

Impact: Individuals may not recognize the need to improve their health literacy skills, leading to less proactive health management.

LITERATURE REVIEW

Blood Transfusion

1. Life-Saving Potential:

Studies such as that by Rossaint et al. (2023) emphasize the critical role of blood transfusion in emergency medical care. Immediate access to a sufficient blood supply is paramount in trauma situations, surgeries, and other life-threatening conditions.

2. Disease Management:

Research by Estcourt (2019) underscores the importance of blood transfusions in managing chronic conditions. Patients with disorders like sickle cell anemia benefit significantly from regular transfusions, improving their overall health and reducing complications.

3. Advancements in Blood Safety:

The work of Udvardy (2023) highlights ongoing efforts to enhance blood safety. Technological advancements, including nucleic acid testing, have contributed to the reduction of transfusion-transmitted infections, ensuring a safer transfusion process.

4. Impact on Maternal Health:

A study conducted by Thurn et al. (2017) explores the significance of blood transfusions in maternal healthcare. Transfusions play a crucial role in managing postpartum hemorrhage, a leading cause of maternal mortality worldwide.

5. Economic and Societal Benefits:

The economic impact of blood transfusions is discussed in the research by Oge (2014). Accessible blood transfusion services contribute to economic stability by reducing the economic burden associated with prolonged illness and complications.

Organ Donation

1. Transplantation Success Rates:

Recent research by Thongprayoon et al. (2022) provides insights into the success rates of organ transplantations. Advances in surgical techniques and immunosuppressive therapies have significantly improved outcomes, reinforcing the life-transforming impact of organ donation.

2. Addressing Organ Shortages:

The work of Nambiar (2018) delves into the persistent issue of organ shortages. Organ donation campaigns and public awareness efforts are discussed as crucial strategies to bridge the gap between demand and supply, ensuring timely access to life-saving transplants.

3. Quality of Life Improvements:

Longitudinal studies, including that by Tucker et al. (2019), demonstrate the long-term improvements in the quality of life for organ transplant recipients. Individuals receiving organs experience not only extended lifespans but also enhanced physical and psychological well-being.

4. Economic and Societal Impacts:

The economic benefits of organ donation are explored in the research conducted by Chen (2021). Organ transplants reduce long-term healthcare costs by replacing the need for ongoing medical treatments, positively impacting both individuals and the healthcare system.

5. Ethical Considerations:

Ethical aspects of organ donation are discussed by Shroff (2009). The research emphasizes the ethical responsibility of society to promote organ donation, balancing the principles of autonomy, beneficence, and justice.

This literature review underscores the multifaceted importance of blood transfusion and organ donation, encompassing medical, economic, and societal dimensions. Building upon the existing body of knowledge, it provides a foundation for understanding the critical role these interventions play in contemporary healthcare.

The Importance of Blood Donation (Giles, 2004)

Blood donation (figure 1) is a selfless act that involves voluntarily giving one's blood to be used for medical treatments and emergencies. It is a fundamental aspect of healthcare systems worldwide, contributing significantly to saving lives and improving health outcomes for numerous patients. The importance of blood donation cannot be overstated, and this chapter explores the various ways in which blood donation plays a critical role in modern medicine and society.

1. Saving Lives in Emergencies

Blood is vital for treating trauma patients, accident victims, and individuals undergoing surgery. In emergencies, every second counts, and having a readily available and adequate blood supply can be the difference between life and death. Blood transfusions are often crucial to stabilize patients and provide them with the necessary support until further medical interventions can be performed.

2. Treating Medical Conditions

Numerous medical conditions and diseases necessitate regular blood transfusions as part of the treatment process. Patients with anaemia, cancer, thalassemia, leukaemia, and certain chronic illnesses often require blood transfusions to improve their health and quality of life. Without a consistent and sufficient blood supply, these individuals would face severe health complications and a diminished quality of life.

3. Supporting Surgical Procedures

Various surgeries, including major operations like organ transplants, heart surgeries, and orthopaedic procedures, often require blood transfusions to replace lost blood during surgery or to support patients in their recovery. A reliable blood supply is critical for surgical teams to carry out complex procedures successfully and ensure the best possible outcomes for patients.

4. Enhancing Maternal and Child Health

Pregnant women experiencing complications during childbirth, such as excessive bleeding, may require blood transfusions to safeguard their health and the health of their newborns. Additionally, blood donations support premature infants and children undergoing treatment for various medical conditions.

5. Cancer Treatment

Cancer patients often undergo chemotherapy, which can cause a significant decrease in red blood cells, white blood cells, and platelets. Blood transfusions can provide the necessary components to help these patients cope with the side effects of treatment and maintain their strength throughout their battle against cancer.

6. Improving Long-term Health Outcomes

A stable and sufficient blood supply allows healthcare professionals to proactively address health challenges and improve long-term health outcomes. Regular blood donations ensure that medical facilities have an adequate supply of blood to meet the needs of their patients, reducing delays in treatment and promoting better health in communities.

7. Natural Disasters and Catastrophes

During natural disasters, accidents, or large-scale emergencies, the demand for blood can skyrocket due to increased injuries and casualties. Blood donations are crucial during these times to meet the sudden surge in demand and save lives effectively.

8. Rare Blood Types and Ethnic Diversity

Blood donations from diverse ethnic backgrounds are vital, as certain diseases and conditions require specific blood types. Some blood types are more common in certain ethnic groups, and having a diverse donor pool ensures that patients receive the most suitable and compatible blood transfusions.

9. Building a Culture of Giving and Community Engagement

Blood donation encourages a culture of giving and community engagement. When individuals donate blood, they contribute to the overall well-being of society and foster a sense of unity and altruism within their communities.

10. Voluntary and Unpaid Donations

The importance of voluntary and unpaid blood donations cannot be emphasized enough. Voluntary donors often have a genuine desire to help others, leading to a more committed and consistent blood supply. Unpaid donations ensure that blood is given for altruistic reasons, free from any financial or commercial influence.

Overall, blood donation is a cornerstone of modern healthcare, significantly impacting emergency medical care, surgical procedures, and the treatment of various medical conditions. Encouraging and promoting regular blood donation within communities is essential to ensure a reliable and sufficient blood supply, ultimately saving countless lives and improving the overall health and well-being of individuals.

Figure 1. Blood Donation

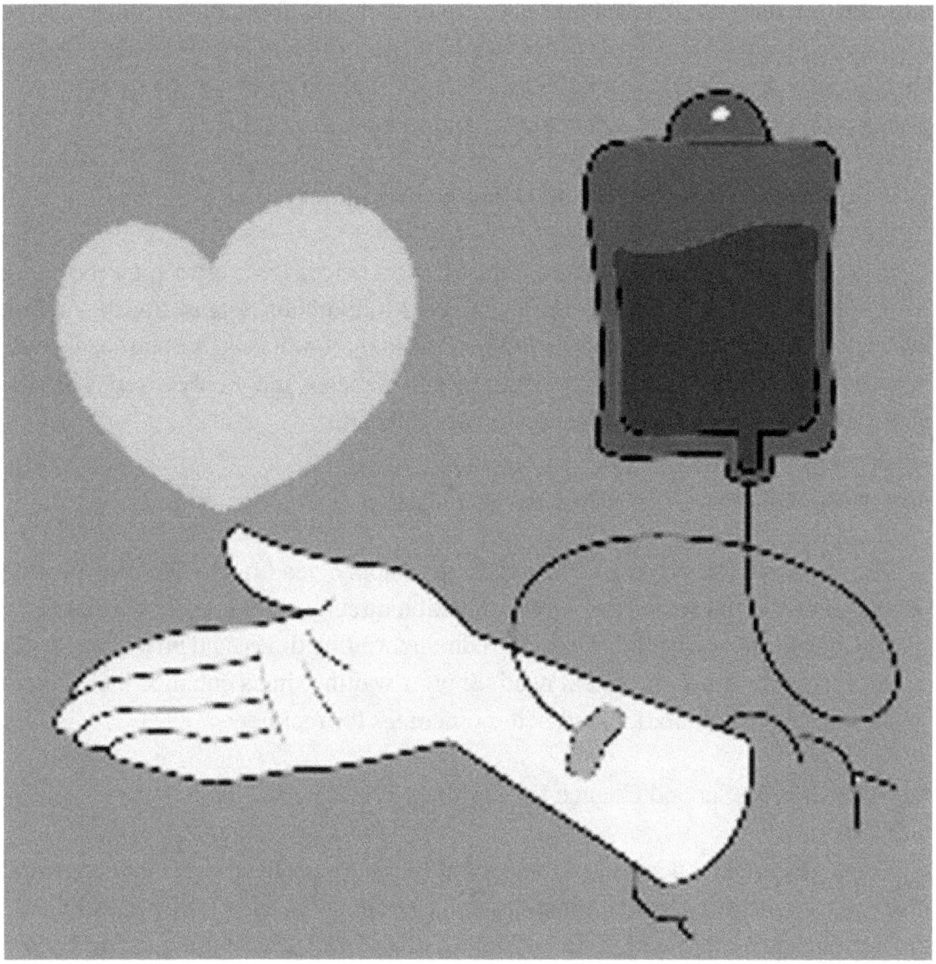

The Importance of Organ Donation

Organ donation is a life-saving and transformative act that involves willingly giving one's organs or tissues to someone in need of a transplant. It is a crucial component of modern medicine, offering hope and a new lease on life to individuals suffering from organ failure or severe medical conditions. This chapter explores the immense significance of organ donation, shedding light on the transformative impact it has on patients, families, and society as a whole.

1. Saving and Enhancing Lives:

Organ donation is a beacon of hope for those suffering from organ failure, providing a lifeline for survival. Transplants can save or dramatically improve the quality of life for recipients suffering from terminal illnesses or severe organ damage. Organs such as the heart, lungs, liver, kidneys, pancreas, and intestines can be transplanted, giving recipients a chance at a healthier and more fulfilling life.

2. Addressing Organ Failure and Chronic Conditions:

Organ failure is a major health concern worldwide, leading to high mortality rates and a reduced quality of life for affected individuals. Organ transplantation offers a definitive solution to organ failure caused by conditions like end-stage renal disease, heart failure, chronic liver disease, and diabetes. It not only extends life but also alleviates symptoms and improves overall health.

3. Reducing Organ Transplant Waiting Lists:

The demand for organs far exceeds the supply, leading to lengthy waiting periods for potential recipients. Organ donation directly addresses this disparity by increasing the pool of available organs, reducing waiting times, and providing timely interventions for those in critical need. Shorter waiting times enhance the chances of successful transplantation and better outcomes for recipients.

4. Providing a Second Chance for Children:

Organ donation is particularly impactful for children suffering from congenital diseases, genetic disorders, or organ failure. Children in need of transplants, such as those requiring a new heart, liver, or kidney, often face a challenging and uncertain future. Organ donation offers these children a second chance at life, enabling them to grow, develop, and experience the joys of childhood.

5. Improving Family and Community Well-being:

Organ donation has a profound impact on the families of both donors and recipients. For the families of donors, it provides solace and comfort in knowing that their loved one's legacy lives on through the lives saved by their donation. On the other hand, for recipients and their families, it brings immense gratitude, joy, and the promise of a brighter future, strengthening community bonds and fostering a culture of compassion and giving.

6. Alleviating Economic Burden:

The financial burden of prolonged medical treatments and dialysis for organ failure can be overwhelming for both individuals and healthcare systems. Organ transplantation, while initially costly, often becomes a cost-effective alternative in the long run. Successful transplants can reduce the need for expensive ongoing treatments and hospitalizations, alleviating the financial strain on patients, their families, and the healthcare system.

7. Advancing Medical Research and Techniques:

Organ transplantation necessitates ongoing advancements in medical research and surgical techniques. The continuous improvement in organ preservation, matching algorithms, immunosuppression drugs, and surgical procedures not only enhances the success rates of transplants but also contributes to advancements in medical science, benefiting patients with a wide array of medical conditions.

8. Promoting a Culture of Giving and Compassion:

Organ donation fosters a culture of altruism, empathy, and giving within society. It encourages individuals to consider the welfare of others and take part in a life-saving endeavour. This cultural shift towards compassion and giving significantly contributes to a more connected and caring community.

9. Raising Awareness about Organ Donation:

The discussion around organ donation encourages education and awareness about the critical need for donors. It prompts individuals to understand the significance of their organs and motivates them to register as donors, ensuring a consistent and ample supply of organs for those in need.

10. Life-Transforming Impact:

Organ donation has the power to transform lives by providing individuals with failing organs a chance for a healthier and more productive life. Transplants are often the only viable treatment for end-stage organ failure.

11. Addressing Organ Shortages:

The demand for organs far exceeds the available supply, leading to lengthy waiting lists and increased mortality rates. Encouraging organ donation helps address these shortages and ensures more timely access to life-saving transplants.

12. Improved Quality of Life:

Organ transplant recipients often experience a significant improvement in their quality of life. They can return to normal activities and contribute to society, highlighting the long-term benefits of organ donation.

13. Advancements in Medical Science:

Organ transplantation has driven advancements in medical science, including surgical techniques, organ preservation, and immunosuppressive medications. Research in this field continues to enhance the success rates and safety of transplant procedures.

14. Economic and Societal Benefits:

Organ donation not only saves lives but also has broader economic and societal benefits. It reduces the economic burden on healthcare systems by decreasing the need for long-term medical treatments and supporting productivity.

Overall, organ donation stands as a beacon of hope, providing the gift of life to countless individuals suffering from organ failure. Its significance lies not only in saving lives but also in transforming communities, fostering empathy, and encouraging a collective effort to support those in need. By promoting awareness, facilitating education, and encouraging organ donation, we can continue to make a profound difference in the lives of patients awaiting a chance at a healthier and happier future.

In the context of donation, health literacy involves understanding the importance of donating blood, organs, or tissues, as well as comprehending the procedures, risks, benefits, and the overall impact on both the donor and the recipient. An empowered and health-literate donor possesses the knowledge and comprehension needed to navigate the donation process, making informed decisions that align with their values and beliefs.

Importance of Blood Transfusion (Sahu, 2014)

Life-Saving Intervention: Blood transfusion is a critical medical intervention that saves millions of lives each year. It is essential in treating various medical conditions such as severe anaemia, trauma, surgery, and certain medical procedures.

Treatment for Medical Conditions: Individuals with chronic conditions like sickle cell anaemia or leukaemia often require regular blood transfusions to manage their health. These treatments improve the quality of life and increase life expectancy.

Emergency Situations: In emergency situations such as accidents, natural disasters, or major surgeries, the availability of an adequate blood supply is crucial for immediate and effective medical care.

Cancer Treatment: Cancer patients undergoing chemotherapy may experience a drop in blood cell count. Blood transfusions provide the necessary support by replenishing red blood cells, platelets, and other components, aiding in the recovery process.

Maternal Health: Complications during childbirth, such as excessive bleeding, may necessitate blood transfusions to save the lives of both mothers and infants. Access to a safe and sufficient blood supply is vital for maternal healthcare.

Blood Transfusion Complication in Some Disease Condition (Ackfeld, 2014)

While blood transfusions are generally considered safe, there can be complications, especially in certain disease conditions. It's important to note that blood transfusions are typically administered when the benefits outweigh the risks, and healthcare professionals carefully evaluate each case. Here are some disease conditions where complications may be of concern:

Haemolytic Reactions: In individuals with conditions such as sickle cell disease or thalassemia, there is a risk of haemolytic reactions. These reactions occur when the body's immune system attacks and destroys the transfused red blood cells.

Iron Overload: Patients with conditions requiring frequent transfusions, such as thalassemia or myelodysplastic syndromes, may develop iron overload over time. This can lead to organ damage, particularly affecting the liver, heart, and endocrine organs.

Infections: Blood transfusions carry a risk of transmitting infections, including viruses (such as HIV, hepatitis B, and hepatitis C) and bacteria. Modern blood banking practices and screening have significantly reduced this risk, but it is not completely eliminated.

Graft-versus-Host Disease (GVHD): GVHD is a rare but serious complication that can occur when the immune cells in donor blood recognize the recipient's tissues as foreign and attack them. This is more common in immunocompromised individuals.

Transfusion-Related Acute Lung Injury (TRALI) (Bux, 2005)

TRALI is a severe respiratory reaction that can occur after a blood transfusion. It is characterized by acute lung injury and can be life-threatening.

Fluid Overload: Patients with heart or kidney conditions may be at risk of fluid overload if large volumes of blood are transfused quickly. Monitoring is crucial to prevent complications related to excessive fluid.

Allergic Reactions: Allergic reactions to components in the blood, such as plasma proteins, can occur. These reactions are usually mild but can occasionally be severe.

Transfusion-Associated Circulatory Overload (TACO)

TACO is a condition in which there is an excessive volume of blood administered, leading to fluid accumulation in the lungs and heart failure. Individuals with heart conditions are at higher risk.

It's crucial for healthcare providers to assess the individual patient's health status, medical history, and specific needs before deciding to administer a blood transfusion. In some cases, alternatives to transfusion, such as medications or other therapeutic approaches, may be considered.

Patients and their families should communicate openly with healthcare providers about any concerns or conditions that might affect the safety of a blood transfusion, and healthcare professionals should provide thorough information about the potential risks and benefits.

CONCLUSION

Blood transfusions are critical in various medical scenarios, such as during childbirth, surgeries, and treatments for severe injuries. In cases of massive blood loss, transfusions can provide the necessary oxygen-carrying red blood cells, ensuring the survival of the patient. Additionally, patients with chronic conditions such as thalassemia or sickle cell disease often require regular transfusions to alleviate symptoms and prevent complications. The availability of a diverse range of blood types is crucial in ensuring that transfusions can be administered promptly and effectively (Lawrence, 2017).Furthermore, blood transfusions have proven to be life-saving in emergency situations, where quick action is essential for survival. In cases of severe trauma or accidents, blood transfusions can stabilize patients, prevent organ failure, and increase the chances of successful surgeries. Without access to compatible blood and adequate supplies, the mortality rates for such cases would be significantly higher.Moving on to organ donation, this procedure involves the transplantation of organs or tissues from one individual (donor) to another (recipient), replacing damaged or failed organs. Organ donation has revolutionized medical practices, offering hope to millions of patients suffering from organ failure or life-threatening conditions. Kidneys, livers, hearts, lungs, and corneas are among the organs that can be transplanted.The importance of organ donation lies in the fact that it can significantly improve the quality of life for recipients, allowing them to resume normal activities and enjoy more years with their loved ones. Moreover, organ transplantation can often be the only treatment option for individuals with end-stage organ failure, offering a chance at survival and recovery.However, the demand for organ transplantation far exceeds the available supply. This scarcity has led to long waiting lists and unfortunate fatalities for many patients. According to the World Health Organization (WHO), as of 2020, over 100,000 solid organ transplants are performed annually, but the need for transplantation is estimated to be 10 times higher. This staggering gap emphasizes the urgent need for more organ donors.

In conclusion, a comprehensive literature review and background on the importance of blood transfusion and organ donation underscore their vital roles in healthcare. Blood transfusions are critical for treating a range of medical conditions and preventing fatalities, while organ donation offers a lifeline to those suffering from organ failure. However, both procedures heavily rely on the benevolence of donors and the availability of compatible matches. Increasing awareness, promoting donation initiatives, and ensuring efficient distribution systems are crucial in bridging the gap between supply and demand. By recognizing the significance of blood transfusion and organ donation, we can collectively work towards enhancing healthcare outcomes and saving lives. Health literacy is an indispensable tool for empowering donors and enhancing their decision-making process in the context of donation. It equips individuals with the knowledge, understanding, and confidence needed to make informed choices regarding blood, organ, and tissue donation. By promoting health literacy, we can cultivate a society of donors who contribute to the well-being and health of others, making a lasting and meaningful impact on countless lives.

REFERENCES

Ackfeld, T., Schmutz, T., Guechi, Y., & Le Terrier, C. (2022). Blood Transfusion Reactions—A Comprehensive Review of the Literature including a Swiss Perspective. *Journal of Clinical Medicine*, *11*(10), 2859. doi:10.3390/jcm11102859 PMID:35628985

Ahern, D., Kreslake, J., Phalen, J., & Bock, B. (2006). What is eHealth (6): Perspectives on the evolution of eHealth research. *Journal of Medical Internet Research*, *8*(1), e4. doi:10.2196/jmir.8.1.e4 PMID:16585029

Baldry, M., Cheal, C., Fisher, B., Gillett, M., & Huet, V. (1986). Giving patients their own records in general practice: experience of patients and staff. Br Med J (Clin Res Ed), 1;292(6520):596-8. . PMID: 3081187; PMCID: PMC1339574. doi:10.1136/bmj.292.6520.596

. Berland, G. K., Elliott, M. N., Morales, L. S., Algazy, J. I., Kravitz, R. L., Broder, M. S., Kanouse, D. E., Muñoz, J. A., Puyol, J.A., Lara, M., Watkins, K. E., Yang, H., McGlynn, E. A. (2001). Health information on the Internet: accessibility, quality, and readability in English and Spanish. JAMA. 23-30;285(20):2612-21. . PMID: 11368735; PMCID: PMC4182102. doi:10.1001/jama.285.20.2612

Bux, J. (2005). Transfusion-related acute lung injury (TRALI): A serious adverse event of blood transfusion. *Vox Sanguinis*, *89*(1), 1–10. doi:10.1111/j.1423-0410.2005.00648.x PMID:15938734

Chen, H. F., Ali, H., Marrero, W. J., Parikh, N, D., Lavieri, M. S., Hutton, D. W. (2021). The Magnitude of the Health and Economic Impact of Increased Organ Donation on Patients with End-Stage Renal Disease. *MDM Policy Pract.* 6;6(2):23814683211063418. . PMID: 34901442; PMCID: PMC8655828. doi:10.1177/23814683211063418

Coughlin, S. S., Vernon, M., Hatzigeorgiou, C., & George, V. (2020). Health Literacy, Social Determinants of Health, and Disease Prevention and Control. *Journal of Environment and Health Sciences*, *6*(1), 3061. PMID:33604453

Cristofori, E., Zeffiro, V., Alvaro, R., D'Agostino, F., Zega, M., Cocchieri, A. (2022). Health Literacy in Patients' Clinical Records of Hospital Settings: A Systematic Review. *SAGE Open Nurs.*7; 8:23779608221078555. . PMID: 35284632; PMCID: PMC8905211. doi:10.1177/23779608221078555

Estcourt, L. J., Hopewell, S., Trivella, M., Hambleton, I. R, Cho, G. (2019). Regular long-term red blood cell transfusions for managing chronic chest complications in sickle cell disease. *Cochrane Database Syst Rev*. 25;2019(10):CD008360. . PMID: 31684693; PMCID: PMC6814284. doi:10.1002/14651858.CD008360.pub5

Ferguson, E., Murray, C., & O'Carroll, R. E. (2019). Blood and organ donation: Health impact, prevalence, correlates, and interventions. *Psychology & Health*, *34*(9), 1073–1104. doi:10.1080/08870446.2019.1603385 PMID:31213077

Fitzpatrick, P. J. (2023). Improving health literacy using the power of digital communications to achieve better health outcomes for patients and practitioners. *Frontiers in Digital Health*, *5*, 1264780. doi:10.3389/fdgth.2023.1264780 PMID:38046643

Giles, M., Mc, C., Clenahan, E., & Cairns, J. M. (2004). An application of the Theory of Planned Behaviour to blood donation: The importance of self-efficacy. *Health Education Research, 19*(4), 380–391. doi:10.1093/her/cyg063 PMID:15155590

Lawrence, T. G., & Panigrahi, A. K. (2017). Blood Transfusion Therapy. *The Medical Clinics of North America, 101*(2), 431–447. doi:10.1016/j.mcna.2016.09.012 PMID:28189180

Liu, C., Wang, D., Liu, C., Jiang, J., Wang, X., Chen, H., Ju, X., & Zhang, X. (2020). What is the meaning of health literacy? A systematic review and qualitative synthesis. *Family Medicine and Community Health, 8*(2), e000351. doi:10.1136/fmch-2020-000351 PMID:32414834

McCray, A. T. (2005). Promoting health literacy. *Journal of the American Medical Informatics Association : JAMIA, 12*(2), 152–163. doi:10.1197/jamia.M1687 PMID:15561782

Moritsugu, K. P. (2013). The power of organ donation to save lives through transplantation. *Public Health Reports (Washington, D.C.), 128*(4), 245–246. doi:10.1177/003335491312800402 PMID:23814318

Nambiar, P., Silibovsky, R., & Belden, K. A. (2018). Infection in Kidney Transplantation. *Contemporary Kidney Transplantation, 27*, 307–327. doi:10.1007/978-3-319-19617-6_22

Oge, T., Kilic, C. H., & Kilic, G. S. (2014). Economic impact of blood transfusions: Balancing cost and benefits. *The Eurasian Journal of Medicine, 46*(1), 47–49. doi:10.5152/eajm.2014.08 PMID:25610294

Rossaint, R., Afshari, A., & Bouillon, B. (2023). The European guideline on management of major bleeding and coagulopathy following trauma: sixth edition. Crit Care, 27, 80. doi:10.1186/s13054-023-04327-7

Sahu, S., Hemlata, V. A., & Verma, A. (2014). Adverse events related to blood transfusion. *Indian Journal of Anaesthesia, 58*(5), 543–551. doi:10.4103/0019-5049.144650 PMID:25535415

Shroff, S. (2009). Legal and ethical aspects of organ donation and transplantation. *Indian Journal of Urology, 25*(3), 348–355. doi:10.4103/0970-1591.56203 PMID:19881131

Thongprayoon, C., Kaewput, W., Pattharanitima, P., Cheungpasitporn, W. (2022). Progress and Recent Advances in Solid Organ Transplantation. *J Clin Med.* 11;11(8):2112. . PMID: 35456205; PMCID: PMC9031939. doi:10.3390/jcm11082112

Thurn, L., Wide-Swensson, D., Hellgren-Wångdahl, M. (2023). Postpartumblödningar med blood transfusioner har ökat [Postpartum hemorrhage and need of blood transfusions]. Lakartidningen. 15; 118:20147. Swedish. PMID: 33720382.

Tucker, E. L., Smith, A. R., Daskin, M. S., Schapiro, H., Cottrell, S. M., Gendron, E. S., Hill-Callahan, P., Leichtman, A. B., Merion, R. M., Gill, S. J., & Maass, K. L. (2019). Life and expectations post-kidney transplant: A qualitative analysis of patient responses. *BMC Nephrology*, *20*(1), 175. doi:10.1186/s12882-019-1368-0 PMID:31096942

Udvardy, M., Illés, Á., Gergely, L., Pinczés, L. I., Magyari, F., Simon, Z. (2023). Transfusion-Transmitted Disorders with Special Attention to Bone Marrow Transplant Patients. *Pathogens.* 1;12(7):901. . PMID: 37513748; PMCID: PMC10383292. doi:10.3390/pathogens12070901

Van den Broucke, S. (2014). Health literacy: a critical concept for public health. *Arch Public Health*, 1;72(1):10. . PMID: 24685171; PMCID: PMC3994208. doi:10.1186/2049-3258-72-10

Compilation of References

Abel, T., & Mcqueen, D. (2020). Critical health literacy and the COVID-19 crisis. *Health Promotion International*, *35*(6), 1612–1613. doi:10.1093/heapro/daaa040 PMID:32239213

Ackfeld, T., Schmutz, T., Guechi, Y., & Le Terrier, C. (2022). Blood Transfusion Reactions—A Comprehensive Review of the Literature including a Swiss Perspective. *Journal of Clinical Medicine*, *11*(10), 2859. doi:10.3390/jcm11102859 PMID:35628985

Adler, N., & Matthews, K. (1994). Health psychology: Why do some people get sick and some stay well? *Annual Review of Psychology*, *45*(1), 229–259. doi:10.1146/annurev.ps.45.020194.001305 PMID:8135503

Agarahari, P., Jain, A., Pandey, S. M., Agrahari, A. K., Yadav, J., Srivastava, R., & Pandey, S. M. (2023). Exploring the Synergistic Association Between Oral Health Status and Oral Health Literacy Among College Students: A Cross-Sectional Study. *Cureus*, *15*(7), 1–8. doi:10.7759/cureus.41885 PMID:37581155

Agarwal, S. (2020). *'Aarogya Setu app launched by GoI in public-private partnership mode'*. The Economic Times. Retrieved from https://economictimes.indiatimes.com/tech/information-tech/aarogya-setu-app-launched-by-goi-in-public-private-partnership-mode/articleshow/78916970.cms

Ahern, D., Kreslake, J., Phalen, J., & Bock, B. (2006). What is eHealth (6): Perspectives on the evolution of eHealth research. *Journal of Medical Internet Research*, *8*(1), e4. doi:10.2196/jmir.8.1.e4 PMID:16585029

Ajzen, I. (1991). The theory of planned behavior. *Organizational Behavior and Human Decision Processes*, *50*(2), 179–211. doi:10.1016/0749-5978(91)90020-T

Allah, H. A., & S, P. M. (2019). The knowledge and perceptions regarding probiotics among the people of al-qassim region, Saudi Arabia. *Journal of Health and Medical Sciences*, *2*(3). Advance online publication. doi:10.31014/aior.1994.02.03.56

Alshammari, T. (2014). Drug safety: The concept, inception and its importance in patients' health. *Saudi Pharmaceutical Journal*, *24*(4), 405–412. doi:10.1016/j.jsps.2014.04.008 PMID:27330371

American Civil Liberties Union (ACLU). (2021). Principles for technology-assisted contact-tracing. ACLU White Paper. Retrieved from https://www.aclu.org/report/aclu-white-paper-principles-technology-assisted-contact-tracing

Anadolu Agency. (2020). Hidden heroes of the fight against coronavirus: Filection teams. Retrieved from https://www.aa.com.tr/tr/koronavirus/koronavirus-ile-mucadelenin-gizli-kahramanlari-filmasyon-ekipleri/1807025

Anasi, S. N. (2012). Access to and dissemination of health information in Africa: The patient and the public. *Journal of Hospital Librarianship*, *12*(2), 120–134. doi:10.1080/15323269.2012.666647

Anson, P. (2021, May 25). *How opioid hysteria affects cancer patients*. Pain News Network. Retrieved August 10, 2023, from https://www.painnewsnetwork.org/stories/2021/5/25/how-opioid-hysteria-affects-cancer-patients

Appel, G., Grewal, L., Rhonda Hadi, R., & Stephen, A. T. (2020). The future of social media in marketing. [January.]. *Journal of the Academy of Marketing Science*, *48*(1), 79–95. doi:10.1007/s11747-019-00695-1 PMID:32431463

Are cancer patients getting the opioids they need to control pain? (2020, September 16). National Cancer Institute at the National Institutes of Health. Retrieved August 10, 2023, from https://www.cancer.gov/news-events/cancer-currents-blog/2020/opioids-cancer-pain-oncologists-decreasing-prescriptions

Arora, P., Mehta, S., & Arora, N. (2021). Effect of Consumers' Immunity Consciousness on Monthly Consumption of Immunity Booster Products.

Arora, P., & Arora, N. (2023). People, Immunity and Nutrition: A Categorization. *International Journal of Innovative Science and Research Technology*, *8*(4).

Arora, S., Prabha, K., Sharanagat, V. S., & Mishra, V. (2020). Consumer awareness and willingness to purchase probiotic food and beverage products: A study of Sonipat district, Haryana. *British Food Journal*, *123*(8), 2805–2817. doi:10.1108/BFJ-06-2020-0469

Arshad, M. S., Saqlain, M., Majeed, A., Imran, I., Saeed, H., Saleem, M. U., Abrar, M. A., Islam, M., Hashmi, F., Akbar, M., Chaudhry, M. O., Ramzan, B., & Rasool, M. F. (2021). Cross-sectional study to assess the healthcare professionals' knowledge, attitude and practices about probiotics use in Pakistan. *BMJ Open*, *11*(7), e047494. doi:10.1136/bmjopen-2020-047494 PMID:34321300

Arthur, J., & Bruera, E. (2022). Managing cancer pain in patients with opioid use disorder or nonmedical opioid use. *JAMA Oncology*, *8*(8), 1104. doi:10.1001/jamaoncol.2022.2150 PMID:35771548

As-Sanie, S., Gantt, A., & Rosenthal, M. S. (2004). Pregnancy prevention in adolescents. *American Family Physician*, *70*(8), 1517–1524. PMID:15526738

Astbury, S., Mostyn, A., Symonds, M. E., & Bell, R. C. (2015). Nutrient availability, the microbiome, and intestinal transport during pregnancy. *Applied Physiology, Nutrition, and Metabolism*, *40*(11), 1100–1106. doi:10.1139/apnm-2015-0117 PMID:26499849

Babalola, S., Lawal, A. S., Mako, I. V., Rimon, J. G. II, Corso, C., Kiragu, K., & Church. (1993). Mobile family planning drama. *Promotion & Education, 1*(4), 42–45. doi:10.1177/175797599300100412 PMID:8186944

Baker, D. W., Gazmararian, J. A., Williams, M. V., Scott, T., Parker, R. M., Green, D., Ren, J., & Peel, J. (2002). Functional health literacy and the risk of hospital admission among Medicare managed care enrollees. *American Journal of Public Health, 92*(8), 1278–1283. doi:10.2105/AJPH.92.8.1278 PMID:12144984

Baker, D. W., Williams, M. V., Parker, R. M., Gazmararian, J. A., & Nurss, J. (1999). Development of a brief test to measure functional health literacy. *Patient Education and Counseling, 38*(1), 33–42. doi:10.1016/S0738-3991(98)00116-5 PMID:14528569

Baker, D. W., Wolf, M. S., Feinglass, J., Thompson, J. A., Gazmararian, J. A., & Huang, J. (2007). Health literacy and mortality among elderly persons. *Archives of Internal Medicine, 167*(14), 1503–1509. doi:10.1001/archinte.167.14.1503 PMID:17646604

Baker, J. A., Canvin, K., & Berzins, K. (2019). The relationship between workforce characteristics and perception of quality of care in mental health: A qualitative study. *International Journal of Nursing Studies, 100*, 103412. doi:10.1016/j.ijnurstu.2019.103412 PMID:31629212

Balamurugan, R., Janardhan, H. P., George, S., Chittaranjan, S. P., & Ramakrishna, B. S. (2008). Bacterial succession in the colon during childhood and adolescence: Molecular studies in a southern Indian village. *The American Journal of Clinical Nutrition, 88*(6), 1643–1647. doi:10.3945/ajcn.2008.26511 PMID:19064526

Baldassarre, M., Palladino, V., Amoruso, A., Pindinelli, S., Mastromarino, P., Fanelli, M., Di Mauro, A., & Laforgia, N. (2018). Rationale of probiotic supplementation during pregnancy and neonatal period. *Nutrients, 10*(11), 1693. doi:10.3390/nu10111693 PMID:30404227

Baldry, M., Cheal, C., Fisher, B., Gillett, M., & Huet, V. (1986). Giving patients their own records in general practice: experience of patients and staff. Br Med J (Clin Res Ed), 1;292(6520):596-8. . PMID: 3081187; PMCID: PMC1339574. doi:10.1136/bmj.292.6520.596

Balfour, M. E., Hahn Stephenson, A., Delany-Brumsey, A., Winsky, J., & Goldman, M. L. (2022). Cops, clinicians, or both? Collaborative approaches to responding to behavioral health emergencies. *Psychiatric Services (Washington, D.C.), 73*(6), 658–669. doi:10.1176/appi.ps.202000721 PMID:34666512

Bano, R., AlShammari, E., Fatima, S. B., & Al-Shammari, N. A. (2013). A comparative study of Knowledge, Attitude, Practice of nutrition and non-nutrition student towards a balanced diet in Hail University. *IOSR Journal of Nursing and Health Science, 2*(3), 29–36. https://www.iosrjournals.org/iosr-jnhs/papers/vol2-issue3/E0232936.pdf?id=8220

Barkataki, I., & Ross, L. (2019). Psychological treatment on the acute ward. *Oxford Textbook of Inpatient Psychiatry, 245*, 245–252. Advance online publication. doi:10.1093/med/9780198794257.003.0028

Barqawi, H. J., Adra, S. F., Ramzi, H. R., Abouaggour, M. A., & Almehairi, S. K. (2021). Evaluating the knowledge, attitudes and practices of the UAE community on microbiota composition and the main factors affecting it: A cross-sectional study. *BMJ Open*, *11*(8), e047869. doi:10.1136/bmjopen-2020-047869 PMID:34404705

Barrett, L. F. (2022). Context reconsidered: Complex signal ensembles, relational meaning, and population thinking in psychological science. *The American Psychologist*, *77*(8), 894–920. doi:10.1037/amp0001054 PMID:36409120

Bashshur, R. L., Shannon, G. W., & Bashshur, N. (2016). The empirical evidence for telemedicine interventions in primary care: An updated systematic review. *Telemedicine Journal and e-Health*, *22*(1), 37–40. PMID:27336754

Bauce, K. (2014). Cultural competence model. In J. J. Fitzpatrick & G. McCarthy (Eds.), *Theories guiding nursing research and practice* (pp. 159–171). Springer., doi:10.1891/9780826164056.0010

Baumgardt, J., & Weinmann, S. (2022). Using Crisis Theory in Dealing with Severe Mental Illness-A Step Toward Normalization? *Frontiers in Sociology*, *7*, 805604. doi:10.3389/fsoc.2022.805604 PMID:35755483

Bauza, V., Sclar, G. D., Bisoyi, A., Owens, A., Ghugey, A., & Clasen, T. (2021). Experience of the COVID-19 Pandemic in Rural Odisha, India: Knowledge, Preventative Actions, and Impacts on Daily Life. International Journal of Environmental Research and Public Health, 18(6), 2863. MDPI AG. Retrieved from doi:10.3390/ijerph18062863

BBC. (2020). Covid-19: China pushes for QR code based global travel system. Retrieved from https://www.bbc.com/news/business-55039662. Posted on October 09, 2020.

Beauchemin, M., & Cogan, J. (2022, June 1). *Addressing opioid misuse in cancer pain management* (Interview by M. A. Farmer) [Transcript]. Columbia University. Retrieved February 2, 2024, from https://www.cancer.columbia.edu/news/ addressing-opioid-misuse-cancer-pain-management

Beauchemin, M. P., Raghunathan, R. R., Accordino, M. K., Cogan, J. C., Kahn, J. M., Wright, J. D., & Hershman, D. L. (2022). New persistent opioid use among adolescents and young adults with sarcoma. *Cancer*, *128*(14), 2777–2785. doi:10.1002/cncr.34238 PMID:35599575

Beck, J. (2015, April 21). What Good Is 'Raising Awareness?'. *The Atlantic*. https://www.theatlantic.com/health/archive/2015/04/what-good-is-raising-awareness/391002/

Benabdellah, A. C., Benghabrit, A., & Bouhaddou, I. (2019). A survey of clustering algorithms for an industrial context. *Procedia Computer Science*, *148*, 291–302. doi:10.1016/j.procs.2019.01.022

Ben-Ari, E. (2023, February 14). Study finds disparities in access to opioids for cancer pain at end of life. *Cancer currents*. https://www.cancer.gov/ news-events/cancer-currents-blog/2023/disparities-opioids-cancer-pain-end-of-life

Bennett, M., Paice, J. A., & Wallace, M. (2018). Pain and opioids in cancer care: Benefits, risks, and alternatives. *American Society of Clinical Oncology Educational Book*, *37*(37), 705–713. doi:10.1200/EDBK_180469 PMID:28561731

Berkman, N. D., Sheridan, S. L., Donahue, K. E., Halpern, D. J., & Crotty, K. (2011). Low health literacy and health outcomes: An updated systematic review. *Annals of Internal Medicine, 155*(2), 97–107. doi:10.7326/0003-4819-155-2-201107190-00005 PMID:21768583

Bernstein, K. S., & Kaplan, R. (2022). *Psychiatric Mental Health Assessment and Diagnosis of Adults for Advanced Practice Mental Health Nurses*. Taylor & Francis., doi:10.4324/9781003137597

Betancourt, J. R., Green, A. R., Carrillo, J. E., & Park, E. R. (2005). Cultural competence and health care disparities: Key perspectives and trends. *Health Affairs, 24*(2), 499–505. doi:10.1377/hlthaff.24.2.499 PMID:15757936

Bish, A., Yardley, L., Nicoll, A., & Michie, S. (2011). Factors associated with uptake of vaccination against pandemic influenza: A systematic review. *Vaccine, 29*(38), 6472–6484. doi:10.1016/j.vaccine.2011.06.107 PMID:21756960

Bohler, R., Thomas, C.P., Clark, T.W., & Horgan, C.M. (2021, February). *Addressing the opioid crisis through social determinants of health: What are communities doing?* Opioid Policy Research Collaborative at Brandeis University.

Borre, Y. E., O'Keeffe, G. W., Clarke, G., Stanton, C., Dinan, T. G., & Cryan, J. F. (2014). Microbiota and neurodevelopmental Windows: Implications for brain disorders. *Trends in Molecular Medicine, 20*(9), 509–518. doi:10.1016/j.molmed.2014.05.002 PMID:24956966

Bowden-Jones, O., & Abdulrahim, D. (2020). *Club Drugs and Novel Psychoactive Substances: The Clinician's Handbook*. Cambridge University Press., doi:10.1017/9781911623106

Brett, J. (2020). How Blockchain Technology Offers 'Computational Trust' For Tracking The Coronavirus Outbreak", Forbes, https://www.forbes.com/sites/jasonbrett/2020/03/23/how-blockchain-technology-offers-computational-trust-for-tracking---the-coronavirus-outbreak/#c56e0351cd06

Browne, P. D., Bolte, A. C., Besseling-van der Vaart, I., Claassen, E., & De Weerth, C. (2021). Probiotics as a treatment for prenatal maternal anxiety and depression: A double-blind randomized pilot trial. *Scientific Reports, 11*(1), 3051. Advance online publication. doi:10.1038/s41598-021-81204-9 PMID:33542275

Bruera, E., & Paice, J. A. (2015). Cancer pain management: Safe and effective use of opioids. *American Society of Clinical Oncology Educational Book*, (35), e593–e599. doi:10.14694/EdBook_AM.2015.35.e593 PMID:25993228

Bugada, D., Lorini, L. F., Fumagalli, R., & Allegri, M. (2020). Genetics and opioids: Towards more appropriate prescription in cancer pain. *Cancers (Basel), 12*(7), 1951. doi:10.3390/cancers12071951 PMID:32708424

Bulls, H. W., Chu, E., Goodin, B. R., Liebschutz, J. M., Wozniak, A., Schenker, Y., & Merlin, J. S. (2021). Framework for opioid stigma in cancer pain. *Pain, 163*(2), e182–e189. doi:10.1097/j.pain.0000000000002343 PMID:34010940

Bux, J. (2005). Transfusion-related acute lung injury (TRALI): A serious adverse event of blood transfusion. *Vox Sanguinis*, *89*(1), 1–10. doi:10.1111/j.1423-0410.2005.00648.x PMID:15938734

Cappelletty, G. (2022). *Into the Maelstrom: Toward a Theory of Chaos and Crisis*. Austin Macauley Publishers.

Caretaker Medical. (2020). Caretaker Medical News Australia's first 'virtual hospital' for COVID-19 patients use Caretaker Medical wireless patient monitor for remote monitoring and reporting. Retrieved from https://www.caretakermedical.net/australias-first-virtual-hospital-for-covid-19-patients-use-caretaker-medical-wireless-patient-monitor-for-remote-monitoring-and-reporting/

Carvalho, N. B., Costa, T. D., Ferreira, M. A., Simiqueli, A. A., & Minim, V. P. (2014). Consumer attitude regarding products containing probiotics. *Ciência Rural*, *44*(7), 1319–1326. doi:10.1590/0103-8478cr20131178

Cascini, F., Pantovic, A., Al-Ajlouni, Y., Failla, G., & Ricciardi, W. (2021). Attitudes, acceptance and hesitancy among the general population worldwide to receive the COVID-19 vaccines and their contributing factors: A systematic review. *EClinicalMedicine*, *40*, 101113. doi:10.1016/j.eclinm.2021.101113 PMID:34490416

Cevik Guner, U., & Kissal, A. (2021). Mothers' knowledge, attitudes and practices regarding probiotic use during pregnancy and for their infants in Turkey. *Public Health Nutrition*, *24*(13), 4297–4304. doi:10.1017/S1368980021000951 PMID:33663639

Chan, E. A., Tsang, P. L., Ching, S. S. Y., Wong, F. Y., & Lam, W. (2019). Nurses' perspectives on their communication with patients in busy oncology wards: A qualitative study. *PLoS One*, *14*(10), e0224178. doi:10.1371/journal.pone.0224178 PMID:31648272

Chauhan, S., Agarwal, N., & Kar, A. K. (2016). Addressing big data challenges in smart cities: A systematic literature review. *Info*, *18*(4), 73–90. doi:10.1108/info-03-2016-0012

Cheetham, A., Picco, L., Barnett, A., Lubman, D. I., & Nielsen, S. (2022). The impact of stigma on people with opioid use disorder, opioid treatment, and policy. *Substance Abuse and Rehabilitation*, *13*, 1–12. doi:10.2147/SAR.S304566 PMID:35115860

Chen, H. F., Ali, H., Marrero, W. J., Parikh, N, D., Lavieri, M. S., Hutton, D. W. (2021). The Magnitude of the Health and Economic Impact of Increased Organ Donation on Patients with End-Stage Renal Disease. *MDM Policy Pract.* 6;6(2):23814683211063418. . PMID: 34901442; PMCID: PMC8655828. doi:10.1177/23814683211063418

Cheng, L., Liu, Y., Wu, C., Wang, S., & Tsai, Y. (2019). Psychobiotics in mental health, neurodegenerative and neurodevelopmental disorders. *Yao Wu Shi Pin Fen Xi*, *27*(3), 632–648. doi:10.1016/j.jfda.2019.01.002 PMID:31324280

Chen, J., & See, K. C. (2020). Artificial Intelligence for COVID-19: Rapid Review. *Journal of Medical Internet Research*, *22*(10), e21476. doi:10.2196/21476 PMID:32946413

Chen, X., Jiang, X., Huang, X., He, H., & Zheng, J. (2020). Association between probiotic yogurt intake and gestational diabetes mellitus: A case-control study. *Iranian Journal of Public Health*. Advance online publication. doi:10.18502/ijph.v48i7.2946 PMID:31497545

Chen, Y., Li, Z., Tye, K. D., Luo, H., Tang, X., Liao, Y., Wang, D., Zhou, J., Yang, P., Li, Y., Su, Y., & Xiao, X. (2019). Probiotic supplementation during human pregnancy affects the gut microbiota and immune status. *Frontiers in Cellular and Infection Microbiology*, *9*, 254. Advance online publication. doi:10.3389/fcimb.2019.00254 PMID:31380297

Chinn, D., & McCarthy, C. (2013). All Aspects of Health Literacy Scale (AAHLS): Developing a tool to measure functional, communicative and critical health literacy in primary healthcare settings. *Patient Education and Counseling*, *90*(2), 247–253. doi:10.1016/j.pec.2012.10.019 PMID:23206659

Choudhary, S. R. & Barman, A. (2014). Holistic Model of subjective well-being a proposed model and exploration of contents. *Zenith International Journal of Multidisciplinary research*, *4*(3), 259-278.

Choudhury, S. M., Arora, T., Alebbi, S., Ahmed, L., Aden, A., Omar, O., & Taheri, S. (2016). How do Qataris source health information? *PLoS One*, *11*(11), e0166250. doi:10.1371/journal.pone.0166250 PMID:27832112

Cho, Y. I., Lee, S. Y. D., Arozullah, A. M., & Crittenden, K. S. (2008). Effects of health literacy on health status and health service utilization amongst the elderly. *Social Science & Medicine*, *66*(8), 1809–1816. doi:10.1016/j.socscimed.2008.01.003 PMID:18295949

Christiano, A., & Neimand, A. (2017, Spring). Stop raising awareness already. *Essentials of Social Innovation*. https://ssir.org/articles/entry/stop_raising_awareness_already#

Chuang, Y. T., Zargoush, M., Ghazalbash, S., Samiedaluie, S., Kuluski, K., & Guilcher, S. (2023). From prediction to decision: Optimizing long-term care placements among older delayed discharge patients. *Production and Operations Management*, *32*(4), 1041–1058. doi:10.1111/poms.13910

Chu, D. M., Antony, K. M., Ma, J., Prince, A. L., Showalter, L., Moller, M., & Aagaard, K. M. (2016). The early infant gut microbiome varies in association with a maternal high-fat diet. *Genome Medicine*, *8*(1), 77. Advance online publication. doi:10.1186/s13073-016-0330-z PMID:27503374

Colombia Mailman School of Public Health. (2020). Mapping the Areas Most Vulnerable to COVID-19 Hospitalizations. https://www.mailman.columbia.edu/public-health-now/news/mapping-areas-most-vulnerable-COVID-19-hospitalizations

Connell, J. (2013). Contemporary medical tourism: Conceptualisation, culture and commodification. *Tourism Management*, *34*, 1–13. doi:10.1016/j.tourman.2012.05.009

Costa, T., & Evans, L. L., Jr. (2022, February 23). *Older workers: Opioid misuse and employment outcomes* [Letter to Robert P. Casey, Jr. & Susan M. Collins]. https://www.gao.gov/assets/gao-22-104491.pdf

Coughlin, S. S., Datta, B., Vernon, M., Hatzigeorgiou, C., & George, V. (2022). Health literacy among cancer survivors. *Medicine*, *101*(9), e29010. doi:10.1097/MD.0000000000029010 PMID:35244079

Coughlin, S. S., Vernon, M., Hatzigeorgiou, C., & George, V. (2020). Health Literacy, Social Determinants of Health, and Disease Prevention and Control. *Journal of Environment and Health Sciences*, *6*(1), 3061. PMID:33604453

Cristofori, E., Zeffiro, V., Alvaro, R., D'Agostino, F., Zega, M., Cocchieri, A. (2022). Health Literacy in Patients' Clinical Records of Hospital Settings: A Systematic Review. *SAGE Open Nurs.*7; 8:23779608221078555. . PMID: 35284632; PMCID: PMC8905211. doi:10.1177/23779608221078555

Curtis, K. M., Tepper, N. K., Jatlaoui, T. C., Berry-Bibee, E., Horton, L. G., Zapata, L. B., ... & Whiteman, M. K. (2016). US medical eligibility criteria for contraceptive use, 2016. *Morbidity and Mortality Weekly Report: Recommendations and Reports, 65*(3), 1-103. DOI: http://dx.doi.org/ icon doi:10.15585/mmwr.rr6503a1external

Da Silva, A. G., Baldaçara, L., Cavalcante, D. A., Fasanella, N. A., & Palha, A. P. (2020). The impact of mental illness stigma on psychiatric emergencies. *Frontiers in Psychiatry*, *11*, 573. doi:10.3389/fpsyt.2020.00573 PMID:32636773

Dalgleish, T., Black, M., Johnston, D., & Bevan, A. (2020). Transdiagnostic approaches to mental health problems: Current status and future directions. *Journal of Consulting and Clinical Psychology*, *88*(3), 179–195. doi:10.1037/ccp0000482 PMID:32068421

Dalton-Locke, C., Johnson, S., Harju-Seppänen, J., Lyons, N., Sheridan Rains, L., Stuart, R., Campbell, A., Clark, J., Clifford, A., Courtney, L., Dare, C., Kelly, K., Lynch, C., McCrone, P., Nairi, S., Newbigging, K., Nyikavaranda, P., Osborn, D., Persaud, K., ... Lloyd-Evans, B. (2021). Emerging models and trends in mental health crisis care in England: A national investigation of crisis care systems. *BMC Health Services Research*, *21*(1), 1–12. doi:10.1186/s12913-021-07181-x PMID:34711222

Davenport, T. H. (1997). *Information Ecology*. Oxford University Press. doi:10.1093/oso/9780195111682.001.0001

David. R. (January 2020). *'India Confirm its first corona virus case'*. CNBC. Retrieved from https://www.cnbc.com/2020/01/30/india-confirms-first-case-of-the-coronavirus.html

Dawe, J. P., McCowan, L. M., Wilson, J., Okesene-Gafa, K. A., & Serlachius, A. S. (2020). Probiotics and maternal mental health: A randomised controlled trial among pregnant women with obesity. *Scientific Reports*, *10*(1), 1291. Advance online publication. doi:10.1038/s41598-020-58129-w PMID:31992802

Deloitte. (2014). L. L. P. (2009). Medical tourism: Update and implications. *Retrieved*, (September), 29.

Demirtaş, T., & Tekiner, H. (2020). Filiation: A Historical Term the COVID-19 Outbreak Recalled in Turkey. *Erciyes Med J*, *42*(3), 354–358. doi:10.14744/etd.2020.54782

Department of Health and Family Welfare, Government of Karnataka. Department of Psychiatry National Institute of Mental Health and Neurosciences, Bangaluru. (2020, July). Caring for Health Care Warriors Mental Health Support during. *COVID*, 19.

Duan, H., Wang, S., & Yang, C. (2020). Coronavirus: Limit short-term economic damage. *Nature*, *578*(7796), 515. doi:10.1038/d41586-020-00522-6 PMID:32099120

Duggan, M., Harris, B., Chislett, W. K., & Calder, R. (2020). *Nowhere else to go: Why Australia's health system results in people with mental illness getting 'stuck' in emergency departments.*

Edwards, D., Carrier, J., Csontos, J., Evans, N., Elliott, M., Gillen, E., & Williams, L. (2023). Crisis responses for children and young people-a systematic review of effectiveness, experiences and service organisation (CAMH-Crisis). *Child and Adolescent Mental Health*. Advance online publication. doi:10.1111/camh.12639 PMID:36785997

Edwards, S. M., Cunningham, S. A., Dunlop, A. L., & Corwin, E. J. (2017). The maternal gut microbiome during pregnancy. *MCN. The American Journal of Maternal Child Nursing*, *42*(6), 310–317. doi:10.1097/NMC.0000000000000372 PMID:28787280

Ekong, I., Chukwu, E., & Chukwu, M. (2020). COVID-19 Mobile Positioning Data Contact Tracing and Patient Privacy Regulations: Exploratory Search of Global Response Strategies and the Use of Digital Tools in Nigeria. *JMIR mHealth and uHealth*, *8*(4), e19139. doi:10.2196/19139 PMID:32310817

Erchul, W. P., & Schulte, A. C. (2019). Gerald Caplan's contributions to professional psychology: Conceptual underpinnings. In *Consultation in community, school, and organizational practice* (pp. 3–40). Taylor & Francis., doi:10.4324/9781315787077-1

Estcourt, L. J., Hopewell, S., Trivella, M., Hambleton, I. R, Cho, G. (2019). Regular long-term red blood cell transfusions for managing chronic chest complications in sickle cell disease. *Cochrane Database Syst Rev*. 25;2019(10):CD008360.. PMID: 31684693; PMCID: PMC6814284. doi:10.1002/14651858.CD008360.pub5

European Center for Disease Prevention and Control (ECDC). (2019). Infection prevention and control for the care of patients with 2019-nCoV in healthcare settings. Retrieved from https://www.ecdc.europa.eu/en/publications-data/infection-prevention-and-control-care-patients-2019-ncov-healthcare-settings

Evans, N., Edwards, D., Carrier, J., Elliott, M., Gillen, E., Hannigan, B., & Williams, L. (2023). Organisation of crisis services. In *Mental health crisis care for children and young people aged 5 to 25 years: the CAMH-Crisis evidence synthesis*. National Institute for Health and Care Research., doi:10.3310/BPPT3407

Eysenbach, G., & Kohler, C. (2003). What is the prevalence of health-related searches on the World Wide Web? Qualitative and quantitative analysis of search engine queries on the internet. [American Medical Informatics Association.]. *AMIA Annual Symposium Proceedings - AMIA Symposium. AMIA Symposium, 2003*, 225. PMID:14728167

Farmer, M. A. (2022, June 1). *Addressing opioid misuse in cancer pain management.* Columbia University Herbert Irving Comprehensive Cancer Center. Retrieved July 12, 2023, from https://www.cancer.columbia.edu/news/addressing-opioid-misuse-cancer- pain-management

Ferguson, E., Murray, C., & O'Carroll, R. E. (2019). Blood and organ donation: Health impact, prevalence, correlates, and interventions. *Psychology & Health*, *34*(9), 1073–1104. doi:10.1080/08870446.2019.1603385 PMID:31213077

Ferretti, L., Wymant, C., Kendall, M., Zhao, L., Nurtay, A., Abeler-Dörner, L., Parker, M., Bonsall, D., & Fraser, C. (2020). Quantifying SARS-CoV-2 transmission suggests epidemic control with digital contact tracing. *Science*, *368*(6491), eabb6936. Advance online publication. doi:10.1126/science.abb6936 PMID:32234805

Fijan, S., Frauwallner, A., Varga, L., Langerholc, T., Rogelj, I., Lorber, M., Lewis, P., & Povalej Bržan, P. (2019). Health professionals' knowledge of probiotics: An international survey. *International Journal of Environmental Research and Public Health*, *16*(17), 3128. doi:10.3390/ijerph16173128 PMID:31466273

Firstpost Staff. (April 09, 2020). *'Media usage during COVID-19 lockdown: Indian users flock to FB and WhatsApp'*. Firstpost. Retrieved from https://www.firstpost.com/health/media-usage-during-covid-19-lockdown-indian-users-flock-to-fb-and-whatsapp-general-news-sites-see-numbers-rise-8242811.html

First-Responder trauma and the opioid crisis. (2020, June). *Catching Up With COSSAP*, 1-3. https://www.cossapresources.org/Content/Documents/Articles/Final_TASC_AHP_First_Responder_Trauma.pdf

Fishbein, M., & Ajzen, I. (1975). *Belief, Attitude, Intention, and Behavior.* Wiley.

Fitzpatrick, P. J. (2023). Improving health literacy using the power of digital communications to achieve better health outcomes for patients and practitioners. *Frontiers in Digital Health*, *5*, 1264780. doi:10.3389/fdgth.2023.1264780 PMID:38046643

Ford, N., Williams, A., Renshaw, M., & Nkum, J. (2005). Communication strategy for implementing community IMCI. *Journal of Health Communication*, *10*(5), 379–401. doi:10.1080/10810730591009817 PMID:16199384

Galanis, P., Vraka, I., Fragkou, D., Bilali, A., & Kaitelidou, D. (2021). Intention of healthcare workers to accept COVID-19 vaccination and related factors: A systematic review and meta-analysis. *Asian Pacific Journal of Tropical Medicine*, *14*(12), 543. doi:10.4103/1995-7645.332808

Gale, N., & Dowswell, G. (2020). Access to healthcare for rural communities: A scoping review of relevant theories and models. *Journal of Rural Studies*, *75*, 191–201.

Gasior, M., Bond, M., & Malamut, R. (2015). Routes of abuse of prescription opioid analgesics: A review and assessment of the potential impact of abuse-deterrent formulations. *Postgraduate Medicine*, *128*(1), 85–96. doi:10.1080/00325481.2016.1120642 PMID:26566680

Geller, S. E., Koch, A. R., Garland, C. E., MacDonald, E. J., Storey, F., & Lawton, B. (2018). A global view of severe maternal morbidity: Moving beyond maternal mortality. *Reproductive Health*, *15*(S1), 98. Advance online publication. doi:10.1186/s12978-018-0527-2 PMID:29945657

Genuis, S. J., & Genuis, R. A. (2016). Preconception care: A new standard of care within maternal health services. *BioMed Research International*, *2016*, 1–30. doi:10.1155/2016/6150976 PMID:27314031

Gilbert, A. (2023, July 6). *After the addiction, opioid users struggle to get back to work.* Bloomberg Law. Retrieved February 2, 2024, from https://news.bloomberglaw.com/daily-labor-report/ after-the-addiction-opioid-users-struggle-to-get-back-to-work

Giles, M., Mc, C., Clenahan, E., & Cairns, J. M. (2004). An application of the Theory of Planned Behaviour to blood donation: The importance of self-efficacy. *Health Education Research*, *19*(4), 380–391. doi:10.1093/her/cyg063 PMID:15155590

Gipson, J. D., Koenig, M. A., & Hindin, M. J. (2008). The effects of unintended pregnancy on infant, child, and parental health: A review of the literature. *Studies in Family Planning*, *39*(1), 18–38. doi:10.1111/j.1728-4465.2008.00148.x PMID:18540521

Goverment, E. T. (2020). *'Digital India: Govt braces for robust, secure tech solutions as Aarogya Setu App opens up source code'*. ET Government.Com. Retrieved from https://government.economictimes.indiatimes.com/news/digital-india/digital-india-govt-braces-for-robust-secure-tech-solutions-as-aarogya-setu-app-opens-up-source-code/76059270

Greenberg, A. J., Haney, D., Blake, K. D., Moser, R. P., & Hesse, B. W. (2018). Differences in access to and use of electronic personal health information between rural and urban residents in the United States. *The Journal of Rural Health*, *34*(S1), s30–s38. doi:10.1111/jrh.12228 PMID:28075508

Greene, D., & King, N. (Hosts), & Noguchi, Y. (Writer). (2018, April 18). Anguished families shoulder the biggest burdens of opioid addiction [Radio broadcast]. In Morning edition. NPR.

Greenhalgh, T. (2015). Health literacy: Towards system level solutions. *British Medical Journal*, *350*(feb24 13), h1026. doi:10.1136/bmj.h1026 PMID:25712067

Grimmer-Somers, K., Johnston, K., Somers, E., Luker, J., Alemao, L. A., & Jones, D. (2010). A holistic client-centred program for vulnerable frequent hospital attenders: Cost efficiencies and changed practices. *Australian and New Zealand Journal of Public Health*, *34*(6), 609–612. doi:10.1111/j.1753-6405.2010.00616.x PMID:21134064

Gruber, J., Prinstein, M. J., Clark, L. A., Rottenberg, J., Abramowitz, J. S., Albano, A. M., Aldao, A., Borelli, J. L., Chung, T., Davila, J., Forbes, E. E., Gee, D. G., Hall, G. C. N., Hallion, L. S., Hinshaw, S. P., Hofmann, S. G., Hollon, S. D., Joormann, J., Kazdin, A. E., ... Weinstock, L. M. (2021). Mental health and clinical psychological science in the time of COVID-19: Challenges, opportunities, and a call to action. *The American Psychologist*, *76*(3), 409–426. doi:10.1037/amp0000707 PMID:32772538

GSMA. (2019). The state of mobile internet connectivity. Retrieved from https://www.gsma.com/mobilefordevelopment/wp-content/uploads/2019/07/GSMA-State-of-Mobile-Internet-Connectivity-Report-2019.pdf

Guy, A., Brown, M., Lewis, S., & Horowitz, M. (2020). The 'patient voice': Patients who experience antidepressant withdrawal symptoms are often dismissed, or misdiagnosed with relapse, or a new medical condition. *Therapeutic Advances in Psychopharmacology*, *10*, 2045125320967183. doi:10.1177/2045125320967183 PMID:33224468

Haggstrom, D. A., Lee, J. L., Dickinson, S. L., Kianersi, S., Roberts, J. L., Teal, E., Baker, L. B., & Rawl, S. M. (2019). Rural and urban differences in the adoption of new health information and medical technologies. *The Journal of Rural Health*, *35*(2), 144–154. doi:10.1111/jrh.12358 PMID:30830983

Hajela, N., Balakrish Nair, G., Ramakrishna, B. S., & Ganguly, N. K. (2014). Probiotic foods: Can their increasing use in India ameliorate the burden of chronic lifestyle disorders? *The Indian Journal of Medical Research*, *139*(1). https://www.ncbi.nlm.nih.gov/pmc/articles/PMC3994739/ PMID:24604038

Hantoushzadeh, S., Golshahi, F., Javadian, P., Khazardoost, S., Aram, S., Hashemi, S., Mirarmandehi, B., & Borna, S. (2011). Comparative efficacy of probiotic yoghurt and clindamycin in treatment of bacterial vaginosis in pregnant women: A randomized clinical trial. *The Journal of Maternal-Fetal & Neonatal Medicine*, *25*(7), 1021–1024. doi:10.3109/14767058.2011.614654 PMID:21854132

Harding, R., Salins, N., Sharan, K., & Ekstrand, M. L. (2022). Health literacy in communication, decision-making and outcomes among cancer patients, their families and clinicians in India: A multicentre cross-sectional qualitative study. *Psycho-Oncology*, *31*(3), 532–540. doi:10.1002/pon.5838 PMID:34687573

Harris, J., Clarke, I., & Riches, S. (2023). Developing'Comprehend, Cope and Connect'Training for Acute and Crisis Mental Health Services: Staff, Patient and Carer Perspectives. *Journal of Psychiatric Intensive Care*, *19*(1), 33–50. doi:10.20299/jpi.2023.004

Harsanyi, H., Cuthbert, C., & Schulte, F. (2023). The stigma surrounding opioid use as a barrier to cancer-pain management: An overview of experiences with fear, shame, and poorly controlled pain in the context of advanced cancer. *Current Oncology (Toronto, Ont.)*, *30*(6), 5835–5848. doi:10.3390/curroncol30060437 PMID:37366920

Hayran, O., & Özer, O. (2018). Organizational health literacy as a determinant of patient satisfaction. *Public Health, 163*, 20–26. doi:10.1016/j.puhe.2018.06.011 PMID:30041046

He, A., Chin, J., & Lomiguen, C. M. (2020). Benefits of probiotic yogurt consumption on maternal health and pregnancy outcomes: A systematic review. *Cureus*. Advance online publication. doi:10.7759/cureus.9408 PMID:32864237

Health, T. L. G.The Lancet Global Health. (2020). Mental health matters. *The Lancet. Global Health, 8*(11), e1352. doi:10.1016/S2214-109X(20)30432-0 PMID:33069297

Hochbaum, G., Rosenstock, I., & Kegels, S. (1952). Health belief model. United States Public Health Service, 1, 78-80.

Holmes, E. A., O'Connor, R. C., Perry, V. H., Tracey, I., Wessely, S., Arseneault, L., Ballard, C., Christensen, H., Cohen Silver, R., Everall, I., Ford, T., John, A., Kabir, T., King, K., Madan, I., Michie, S., Przybylski, A. K., Shafran, R., Sweeney, A., ... Bullmore, E. (2020). Multidisciplinary research priorities for the COVID-19 pandemic: A call for action for mental health science. *The Lancet. Psychiatry, 7*(6), 547–560. doi:10.1016/S2215-0366(20)30168-1 PMID:32304649

Housten, A. J., Gunn, C. M., Paasche-Orlow, M. K., & Basen-Engquist, K. M. (2020). Health literacy interventions in cancer: A systematic review. *Journal of Cancer Education, 36*(2), 240–252. doi:10.1007/s13187-020-01915-x PMID:33155097

Howard, D. H., Gazmararian, J., & Parker, R. (2005). The impact of low health literacy on the medical costs of Medicare managed care enrollees. *The American Journal of Medicine, 118*(4), 371–377. doi:10.1016/j.amjmed.2005.01.010 PMID:15808134

https://en.wikipedia.org/wiki/Drugs.com (Accessed: 8th May to 26th July 2023)

https://en.wikipedia.org/wiki/WebMD (Accessed: 8th May to 26th July 2023)

https://www.drugs.com/ (Accessed: 8th May to 26th July 2023)

https://www.thehoth.com/hoth-x/ (Accessed: 8th May to 26th July 2023)

https://www.webmd.com/ (Accessed: 8th May to 26th July 2023)

Huey, C. W. T., & Palaganas, J. C. (2020). What are the factors affecting resilience in health professionals? A synthesis of systematic reviews. *Medical Teacher, 42*(5), 550–560. doi:10.1080/0142159X.2020.1714020 PMID:31984844

ICMR. (2011). ICMR-DBT guidelines for evaluation of probiotics in food. *The Indian Journal of Medical Research, 134*(1). https://pubmed.ncbi.nlm.nih.gov/21808130/ PMID:21808130

Improving opioid misuse prevention literacy between older adults and health care providers [Video]. (2019, April 2). YouTube. https://www.youtube.com/watch?v=9m7NYDUlCzc&t=10s

India Medical Tourism Market. (2022, October). Retrieved September 20, 2023, from https://www.futuremarketinsights.com/reports/india-medical-tourism-market#:~:text=The%20Indian%20medical%20tourism%20industry%20is%20estimated%20to,a%20healthy%2019%25%20CAGR%20from%202022%20to%202032

India's COVID vaccination programme one of world's most successful: Govt. (2022, January 2). *Business Standard.* Retrieved March 18, 2022, from https://www.business-standard.com/article/current-affairs/india-s-COVID-vaccination-programme-one-of-world-s-most-successful-govt-122010200558_1.html

International Bar Association. (2020). Guidelines and Regulations to Provide Insights on Public Policies to Ensure Artificial Intelligence's Beneficial Use as a Professional Tool. Retrieved from https://www.ibanet.org/MediaHandler?id=f5099a33-1e70-4a32-839d-589236b7568d

Ishikawa, H., Takeuchi, T., & Yano, E. (2008). Measuring functional, communicative, and critical health literacy among diabetic patients. *Diabetes Care*, *31*(5), 874–879. doi:10.2337/dc07-1932 PMID:18299446

Ishikawa, H., & Yano, E. (2008). Patient health literacy and participation in the healthcare process. *Health Expectations*, *11*(2), 113–122. doi:10.1111/j.1369-7625.2008.00497.x PMID:18494956

Islam, M. M., & Mcrae, I. S. (2014). An inevitable wave of prescription drug monitoring programs in the context of prescription opioids: Pros, cons and tensions. *BMC Pharmacology & Toxicology*, *15*(1), 46. Advance online publication. doi:10.1186/2050-6511-15-46 PMID:25127880

Jacobs, W., Amuta, A. O., & Jeon, K. C. (2017). Health information seeking in the digital age: An analysis of health information seeking behavior among US adults. *Cogent Social Sciences*, *3*(1), 1302785. doi:10.1080/23311886.2017.1302785

Jayaweera, M., Perera, H., Gunawardana, B., & Manatunge, J. (2020). Transmission of COVID-19 virus by droplets and aerosols: A critical review on the unresolved dichotomy. *Environmental Research*, *188*, 109819. doi:10.1016/j.envres.2020.109819 PMID:32569870

Jin, X., & Han, J. (2011). *K*-Means Clustering. In C. Sammut & G. I. Webb (Eds.), *Encyclopedia of Machine Learning*. Springer., doi:10.1007/978-0-387-30164-8_425

Johns Hopkins Center for Health Security. (2020), "Modernizing and Expanding Outbreak Science to Support Better Decision Making During Public Health Crises: Lessons for COVID-19 and Beyond". https://www.centerforhealthsecurity.org/our-work/publications/modernizing-and-expanding-outbreak-science-to-support-better-decision-making-during-public-health-crises

Kabeerdoss, J., Ferdous, S., Balamurugan, R., Mechenro, J., Vidya, R., Santhanam, S., Jana, A. K., & Ramakrishna, B. S. (2013). Development of the gut microbiota in southern Indian infants from birth to 6 months: A molecular analysis. *Journal of Nutritional Science*, *3*, e2. Advance online publication. doi:10.1017/jns.2013.6 PMID:25191566

Kahn, P. J. (2020). *Digital Contact Tracing for Pandemic Response*. Johns Hopkins University Press. doi:10.1353/book.75831

Kain, E. (2011, June 29). *The war on drugs is a war on minorities and the poor*. Forbes. Retrieved August 5, 2023, from https://www.forbes.com/sites/erikkain/2011/06/28/the-war-on-drugs-is-a-war-on-minorities-and-the-poor/?sh=258062dc624c

Karina, M. (2020). How AI is helping scientists in the fight against COVID-19, from robots to predicting the future. Retrieved from https://www.geekwire.com/2020/ai-helping-scientists-fightcovid-19-robots-predicting-future/amp/

Kaunain Sheriff, M. (2021, September 10). Explained: What latest govt data reveals on COVID-19 vaccine effectiveness, preventing mortality. The Indian Express. https://indianexpress.com/article/explained/govt-data-COVID-19-vaccine-effectiveness-preventing-mortality-7499460/

Kelley, M. S., Su, D., & Britigan, D. H. (2016). Disparities in health information access: Results of a county-wide survey and implications for health communication. *Health Communication*, *31*(5), 575–582. doi:10.1080/10410236.2014.979976 PMID:26452300

Kelly, B. (2022). *In search of madness: A psychiatrist's travels through the history of mental illness*. Gill & Macmillan Ltd.

Khalesi, S., Vandelanotte, C., Thwaite, T., Russell, A. M., Dawson, D., & Williams, S. L. (2020). Awareness and attitudes of gut health, probiotics and prebiotics in Australian adults. *Journal of Dietary Supplements*, *18*(4), 418–432. doi:10.1080/19390211.2020.1783420 PMID:32588677

Koley, T. K., & Dhole, M. (2021). [*Pandemic: The Deadly Coronavirus Outbreak'*. Routledge. Newyork Ministry of Health and Family Welfare, Government of India. Retrieved from https://www.mohfw.gov.in/]. *COVID*, *19*

Krieger, C. (n.d.). *What are opioids and why are they dangerous?* Mayo Clinic. Retrieved July 13, 2023, from https://www.mayoclinic.org/diseases-conditions/prescription-drug- abuse/expert-answers/what-are-opioids/faq-20381270

Kumar, R. (2019, April). Health literacy a must to empower patients. Retrieved October 2023, from The Tribune: https://www.tribuneindia.com/news/archive/comment/health-literacy-a-must-to-empower-patients-752945

Kumar, A., & Nayar, K. R. (2021). COVID 19 and its mental health consequences. *Journal of Mental Health (Abingdon, England)*, *30*(1), 1–2. doi:10.1080/09638237.2020.1757052 PMID:32339041

Kumar, P., Kumar, M., Bedi, O., Gupta, M., Kumar, S., Jaiswal, G., Rahi, V., Yedke, N. G., Bijalwan, A., Sharma, S., & Jamwal, S. (2021). Role of vitamins and minerals as immunity boosters in COVID-19. *Inflammopharmacology*, *29*(4), 1001–1016. doi:10.1007/s10787-021-00826-7 PMID:34110533

Kunter, M., (2006). The health literacy of America's adults: Result from the 2003 National Assessment of Adult Literacy. *Education*, *6*, 1–59.

Lambert, S. D., & Loiselle, C. G. (2007). Health Information—Seeking Behavior. *Qualitative Health Research*, *17*(8), 1006–1019. doi:10.1177/1049732307305199 PMID:17928475

Lam, P., & Yang, W. (2017). A Study of the Costs and Benefits of Smart City Projects Including the Scenario of Public-Private Partnerships. *World Academy of Science, Engineering and Technology, International Journal of Civil, Environmental, Structural. Construction and Architectural Engineering*, *11*, 600–605.

Landge, R. R., & Petare, P. (2021). Study on Consumer Behaviour in COVID Pandemic with respect to OTC medicine. *International Research Journal of Humanities and Interdisciplinary Studies*, *2*(5), 104–113.

Lawrance, E. L., Thompson, R., Newberry Le Vay, J., Page, L., & Jennings, N. (2022). The impact of climate change on mental health and emotional wellbeing: A narrative review of current evidence, and its implications. *International Review of Psychiatry (Abingdon, England)*, *34*(5), 443–498. doi:10.1080/09540261.2022.2128725 PMID:36165756

Lawrence, T. G., & Panigrahi, A. K. (2017). Blood Transfusion Therapy. *The Medical Clinics of North America*, *101*(2), 431–447. doi:10.1016/j.mcna.2016.09.012 PMID:28189180

Levy, H., & Janke, A. (2016). Health literacy and access to care. *Journal of health communication*, *21*(sup1), 43-50.

Liang, X., Li, Z., Tye, K. D., Chen, Y., Luo, H., & Xiao, X. (2020). The effect of probiotic supplementation during pregnancy on the interaction network of vaginal microbiome. *Journal of Obstetrics and Gynaecology Research*, *47*(1), 103–113. doi:10.1111/jog.14434 PMID:32885568

Li, L. Q. L., & Xu, Z. (2020). Artificial intelligence distinguishes COVID-19 from community acquired pneumonia on chest CT. *Radiology*. Advance online publication. doi:10.1148/radiol.2020200905 PMID:32191588

Lindholm, S. K., & Wickström, A. (2020). 'Looping effects' related to young people's mental health: How young people transform the meaning of psychiatric concepts. *Global Studies of Childhood*, *10*(1), 26–38. doi:10.1177/2043610619890058

Liu, C., Wang, D., Liu, C., Jiang, J., Wang, X., Chen, H., Ju, X., & Zhang, X. (2020). What is the meaning of health literacy? A systematic review and qualitative synthesis. *Family Medicine and Community Health*, *8*(2), e000351. doi:10.1136/fmch-2020-000351 PMID:32414834

Local is better than national. (2017). *A Better Way*. Retrieved August 5, 2023, from https://www.betterway.network/local-is-better-than-national

Loideain, N. N. (2019). A port in the data-sharing storm: The GDPR and the Internet of things. *Journal of Cyber Policy*, *4*(2), 178–196. doi:10.1080/23738871.2019.1635176

Lotta, G., Fernandez, M., & Corrêa, M. (2021). The vulnerabilities of the Brazilian health workforce during health emergencies: Analysing personal feelings, access to resources and work dynamics during the COVID-19 pandemic. *The International Journal of Health Planning and Management*, *36*(S1), 42–57. doi:10.1002/hpm.3117 PMID:33502795

Lunt, N., & Carrera, P. (2010). Medical tourism: Assessing the evidence on treatment abroad. *Maturitas*, *66*(1), 27–32. doi:10.1016/j.maturitas.2010.01.017 PMID:20185254

Lustria, M. L. A., Smith, S. A., & Hinnant, C. C. (2011). Exploring digital divides: An examination of eHealth technology use in health information seeking, communication and personal health information management in the USA. *Health Informatics Journal*, *17*(3), 224–243. doi:10.1177/1460458211414843 PMID:21937464

M'Jamtu-Sie, N. (2003). Disseminating health information in Sierra Leone: The challenge. *Information Development*, *19*(4), 250–254. doi:10.1177/026666690301900404

Macaulay, T. (2020), "AI sent first coronavirus alert, but underestimated the danger", The Next Web, https://thenextweb. com/neural/2020/02/21/ai-sent-first-coronavirus-alert-but-underestimated-the-danger/

MacLeod, M. L. P., Kulig, J. C., Stewart, N. J., Anguish, P., Andrews, M. E., Banner, D., & Karunanayake, C. (2020). Rural women's health knowledge: Implications for healthcare delivery in rural communities. *Health & Place*, *65*, 102417.

Maconick, L., Ikhtabi, S., Broeckelmann, E., Pitman, A., Barnicot, K., Billings, J., Osborn, D., & Johnson, S. (2023). Crisis and acute mental health care for people who have been given a diagnosis of a 'personality disorder': A systematic review. *BMC Psychiatry*, *23*(1), 720. doi:10.1186/s12888-023-05119-7 PMID:37798701

Malhotra, N., & Dave, K. (2022). An assessment of competitiveness of medical tourism industry in India: A case of Delhi NCR. *International Journal of Global Business and Competitiveness*, *17*(2), 215–228. doi:10.1007/s42943-022-00060-0

Maslowsky, J., Frost, S., Hendrick, C. E., Cruz, F. O. T., & Merajver, S. D. (2016). Effects of postpartum mobile phone-based education on maternal and infant health in Ecuador. *International Journal of Gynaecology and Obstetrics: the Official Organ of the International Federation of Gynaecology and Obstetrics*, *134*(1), 93–98. doi:10.1016/j.ijgo.2015.12.008 PMID:27126905

Maternal Health Task Force. (2018, June 27). *The sustainable development goals and maternal mortality*. https://www.mhtf.org/topics/the-sustainable-development-goals-and-maternal-mortality/

Mayer, E. A., Knight, R., Mazmanian, S. K., Cryan, J. F., & Tillisch, K. (2014). Gut microbes and the brain: Paradigm shift in neuroscience. *The Journal of Neuroscience : The Official Journal of the Society for Neuroscience*, *34*(46), 15490–15496. doi:10.1523/JNEUROSCI.3299-14.2014 PMID:25392516

McCormack, L., Bann, C., Squiers, L., Berkman, N. D., Squire, C., Schillinger, D., Ohene-Frempong, J., & Hibbard, J. (2010). Measuring health literacy: A pilot study of a new skills-based instrument. *Journal of Health Communication*, *15*(sup2, S2), 51–71. doi:10.1080/10810730.2010.499987 PMID:20845193

McCray, A. T. (2005). Promoting health literacy. *Journal of the American Medical Informatics Association : JAMIA*, *12*(2), 152–163. doi:10.1197/jamia.M1687 PMID:15561782

McCurry, M. K., Avery-Desmarais, S., Schuler, M., Tyo, M., Viveiros, J., & Kauranen, B. (2022). Perceived stigma, barriers, and facilitators experienced by members of the opioid use disorder community when seeking healthcare. *Journal of Nursing Scholarship*, *55*(3), 701–710. doi:10.1111/jnu.12837 PMID:36317787

McDonald, B., & McCoy, K. D. (2019). Maternal microbiota in pregnancy and early life. *Science*, *365*(6457), 984–985. doi:10.1126/science.aay0618 PMID:31488675

McGorry, P. D., Mei, C., Chanen, A., Hodges, C., Alvarez-Jimenez, M., & Killackey, E. (2022). Designing and scaling up integrated youth mental health care. *World Psychiatry; Official Journal of the World Psychiatric Association (WPA)*, *21*(1), 61–76. doi:10.1002/wps.20938 PMID:35015367

Medical Tourism market. (2022, October). Retrieved October 15, 2023, from https://www.transparencymarketresearch.com/medical-tourism.html#:~:text=The%20global%20market%20for%20medical%20tourism%20was%20valued,US%24%2072.8%20Bn%20by%20the%20end%20of%202031

Mercadante, S. (1999). Opioid rotation for cancer pain. *Cancer*, *86*(9), 1856–1866. doi:10.1002/(SICI)1097-0142(19991101)86:9<1856::AID-CNCR30>3.0.CO;2-G PMID:10547561

Midway, S. R. (2020). Principles of effective data visualization. *Patterns (New York, N.Y.)*, *1*(9), 100141. Advance online publication. doi:10.1016/j.patter.2020.100141 PMID:33336199

Mikolajczak, C. (2015, June 1). Local initiatives or national policies: What's best for our planet? *Cafe Babel*. https://cafebabel.com/en/article/local-initiatives-or-national-policies-whats-best-for-our-planet-5ae00a0ff723b35a145e5d48/

Ministry of Education, Culture, Sports, Science and Technology (2019) *The Japanese Courses of Study Commentary for Special Educational Schools*, Kairyudo P ublication. Tokyo. (originally in Japanese).

Mirchandani, P. (2020). Health Care Supply Chains: COVID-19 Challenges and Pressing Actions. *Annals of Internal Medicine*, *173*(4), 300–301. doi:10.7326/M20-1326 PMID:32369540

Mirghafourvand, M., Homayouni Rad, A., Mohammad Alizadeh Charandabi, S., Fardiazar, Z., & Shokri, K. (2016). The effect of probiotic yogurt on constipation in pregnant women: A randomized controlled clinical trial. *Iranian Red Crescent Medical Journal*, *18*(11). Advance online publication. doi:10.5812/ircmj.39870 PMID:28203450

Mitchell, J. T. (2021). Continuum of care for disasters and catastrophes. *International Review of Psychiatry (Abingdon, England)*, *33*(8), 728–739. doi:10.1080/09540261.2022.2030678 PMID:35412427

Mithra, P., Unnikrishnan, B., Rekha, T., Nithin, K., Mohan, K., Kulkarni, V., Holla, R., & Agarwal, D. (2014). Compliance with iron-folic acid (IFA) therapy among pregnant women in an urban area of south India. *African Health Sciences*, *14*(1), 255–260. doi:10.4314/ahs.v14i1.39 PMID:26060488

Mohamed Arsaath, N., & Gheena, S. (2020). Awareness on the possible role of Ayurveda as an immunity booster in the covid19 pandemic. *International Journal of Research in Pharmaceutical Sciences*, 567-574.

Moncrieff, J., Gupta, S., & Horowitz, M. A. (2020). Barriers to stopping neuroleptic (antipsychotic) treatment in people with schizophrenia, psychosis or bipolar disorder. *Therapeutic Advances in Psychopharmacology*, *10*, 2045125320937910. doi:10.1177/2045125320937910 PMID:32670542

Montenegro, C., Dominguez, M. I., Moller, J. G., Thomas, F., & Ortiz, J. U. (2023). Moving psychiatric deinstitutionalization forward: A scoping review of barriers and facilitators. Cambridge Prisms. *Global Mental Health (Cambridge, England)*, *10*, e29. doi:10.1017/gmh.2023.18 PMID:37808271

Morant, N., Davidson, M., Wackett, J., Lamb, D., Pinfold, V., Smith, D., Johnson, S., Lloyd-Evans, B., & Osborn, D. P. (2021). Acute day units for mental health crises: A qualitative study of service user and staff views and experiences. *BMC Psychiatry*, *21*(1), 1–12. doi:10.1186/s12888-021-03140-2 PMID:33691668

Morganstein, J. C., & Ursano, R. J. (2020). Ecological disasters and mental health: Causes, consequences, and interventions. *Frontiers in Psychiatry*, *11*, 1. doi:10.3389/fpsyt.2020.00001 PMID:32116830

Moritsugu, K. P. (2013). The power of organ donation to save lives through transplantation. *Public Health Reports (Washington, D.C.)*, *128*(4), 245–246. doi:10.1177/003335491312800402 PMID:23814318

Moseley, S. (2020). 5 Steps for Secure Video Conferencing. https://highfive.com/blog/5-steps-for-secure-video-conferencing. (Access Date 12 March 2022)

Mukul. P. (May 14, 2020). *'Aarogya Setu: Who can access your data, and when?'*.The Indian Express. Retrieved from https://indianexpress.com/article/explained/coronavirus-aarogya-setu-who-all-can-access-your-data-and-when-6407175/

Murayama, T. (2016). Key Issues of Health Literacy: A Literature Review. *The Journal of East Asian Educational Research*, *2*, 83–91.

Murphy, P. W., Davis, T. C., Long, S. W., Jackson, R. H., & Decker, B. C. (1993). Rapid estimate of adult literacy in medicine (REALM): A quick reading test for patients. *Journal of Reading*, *37*(2), 124–130.

Mwangakala, H. A. (2021). Accessibility of maternal health information and its influence on maternal health preferences in rural Tanzania: A case study of Chamwino District. *South African Journal of Information Management*, *23*(1), 1–9. doi:10.4102/sajim.v23i1.1353

Naeem, S. B., Bhatti, R., & Khan, A. (2020). An exploration of how fake news is taking over social media and putting public health at risk. *Health Information and Libraries Journal*. Advance online publication. doi:10.1111/hir.12320 PMID:32657000

Nakayama, K. (2016). What is Health Literacy? Fukuda, H. & Eguchi, Y. (eds.) Health Literacy: New Key Word for Health Education. Taishukan Co. Ltd., 1-22. (originally in Japanese)

Nakayama, K. (2022) Health Literacy for Info-pro, *Information Science & Technology, 72(4),* 122-127.(originally in Japanese)

Nakayama, K., Osaka, W., Togari, T., Ishikawa, H., Yonekura, Y., Sekido, A., & Matsumoto, M. (2015). Comprehensive health literacy in Japan is lower than in Europe: A validated Japanese-language assessment of health literacy. *BMC Public Health*, *15*(505), 505. doi:10.1186/s12889-015-1835-x PMID:26001385

Nambiar, P., Silibovsky, R., & Belden, K. A. (2018). Infection in Kidney Transplantation. *Contemporary Kidney Transplantation*, *27*, 307–327. doi:10.1007/978-3-319-19617-6_22

Nankani, M. (2022, January). COVID Has Exposed the Low Health Literacy in India. We Must Up the Communication Game. Retrieved September 2023, from News18: https://www.news18.com/news/opinion/covid-has-exposed-the-low-health-literacy-in-india-we-must-up-the-communication-game-4693484.html

Naushad, V. A., Bierens, J. J., Nishan, K. P., Firjeeth, C. P., Mohammad, O. H., Maliyakkal, A. M., ChaliHadan, S., & Schreiber, M. D. (2019). A systematic review of the impact of disaster on the mental health of medical responders. *Prehospital and Disaster Medicine*, *34*(6), 632–643. doi:10.1017/S1049023X19004874 PMID:31625487

Neelima, M., Chandrashekar, B. R., Thetakala, R. K., Sai, Y., Arzu, F., & Sali, M. N. M. (2018). Rapid estimate of adult literacy in medicine and dentistry-20 and oral health status among adolescents, India: A cross-sectional study. *Journal of Education and Health Promotion*, 7. PMID:30693296

News Editorials. India: [updated 2021 Nov 27]. Available from: https://www.drishtiias.com/daily-news-editorials/nfhs-5-a-closer-look

Newton-Howes, G., & Gordon, S. (2022). The need for a rights-based approach to acute models of care. *World Psychiatry; Official Journal of the World Psychiatric Association (WPA)*, *21*(2), 240–241. doi:10.1002/wps.20965 PMID:35524606

Nguyen, H. C., Nguyen, M. H., Do, B. N., Tran, C. Q., Nguyen, T. T., Pham, K. M., Pham, L. V., Tran, K. V., Duong, T. T., Tran, T. V., Duong, T. H., Nguyen, T. T., Nguyen, Q. H., Hoang, T. M., Nguyen, K. T., Pham, T. T. M., Yang, S.-H., Chao, J. C.-J., & Duong, T. V. (2020). People with suspected COVID-19 symptoms were more likely depressed and had lower health-related quality of life: The potential benefit of health literacy. *Journal of Clinical Medicine*, *9*(4), 965. doi:10.3390/jcm9040965 PMID:32244415

Nguyen, H. T., Do, B. N., Pham, K. M., Kim, G. B., Dam, H. T. B., Nguyen, T. T., Nguyen, T. T. P., Nguyen, Y. H., Sørensen, K., Pleasant, A., & Duong, T. V. (2020). Fear of COVID-19 Scale—Associations of Its Scores with Health Literacy and Health-Related Behaviors among Medical Students. *International Journal of Environmental Research and Public Health*, *17*(11), 4164. doi:10.3390/ijerph17114164 PMID:32545240

NHP INDIA -National Health Portal. Retrieved from https://www.nhp.gov.in/

Nielsen-Bohlman, L., Panzer, A., & Kindig, D. (2004). *Health literacy: A prescription to end confusion*. National Academy Press. doi:10.17226/10883

Norman, P. A. U. L., & Conner, P. (2005). Predicting health behaviour: a social cognition approach. Predicting health behaviour, 1(478), 17-8.

Nutbeam, D. (2000). Health literacy as a public health goal: A challenge for contemporary health education and communication strategies into the 21st century. *Health Promotion International*, *15*(3), 259–267. doi:10.1093/heapro/15.3.259

Nutbeam, D. (2008). The evolving concept of health literacy. *Social Science & Medicine*, *67*(12), 2072–2078. doi:10.1016/j.socscimed.2008.09.050 PMID:18952344

O'Sullivan, K., Clark, S., McGrane, A., Rock, N., Burke, L., Boyle, N., Joksimovic, N., & Marshall, K. (2021). A qualitative study of child and adolescent mental health during the COVID-19 pandemic in Ireland. *International Journal of Environmental Research and Public Health*, *18*(3), 1062. doi:10.3390/ijerph18031062 PMID:33504101

Obeidat, S. (2020), "How Artificial Intelligence Is Helping Fight The COVID-19 Pandemic", Entrepreneur, (30 March 2020), https://www.entrepreneur.com/article/348368

Observer Research Foundation. India: [updated 2020 Jan 14]. Available from: https://www.orfonline.org/research/theres-a-need-to-end-teenage-pregnancies-in-india-its-harming-the-national-economy-60307/

OECD. (2020). Beyond containment: Health systems responses to COVID-19 in the OECD", (16 April 2020), https://www.oecd.org/coronavirus/policy-responses/beyond-containment-health-systems-responses-to-COVID -19-in-the-oecd/

Ogasawara, R., Katsumata, N., Toyooka, T., Akaishi, Y., Yokoyama, T., & Kadokura, G. (2018). Reliability of Cancer Treatment Information on the Internet: Observational Study. *JMIR Cancer*, *4*(2), e10031. doi:10.2196/10031 PMID:30559090

Oge, T., Kilic, C. H., & Kilic, G. S. (2014). Economic impact of blood transfusions: Balancing cost and benefits. *The Eurasian Journal of Medicine*, *46*(1), 47–49. doi:10.5152/eajm.2014.08 PMID:25610294

Okan, O., Bollweg, T. M., Berens, E. M., Hurrelmann, K., Bauer, U., & Schaeffer, D. (2020). Coronavirus-related health literacy: A cross-sectional study in adults during the COVID-19 infodemic in Germany. *International Journal of Environmental Research and Public Health*, *17*(15), 5503. doi:10.3390/ijerph17155503 PMID:32751484

Oliver-Williams, C., Brown, E., Devereux, S., Fairhead, C., & Holeman, I. (2017). Using mobile phones to improve vaccination uptake in 21 low-and middle-income countries: Systematic review. *JMIR mHealth and uHealth*, *5*(10), e7792. doi:10.2196/mhealth.7792 PMID:28978495

Open database: National Family Health Survey (NFHS5) certified by the Ministry of Health and Family Welfare (MoHFW), India http://rchiips.org/nfhs/data1.shtml

Open, A. I. (n.d.). ChatGPT: Improving Grammar and Statements. https://chat.openai.com/c/fccd4b4f-78bc-44f8-9f8e-734ba032ea62

Ormond, M., & Sulianti, D. (2017). More than medical tourism: Lessons from Indonesia and Malaysia on South–South intra-regional medical travel. *Current Issues in Tourism*, *20*(1), 94–110. doi:10.1080/13683500.2014.937324

Osborne, R. H., Batterham, R. W., Elsworth, G. R., Hawkins, M., & Buchbinder, R. (2013). The grounded psychometric development and initial validation of the Health Literacy Questionnaire (HLQ). *BMC Public Health*, *13*(1), 1–17. doi:10.1186/1471-2458-13-658 PMID:23855504

Otuto Amarauche, C. (2015). Assessing the awareness and knowledge on the use of probiotics by healthcare professionals in Nigeria. *Journal of Young Pharmacists : JYP*, *8*(1), 53–55. doi:10.5530/jyp.2016.1.12

Overview United States (OECD Economic Surveys). (2018, June). OECD.

Paakkari, L., & Okan, O. (2020). COVID-19: Health literacy is an underestimated problem. *The Lancet. Public Health*, *5*(5), e249–e250. doi:10.1016/S2468-2667(20)30086-4 PMID:32302535

Page, R., & Blanchard, E. (2019). Opioids and cancer pain: Patients' needs and access challenges. *Journal of Oncology Practice / American Society of Clinical Oncology*, *15*(5), 229–231. doi:10.1200/JOP.19.00081 PMID:31013181

Parker, R. M., Baker, D. W., Williams, M. V., & Nurss, J. R. (1995). The test of functional health literacy in adults: A new instrument for measuring patients' literacy skills. *Journal of General Internal Medicine*, *10*(10), 537–541. doi:10.1007/BF02640361 PMID:8576769

Patkar, A., & Berry, A. K. (2020). Awareness of COVID-19, preventive strategies for the same and factors affecting immunity in adult community dwellers with no medical background-a questionnaire based study. *International Journal of Health Sciences and Research*, *10*(7), 287–295.

Patwardhan, B., & Mashelkar, R. A. (2009). Traditional medicine-inspired approaches to drug discovery: Can Ayurveda show the way forward? *Drug Discovery Today*, *14*(15-16), 804–811. doi:10.1016/j.drudis.2009.05.009 PMID:19477288

Pavli, A., Theodoridou, M., & Maltezou, H. C. (2021). Post-COVID syndrome: Incidence, clinical spectrum, and challenges for primary healthcare professionals. *Archives of Medical Research*, *52*(6), 575–581. doi:10.1016/j.arcmed.2021.03.010 PMID:33962805

Pengput, A., & Schwartz, D. G. (2022). Telemedicine in Southeast Asia: A systematic review. *Telemedicine Journal and e-Health*, *28*(12), 1711–1733. doi:10.1089/tmj.2021.0516 PMID:35417250

Perry, E. L. (2014). Health literacy in adolescents: An integrative review. *Journal for Specialists in Pediatric Nursing*, *19*(3), 210–218. doi:10.1111/jspn.12072 PMID:24612548

Pettoello-Mantovani, M., Çullu Çokuğraş, F., Vural, M., Mestrovic, J., Nigri, L., Piazzolla, R., Giardino, I., Conoscitore, M., & Namazova-Baranova, L. (2019). Pilot study for the understanding and use of probiotics by different paediatric healthcare professionals working in different European countries. *Italian Journal of Pediatrics*, *45*(1), 57. Advance online publication. doi:10.1186/s13052-019-0648-4 PMID:31053146

Pike, E., Tillson, M., Webster, J. M., & Staton, M. (2019). A mixed-methods assessment of the impact of the opioid epidemic on first responder burnout. *Drug and Alcohol Dependence*, *205*, 107620. doi:10.1016/j.drugalcdep.2019.107620 PMID:31675545

Pilav, S., Easter, A., Silverio, S. A., De Backer, K., Sundaresh, S., Roberts, S., & Howard, L. M. (2022). Experiences of perinatal mental health care among minority ethnic women during the COVID-19 pandemic in London: A qualitative study. *International Journal of Environmental Research and Public Health*, *19*(4), 1975. doi:10.3390/ijerph19041975 PMID:35206163

Pollard, K. (2012). Medical tourism: Key facts. *Treatment Abroad*. The Foam Company (intuitionconnect.com).

Pop-Jordanova, N. (2021). Grief: Aetiology, symptoms and management. *prilozi*, 42(2), 9-18. doi:10.2478/prilozi-2021-0014

Prasad. R, Bindu Shajan Parappadan, Shelar Jyoti, Koshy Jacob; (Edited by George. P.J); The Hindu (2020); *'The Pandemic Notebook'.* Retrieved from https://www.thehindu.com/news/resources/the-hindus-e-book-on-covid-19-in-multiple-indian-languages/article31174374.ece

Prince, L. Y., Mears, S. C., Watson, J. C., & Hadden, K. B. (2019). Health Literacy Evaluation of Opioid Patient Education Materials for Orthopaedic Surgery. *Journal of Surgical Orthopaedic Advances*, *28*(3), 232–236. PMID:31675301

Qin, W., Yu, P. S., Chen, J. J., Mehta, G., & Kuo, G. M. (2015). The effect of health literacy on medication knowledge and medication discrepancy in Chinese Americans. *The Journal of Pharmacy Technology*, *31*(6), 262–269. doi:10.1177/8755122515588370 PMID:34860950

Qu, J. M., Cao, B., & Chen, R. C. (2020). 'COVID-19: The Essentials of Prevention and Treatment'. Shanghai Jiao Tong University Press, Published by Elsevier Inc.

Rade, Babic, Zoran, Milosevic & Gordana, (2012). "Web technology in health system" Acta facultatis medicae naissensis. UDC: 616-073:621.3929 (2):81-87. Doi:10.2478/v10283-012-0011-9

Radez, J., Reardon, T., Creswell, C., Lawrence, P. J., Evdoka-Burton, G., & Waite, P. (2021). Why do children and adolescents (not) seek and access professional help for their mental health problems? A systematic review of quantitative and qualitative studies. *European Child & Adolescent Psychiatry*, *30*(2), 183–211. doi:10.1007/s00787-019-01469-4 PMID:31965309

Raghuwanshi, S., Misra, S., Sharma, R., & Bisen, P. S. (2015). Indian perspective for probiotics: A review. *Indian Journal of Dairy Science*, *68*(3). https://www.researchgate.net/publication/280704426_Indian_perspective_for_probiotics_A_review

Rai, R. K., (2021). 'Impact of social media advertisements on the transmission dynamics of COVID-19 pandemic in India'. Journal of Applied Mathematics and Computing. Springer. Retrieved from: https://link.springer.com/content/pdf/10.1007/s12190-021-01507-y.pdf

Ratsika, A., Codagnone, M. C., O'Mahony, S., Stanton, C., & Cryan, J. F. (2021). Priming for life: Early life nutrition and the microbiota-gut-Brain Axis. *Nutrients*, *13*(2), 423. doi:10.3390/nu13020423 PMID:33525617

Real Stories. (2020, December 3). Centers for Disease Control and Prevention. Retrieved July 13, 2023, from https://www.cdc.gov/rxawareness/stories/index.html

Reference Manual for Male Sterilization. Family Planning Division Ministry of Health and Family Welfare Government of India. [updated October 2019]. Available from: https://nhm.gov.in/images/pdf/programmes/family-planing/guidelines/Reference_Manual_for_Male_Sterilization-NSV-Oct_2013.pdf

Research and Markets. (2023, May). Asia Pacific Medical Tourism Market 2022-2032 by specialty type (Cosmetic, cardiac, orthopedic, dental, fertility, organ transplant, Bariatric), tourism type, consumer group, tour type, and country: trend forecast and growth opportunity. Retrieved October 10, 2023, from https://www.researchandmarkets.com/reports/5681816/asia-pacific-medical-tourism-market-2022-2032-by#:~:text=Asia%20Pacific%20medical%20tourism%20market%20will%20grow%20by,growing%20lifestyle-related%20disorders%20along%20with%20the%20aging%20population

Reyes-Mota, A. R., Cerda-Molina, A. L., Mayagoitia-Novales, L., Viveros-Sandoval, M. E., & Borráz-León, J. I. (2021). Reduced cortisol response to traumatic images, self-esteem and stress levels in emergency medical technicians from the Red Cross. *Personality and Individual Differences*, *179*, 110929. doi:10.1016/j.paid.2021.110929

Ribandar, H. (2020). What COVID-19 teaches us about the way forward for digital health solutions in LMICs.? Retrieved from https://www.linkedin.com/pulse/what-covid-19-teaches-us-way-forward-digital-health-solutions-riband/?trackingId=rlxXqseQ%2BhYmY6b3Yat9kw%3D%3D

Robertson, A. (2020). Facebook will add anti-misformation posts to your News Feed if you liked fake coronavirus news", The Verge, https://www.theverge.com/2020/4/16/21223456/facebook-coronavirus-misformation-fake-news- warning-update-who.

Robin, M., Bellone, L., Belbèze, J., Kazemian, K., Radjack, R., & Corcos, M. (2023). Three-level containment model of hospitalized adolescents with borderline pathology: A holistic therapeutic perspective. *Frontiers in Psychiatry*, *14*, 1110788. doi:10.3389/fpsyt.2023.1110788 PMID:37608992

Rogers, A. H., Bakhshaie, J., Orr, M. F., Ditre, J. W., & Zvolensky, M. J. (2019). Health literacy, opioid misuse, and pain experience among adults with chronic pain. *Pain Medicine*, *21*(4), 670–676. doi:10.1093/pm/pnz062 PMID:30938818

Rosenbaum, L. (2020). The untold toll—The pandemic's effects on patients without Covid-19. *The New England Journal of Medicine, 382*(24), 2368–2371. doi:10.1056/NEJMms2009984 PMID:32302076

Rosoff, D. B., Smith, G. D., & Lohoff, F. W. (2021). Prescription opioid use and risk for major depressive disorder and anxiety and stress-related disorders. *JAMA Psychiatry, 78*(2), 151. doi:10.1001/jamapsychiatry.2020.3554 PMID:33175090

Rossaint, R., Afshari, A., & Bouillon, B. (2023). The European guideline on management of major bleeding and coagulopathy following trauma: sixth edition. Crit Care, 27, 80. doi:10.1186/s13054-023-04327-7

Rudd, R. E., & Anderson, J. E. (2006). *The Health Literacy Environment of Hospitals and Health Centers. Partners for Action: Making Your Healthcare Facility Literacy-Friendly. National Center for the study of adult learning and literacy*. NCSALL.

Rudd, R., Kirsch, I., & Yamamoto, K. (2004). *Literacy and health in America. Policy information report*. Educational Testing Service.

Rutten, N., Van der Gugten, A., Uiterwaal, C., Vlieger, A., Rijkers, G., & Van der Ent, K. (2015). Maternal use of probiotics during pregnancy and effects on their offspring's health in an unselected population. *European Journal of Pediatrics, 175*(2), 229–235. doi:10.1007/s00431-015-2618-1 PMID:26319129

Sahu, S., Hemlata, V. A., & Verma, A. (2014). Adverse events related to blood transfusion. *Indian Journal of Anaesthesia, 58*(5), 543–551. doi:10.4103/0019-5049.144650 PMID:25535415

Saluja, S. (2023, July). Enhancing health literacy: A call to action in the post-pandemic era. Retrieved October 2023, from The Times of India: https://timesofindia.indiatimes.com/blogs/voices/enhancing-health-literacy-a-call-to-action-in-the-post-pandemic-era/

Samanta, A. K., Kolte, A. P., Senani, S., Sridhar, M., & Jayapal, N. (2011). Prebiotics in ancient Indian diets. *Current Science, 101*(1).

Sameer, A. S., Khan, M. A., Nissar, S., & Banday, M. Z. (2020). Assessment of mental health and various coping strategies among general population living under imposed COVID-lockdown across world: A cross-sectional study. *Ethics, Medicine, and Public Health, 15*, 100571. doi:10.1016/j.jemep.2020.100571 PMID:32838000

Sampaio, M. L., & Bispo Júnior, J. P. (2021). Towards comprehensive mental health care: Experiences and challenges of psychosocial care in Brazil. *BMC Public Health, 21*(1), 1–12. doi:10.1186/s12889-021-11397-1 PMID:34238266

Sanchez-Comas, A., Synnes, K., & Hallberg, J. (2020). Hardware for Recognition of Human Activities: A Review of Smart Home and AAL Related Technologies. *Sensors (Basel), 20*(15), 4227. doi:10.3390/s20154227 PMID:32751345

Sanders, M. E., Merenstein, D. J., Ouwehand, A. C., Reid, G., Salminen, S., Cabana, M. D., Paraskevakos, G., & Leyer, G. (2016). Probiotic use in at-risk populations. *Journal of the American Pharmacists Association*, *56*(6), 680–686. doi:10.1016/j.japh.2016.07.001 PMID:27836128

Santana, S., Brach, C., Harris, L., Ochiai, E., Blakey, C., Bevington, F., Kleinman, D., & Pronk, N. (2021). Practice full report: Updating health literacy for healthy people 2030: Defining its importance for a new decade in public health. *Journal of Public Health Management and Practice*, *27*(6, Supplement 6), S258–S264. doi:10.1097/PHH.0000000000001324 PMID:33729194

Sarkar, A., Lehto, S. M., Harty, S., Dinan, T. G., Cryan, J. F., & Burnet, P. W. (2016). Psychobiotics and the manipulation of bacteria–gut–Brain signals. *Trends in Neurosciences*, *39*(11), 763–781. doi:10.1016/j.tins.2016.09.002 PMID:27793434

Savalescu, J., Davies, L. W., Roache, R., Davies, W., & Loebel, J. P. (Eds.). (2020). Psychiatry reborn: Biopsychosocial psychiatry in modern medicine. International Perspectives in. doi:10.1093/med/9780198789697.001.0001

Savenije, A., van Lawick, J., & Reijmers, E. (2022). *Systemic Perspectives in Mental Health, Social Work and Youth Care: A Relational Compass*. Taylor & Francis., doi:10.4324/9781003272038

Sawada, S. Health Belief Model, https://www.e-healthnet.mhlw.go.jp/information/dictionaries/exercise, (Last Accessed on 9th, October, 2023.) (originally in Japanese)

Scantlebury, A., Booth, A., & Hanley, B. (2017). Experiences, practices and barriers to accessing health information: A qualitative study. *International Journal of Medical Informatics*, *103*, 103–108. doi:10.1016/j.ijmedinf.2017.04.018 PMID:28550995

Schillinger, D., Grumbach, K., Piette, J., Wang, F., Osmond, D., Daher, C., & Bindman, A. B. (2002). Association of health literacy with diabetes outcomes. *Journal of the American Medical Association*, *288*(4), 475–482. doi:10.1001/jama.288.4.475 PMID:12132978

Schober, P., Boer, C., & Schwarte, L. A. (2018). Correlation coefficients: Appropriate use and interpretation. *Anesthesia and Analgesia*, *126*(5), 1763–1768. doi:10.1213/ANE.0000000000002864 PMID:29481436

Scott, T. (2020), "Coronavirus: Can artificial intelligence be smart enough to detect fake news?", MarketPlace, https:// www.marketplace.org/2020/02/12/coronavirus-can-artificial-intelligence-be -smart-enough-to-detect-fake-news/

Scott, E. (2023). *The One Thing We've Never Spoken about: Exposing Our Untold Mental Health Crisis*. Pantera Press.

Scott, J. T., & Thompson, D. R. (2003). Assessing the information needs of post-myocardial infarction patients: A systematic review. *Patient Education and Counseling*, *50*(2), 167–177. doi:10.1016/S0738-3991(02)00126-X PMID:12781932

Scott, R. E., & Mars, M. (2015). Telehealth in the developing world: Current status and future prospects. *Smart Homecare Technology and Telehealth*, *3*(1), 25–37. doi:10.2147/SHTT.S75184

Scott, R. E., Mars, M., & Bärnighausen, T. (2020). Virtual health interventions during the COVID-19 pandemic: A systematic review. *Journal of Medical Internet Research, 22*(12), e22796.

Security, J. (2020). Can governments track the pandemic and still protect privacy? Retrieved from https://www.justsecurity.org/69549/can-governments-track-the-pandemic-and-still-protect-privacy/

SengJ. J. B.YeamC. T.HuangW. C.TanN. C.LowL. L. (2020). Pandemic related Health literacy-A Systematic Review of literature in COVID-19, SARS and MERS pandemics. medRxiv. doi:10.1101/2020.05.07.20094227

Sentell, T., Vamos, S., & Okan, O. (2020). Interdisciplinary perspectives on health literacy research around the world: More important than ever in a time of COVID-19. *International Journal of Environmental Research and Public Health, 17*(9), 3010. doi:10.3390/ijerph17093010 PMID:32357457

Shah, P., Thornton, I., & Turrin, D. (2024). Informed Consent. In: StatPearls [Internet]. Treasure Island (FL): StatPearls Publishing; 2024 Jan-. Available from: https://www.ncbi.nlm.nih.gov/books/NBK430827/

Sharan, S. (2020). *Lockdown: India Under Siege From Corona*. Published by RosettaBooks.

Sharma, R., Gupta, S., Gupta, D., & Kushwaha, P. K. (2019). Awareness and knowledge about probiotics among college students. *Journal of Pure & Applied Microbiology, 13*(4), 2201–2208. doi:10.22207/JPAM.13.4.33

Sharma, S., & Thapa, R. (2023). Socioeconomic Factors and Their Interaction with Environmental Education and Biodiversity Conservation: Effects on Mental Health and Community Empowerment. *AI. IoT and the Fourth Industrial Revolution Review, 13*(7), 75–90.

Sharton, B. R. (2020). How Organizations Can Ramp Up Their Cybersecurity Efforts Right Now. Harvard Business Review, (May 1, 2020), https://hbr.org/2020/05/how-organizations-can-ramp-up-their-cybersecurity-efforts -right-now?ab=hero-subleft-3.

Shroff, S. (2009). Legal and ethical aspects of organ donation and transplantation. *Indian Journal of Urology, 25*(3), 348–355. doi:10.4103/0970-1591.56203 PMID:19881131

Sigurdsson, S. O., Ring, B. M., O'Reilly, K., & Silverman, K. (2012). Barriers to employment among unemployed drug users: Age predicts severity. *The American Journal of Drug and Alcohol Abuse, 38*(6), 580–587. doi:10.3109/00952990.2011.643976 PMID:22242680

Siltrakool, B. (2017). *Assessment of Community Pharmacists' Knowledge, Attitude and Practice Regarding Non-Prescription Antimicrobial Use and Resistance in Thailand* [Master's thesis]. https://www.researchgate.net/publication/322675323_Assessment_of_Community_Pharmacists%27_Knowledge_Attitude_and_Practice_Regarding_Non-Prescription_Antimicrobial_Use_and_Resistance_in_Thailand

Simpson, S. H. (2015). Creating a data analysis plan: What to consider when choosing statistics for a study. *The Canadian Journal of Hospital Pharmacy*, *68*(4), 311. doi:10.4212/cjhp.v68i4.1471 PMID:26327705

Sinaga, K. P., & Yang, M. S. (2020). Unsupervised K-means clustering algorithm. *IEEE Access : Practical Innovations, Open Solutions*, *8*, 80716–80727. doi:10.1109/ACCESS.2020.2988796

Sokey, P. P., Adjei, E., & Ankrah, E. (2018). Media use for health information dissemination to rural communities by the Ghana Health Service. *Journal of Information Science. Systems and Technology*, *2*(1), 1–18.

Soni, R., Tank, K., & Jain, N. (2018). Knowledge, attitude and practice of health professionals about probiotic use in Ahmedabad, India. *Nutrition & Food Science*, *48*(1), 125–135. doi:10.1108/NFS-02-2017-0032

Sørensen, K., Pelikan, J. M., Röthlin, F., Ganahl, K., Slonska, Z., Doyle, G., Fullam, J., Kondilis, B., Agrafiotis, D., Uiters, E., Falcon, M., Mensing, M., Tchamov, K., Broucke, S., & Brand, H. (2015). Health literacy in Europe: Comparative results of the European health literacy survey (HLS-EU). *European Journal of Public Health*, *25*(6), 1053–1058. doi:10.1093/eurpub/ckv043 PMID:25843827

Sørensen, K., Van den Broucke, S., Pelikan, J. M., Fullam, J., Doyle, G., Slonska, Z., Kondilis, B., Stoffels, V., Osborne, R. H., & Brand, H. (2013). Measuring health literacy in populations: Illuminating the design and development process of the European Health Literacy Survey Questionnaire (HLS-EU-Q). *BMC Public Health*, *13*(1), 1–10. doi:10.1186/1471-2458-13-948 PMID:24112855

Spencer, S. J., Korosi, A., Layé, S., Shukitt-Hale, B., & Barrientos, R. M. (2017). Food for thought: How nutrition impacts cognition and emotion. *npj Science of Food, 1*(1). doi:10.1038/s41538-017-0008-y

Stanghellini, G. (2023). Logics of Discovery II: Lessons from Poetry-Parataxis as a Method That Can Complement the Narrative Compulsion in Vogue in Contemporary Mental Health Care. *Brain Sciences*, *13*(10), 1368. doi:10.3390/brainsci13101368 PMID:37891737

Statista. (2023, September 26). Medical tourism worldwide as of 2023, by procedure. Retrieved from https://www.statista.com/statistics/1414337/share-medical-tourism-worldwide-by-medical-procedure/

Stigma and discrimination. (2022, June 1). National Institute on Drug Abuse. Retrieved February 2, 2024, from https://nida.nih.gov/research-topics/ stigma-discrimination

Stuart, G. S., & Ramesh, S. S. (2018). Interval female sterilization. *Obstetrics and Gynecology*, *131*(1), 117–124. doi:10.1097/AOG.0000000000002376 PMID:29215509

Stuijfzand, S., Deforges, C., Sandoz, V., Sajin, C. T., Jaques, C., Elmers, J., & Horsch, A. (2020). Psychological impact of an epidemic/pandemic on the mental health of healthcare professionals: A rapid review. *BMC Public Health*, *20*(1), 1–18. doi:10.1186/s12889-020-09322-z PMID:32787815

Suganya, R., & Hamsalakshmi, R. (2017). A study on customer buying behaviour of selected Ayurveda healthcare products. *International Journal of Advanced Research and Development, 2*(2), 13–18.

Sutton, J., & Austin, Z. (2015). Qualitative research: Data collection, analysis, and management. *The Canadian Journal of Hospital Pharmacy, 68*(3), 226. doi:10.4212/cjhp.v68i3.1456 PMID:26157184

Swartwout, B., & Luo, X. M. (2018). Implications of probiotics on the maternal-neonatal interface: Gut microbiota, Immunomodulation, and autoimmunity. *Frontiers in Immunology, 9*, 2840. Advance online publication. doi:10.3389/fimmu.2018.02840 PMID:30559747

Synthetic opioids [Leaflet]. (2020). Department of Justice.

Szwajcer, E. M., Hiddink, G. J., Koelen, M. A., & Van Woerkum, C. (2005). Nutrition-related information-seeking behaviours before and throughout the course of pregnancy: Consequences for nutrition communication. *European Journal of Clinical Nutrition, 59*(S1, Suppl. 1), s57–s65. https://www.nature.com/ejcn/journal/v59/n1s/pdf/1602175a.pdf. doi:10.1038/sj.ejcn.1602175 PMID:16052197

Tang, P. C., Newcomb, C., Gorden, S., & Kreider, N. (1997). Meeting the information needs of patients: results from a patient focus group. In *Proceedings of the AMIA Annual Fall Symposium* (p. 672). American Medical Informatics Association.

Thomsen, D. K., Holm, T., Jensen, R., Lind, M., & Pedersen, A. M. (2023). *Storying mental illness and personal recovery*. Cambridge University Press., doi:10.1017/9781108907606

Thongprayoon, C., Kaewput, W., Pattharanitima, P., Cheungpasitporn, W. (2022). Progress and Recent Advances in Solid Organ Transplantation. *J Clin Med.* 11;11(8):2112. . PMID: 35456205; PMCID: PMC9031939. doi:10.3390/jcm11082112

Thurn, L., Wide-Swensson, D., Hellgren-Wångdahl, M. (2023). Post partumblödningar med blood transfusioner har ökat [Postpartum hemorrhage and need of blood transfusions]. Lakartidningen. 15; 118:20147. Swedish. PMID: 33720382.

Tomar H., Krishnamoorthy B. (2021). Post-COVID Emergent Trends in Consumer Buying Behaviour for Pharma-OTC Sector. Advanced Journal of Graduate Research, 1-60.

Treatment for U.S. opioid addicts often inadequate, researchers say [TV program]. (2013, August 5). In News hour. PBS.

Tripp, J., & Viner, R. (2005). Sexual health, contraception, and teenage pregnancy. *BMJ (Clinical Research Ed.), 330*(7491), 590–593. doi:10.1136/bmj.330.7491.590 PMID:15761001

TRT. (2020). What is fillation? How does filyasyo process in Turkey? Retrieved from https://www.trthaber.com/haber/infografik/filyasyon-nedir-turkiyede-filyasyon-sureci-nasil-isliyor-476210.html. Posted on June 17, 2020.

Truong, M., & Fenton, S. H. (2022). Understanding the Current Landscape of Health Literacy Interventions within Health Systems. *Perspectives in Health Information Management*, *19*(Spring), 1h. PMID:35692852

Tucker, E. L., Smith, A. R., Daskin, M. S., Schapiro, H., Cottrell, S. M., Gendron, E. S., Hill-Callahan, P., Leichtman, A. B., Merion, R. M., Gill, S. J., & Maass, K. L. (2019). Life and expectations post-kidney transplant: A qualitative analysis of patient responses. *BMC Nephrology*, *20*(1), 175. doi:10.1186/s12882-019-1368-0 PMID:31096942

Turkish Ministry of Health. (2021). What is HPP Code? Retrieved from https://hayatevesigar.saglik.gov.tr/hes.html

Turner, L. (2012). Beyond medical tourism: Canadian companies marketing medical travel. *Globalization and Health*, *8*(1), 1–11. doi:10.1186/1744-8603-8-16 PMID:22703873

U.S. Congress Congressional Budget Office. (2022, September). *The opioid crisis and recent federal policy responses*. Government Publishing Office.

U.S. Department of Health and Human Services, Office of Disease Prevention and Health Promotion. (2021)Healthy People 2030, https://health.gov/healthypeople, last accessed on 24th, May, 2023.

U.S. Department of Health and Human Services. (2012) Healthy People 2020, https://wayback.archive-it.org/5774/20220413183808/https://www.healthypeople.g ov/2020/dat a-search, last accessed on 22nd, May, 2023.

Udvardy, M., Illés, Á., Gergely, L., Pinczés, L. I., Magyari, F., Simon, Z. (2023). Transfusion-Transmitted Disorders with Special Attention to Bone Marrow Transplant Patients. *Pathogens.* 1;12(7):901. . PMID: 37513748; PMCID: PMC10383292. doi:10.3390/pathogens12070901

Understanding the opioid overdose epidemic. (2023, August 8). Centers for Disease Control and Prevention. Retrieved August 17, 2023, from https://www.cdc.gov/opioids/basics/epidemic.html

UNICEF. (n.d.). *Maternal health*. https://www.unicef.org/india/what-we-do/maternal-health

United Nations Statistics Division. (2016). — *SDG indicators*. https://unstats.un.org/sdgs/report/2016/

United Nations. (2020). Digital technologies critical in facing COVID-19 pandemic? Retrieved from https://www.un.org/development/desa/en/news/policy/digital-technologies-critical-in-facing-covid-19-pandemic.html

Van den Broucke, S. (2014). Health literacy: a critical concept for public health. *Arch Public Health*, 1;72(1):10. . PMID: 24685171; PMCID: PMC3994208. doi:10.1186/2049-3258-72-10

Vannatta, K., Gartstein, M. A., Short, A., & Noll, R. B. (1998). A controlled study of peer relationships of children surviving brain tumors: Teacher, peer, and self ratings. *Journal of Pediatric Psychology*, *23*(5), 279–287. doi:10.1093/jpepsy/23.5.279 PMID:9782676

Wagner, T. (2023, March 22). *Opioid overdose: A deadly cross-roads of health literacy and patient safety*. https://www.safercaretexas.org/opioid-overdose-a-deadly-cross-roads-of- health-literacy-and-patient-safety/

Wagner, K. D., Bovet, L. J., Haynes, B., Joshua, A., & Davidson, P. J. (2016). Training law enforcement to respond to opioid overdose with naloxone: Impact on knowledge, attitudes, and interactions with community members. *Drug and Alcohol Dependence*, *165*, 22–28. doi:10.1016/j.drugalcdep.2016.05.008 PMID:27262898

Wallis, L., Blessing, P., Dalwai, M., & Shin, S. D. (2017). Integrating mHealth at point of care in low- and middle-income settings: the system perspective. *Global health action*, 10(sup3), 1327686. . doi:10.1080/16549716.2017.1327686

Wang, C., Horby, P. W., Hayden, F. G., & Gao, G. F. (2020). A novel coronavirus outbreak of global health concern. *Lancet*, *395*(10223), 470–473. doi:10.1016/S0140-6736(20)30185-9 PMID:31986257

Wang, H. Y. (2012). Value as a medical tourism driver. *Managing Service Quality*, *22*(5), 465–491. doi:10.1108/09604521211281387

Wang, L., Lin, Z. Q., & Wong, A. (2020). COVID-Net: A tailored deep convolutional neural network design for detection of COVID-19 cases from chest X-ray images. *Scientific Reports*, *10*(1), 19549. doi:10.1038/s41598-020-76550-z PMID:33177550

WangQ.Santos FerreiraD. L.NelsonS. M.SattarN.Ala-KorpelaM.LawlorD. A. (2017). Metabolic characterization of menopause: Cross-sectional and longitudinal evidence. doi:10.1101/195909

Warner, D., & Procaccino, J. D. (2004). Toward wellness: Women seeking health information. *Journal of the American Society for Information Science and Technology*, *55*(8), 709–730. doi:10.1002/asi.20016

Watson, R. (2011). Europeans with poor "health literacy" are heavy users of health services. *British Medical Journal*, *343*(nov29 4), d7741. doi:10.1136/bmj.d7741 PMID:22127773

Weiss, B. D., Mays, M. Z., Martz, W., Castro, K. M., DeWalt, D. A., Pignone, M. P., ... Hale, F. A. (2005). Quick assessment of literacy in primary care: The newest vital sign. *Annals of Family Medicine*, *3*(6), 514–522. doi:10.1370/afm.405 PMID:16338915

Whitelaw, S., Mamas, M. A., Topol, E., & Van Spall, H. (2020). Applications of digital technology in COVID-19 pandemic planning and response. *The Lancet. Digital Health*, *2*(8), e435–e440. doi:10.1016/S2589-7500(20)30142-4 PMID:32835201

WHO. (2015). *Strategies toward ending preventable maternal mortality (EPMM)*. World Health Organization. https://www.who.int/reproductivehealth/topics/maternal_perinatal/epmm/en/

WHO. (2019, September 19). *Maternal mortality*. https://www.who.int/news-room/fact-sheets/detail/maternal-mortality

Williams, P., Nicholas, D., Huntington, P., & McLean, F. (2002). Surfing for health: user evaluation of a health information website. Part one: background and literature review. *Health Information and Libraries Journal*, *19*(2), 98–108. doi:10.1046/j.1471-1842.2002.00374_2.x PMID:12389607

Williams, R., Ntontis, E., Alfadhli, K., Drury, J., & Amlôt, R. (2021). A social model of secondary stressors in relation to disasters, major incidents and conflict: Implications for practice. *International Journal of Disaster Risk Reduction*, *63*, 102436. doi:10.1016/j.ijdrr.2021.102436

Wood, S. P. (2018, June 8). *Prescription monitoring programs: Helpful or harmful?* https://www.health.harvard.edu/blog/prescription-monitoring-programs-helpful-or-harmful-2018060814001#:~:text=Good%20intentions%20aside%2C%20there%20are%20some%20unintended%20and,than%20good%2C%20including%20taking%20away%20much%20needed%20medications

World Health Organiation. (April 2020). *'Doing What Matter in Time of Stress: An Illustration Guide'*. Retrieved from https://www.who.int/publications/i/item/9789240003927?gclid=EAIaIQobChMIyPG8ueOB7wIVgjMrCh1iRQnJEAAYASAAEgJFNvD_BwE

World Health Organisation. *'Healthy at Home'*. Retrieved from https://www.who.int/campaigns/connecting-the-world-to-combat-coronavirus/healthyathome#:~:text=The%20COVID%2D19%20pandemic%20means,during%20this%20period%20of%20confinement

World Health Organization. (2022). *World mental health report: transforming mental health for all.*

Wynia, M. K., & Osborn, C. Y. (2010). Health literacy and communication quality in health care organizations. *Journal of health communication*, 15 Suppl 2(Suppl 2), pp.102–115.

Yennurajalingam, S., Arthur, J., Reddy, S., Edwards, T., Lu, Z., Rozman de Moraes, A., Wilson, S. M., Erdogan, E., Joy, M. P., Ethridge, S. D., Kuriakose, L., Malik, J. S., Najera, J. M., Rashid, S., Qian, Y., Kubiak, M. J., Nguyen, K., PharmD, Wu, J., ... Bruera, E. (2021). Frequency of and factors associated with nonmedical opioid use behavior among patients with cancer receiving opioids for cancer pain. *JAMA Oncology*, *7*(3), 404–411. doi:10.1001/jamaoncol.2020.6789 PMID:33410866

Yilmaz-Ersan, L., Ozcan, T., & Akpinar-Bayizit, A. (2020). Assessment of socio-demographic factors, health status and the knowledge on probiotic dairy products. *Food Science and Human Wellness*, *9*(3), 272–279. doi:10.1016/j.fshw.2020.05.004

Zhang, J. K., & Xu, W. (n.d.). Web Service-based Healthcare Information System (WSHIS): A Case Study for System Interoperability Concern in Healthcare Field. *2006 International Conference on Biomedical and Pharmaceutical Engineering*, Singapore, 2006, pp. 588-594.

Zhao, X., Fan, J., Basnyat, I., & Hu, B. (2020). Online health information seeking using "# COVID-19 patient seeking help" on Weibo in Wuhan, China: Descriptive study. *Journal of Medical Internet Research*, *22*(10), e22910. doi:10.2196/22910 PMID:33001838

Zhu, N., Zhang, D., Wang, W., Li, X., Yang, B., Song, J., Zhao, X., Huang, B., Shi, W., Lu, R., Niu, P., Zhan, F., Ma, X., Wang, D., Xu, W., Wu, G., Gao, G. F., & Tan, W. (2020). A Novel Coronavirus from Patients with Pneumonia in China, 2019. *The New England Journal of Medicine*, *382*(8), 727–733. doi:10.1056/NEJMoa2001017 PMID:31978945

Zintel, S., Flock, C., Arbogast, A. L., Forster, A., von Wagner, C., & Sieverding, M. (2022). Gender differences in the intention to get vaccinated against COVID-19: A systematic review and meta-analysis. *Journal of Public Health*, •••, 1–25. PMID:35018277

About the Contributors

Vassilios Papalois is Professor of transplantation surgery and consultant transplant and general surgeon at Hammersmith Hospital. He leads a Transplant Centre of Excellence focusing on high risk and extended criteria kidney and pancreas transplantation. Professor Papalois was trained in general and transplant surgery at St Mary's Hospital and in the department of surgery at the University of Minnesota (post-PhD fellowship and clinical fellowship) which is one of the biggest transplant programmes in the world and has led in the field of transplantation for the last 50 years. Professor Papalois is clinical lead for medico-legal issues at Imperial College Healthcare NHS Trust, chairs the Ethics Committee of the Avon and Somerset Constabulary and he is a member of the Research Ethics Committee of the UK Ministry of Defence. He is the Secretary General of the European Union of Medical Specialists (UEMS), the Secretary General of the European Society of Organ Transplantation (ESOT), a member of the Executive Board of the Association of Surgeons of Great Britain and Ireland (ASGBI), a member of Council of the British Transplantation Society (BTS) and the European Society of Surgery (ESS). Professor Papalois organises a series of advanced international courses annually on transplant training, clinical ethics and health policy and has given more than 100 lectures in international forums as an invited speaker. He has been awarded a Bronze National Award for Clinical Excellence by the UK Department of Health, a Senior Clinical Investigator Award by the European Society for Organ Transplantation and a Teaching Excellence Award by Imperial College London.

Kyriaki-Barbara Papalois completed her BSc in Biomedical Sciences at Queen Mary University of London and has undertaken research projects in the Blizard Institute and Barts Cancer Institute. She completed her medical training at Barts and the London School of Medicine and Dentistry and is currently working as an Academic Foundation doctor in the Royal Berkshire Hospital in Thames Valley Oxford. Dr Papalois is hoping to train in Obstetrics and Gynaecology and has held multiple leadership positions in regional and national organisations including the Association of Surgeons of Great Britain and Ireland (ASGBI), the Moynihan

Academy (MA), Institute of Medical Ethics (IME), British Undergraduate Society of Obstetrics and Gynaecology (BUSOG) as the Mentorship Coordinator and Thames Valley BUSOG representative.

***

Nidhi Arora is a technophile and a fervent scholar with deep expertise in information technology. She has been a dedicated enthusiast in exploring fundamentals of high-end technologies and has written many research papers in National and International journals

Poonam Arora has rich and vivid experience of more than 18 years in imparting knowledge in the field of Data Sciences, Quantitative Techniques, Research, Analytical Skill Building, and HR. She is a research enthusiast and an active researcher who has more than 50 publications to her credit. She has been the recipient of numerous academic achievement awards for her contribution to research in management. She is a passionate number cruncher and is inclined towards innovating ways to analyze data and apply the knowledge in research surveys. She is an active member of data analytics communities and is associated with editorial advisory boards in numerous national and international peer-reviewed journals and publications. She is currently associated as an Associate Professor with St. Kabir Institute of Professional Studies, Ahmedabad.

Susmita Chakrabarty is a lPhD Scholar (Corresponding Author) Centurion University of Technology and Management, Bhubaneswar-752050, India received MSc degree in Medical Laboratory Technology at CUTM, Odisha, India, in 2019. She is currently pursuing a Ph.D. in Applied and Clinical Microbiology. She had been served as an Assistant Professor, Central Laboratory and OPD in-charge in Department of Medical Laboratory Technology and Center for Medical Diagnostics at CUTM, Odisha, India from 2020-2022 and currently working as an Assistant Professor at DRIEMS School of Paramedical, Tangi, Cuttack, Odisha Since 2023. She has 4 years of Clinical along with 3.6 years of teaching, training, and skill experience. Her research and skill areas include Clinical Microbiology, Pathology and Hematology and Clinical Biochemistry development. She has 15+ numbers of publications in SCIE, SCOPUS, and UGC-Care indexed Journals, Conferences, and Books. She can be contacted at email: susmitachakrabarty566@gmail.com

Lakshmi D is presently designated as a Senior Associate Professor in the School of Computing Science and Engineering (SCSE) and assistant Director, at the Centre for Innovation in Teaching & Learning (CITL) at VIT Bhopal. From 2016 to 2021

served as an Educational Research Officer, at Vishnu Educational Development and Innovation Centre (VEDIC) Shri Vishnu Educational Society, Hyderabad She has 26 years of teaching experience. She has addressed innumerable guest lectures, acted as a session chair, and was invited as a keynote speaker at several international conferences. She has conducted FDPs that cover approximately ~1,00,000 plus faculty members including JNTU, TEQIP, SERB, SWAYAM, DST, AICTE, MHRD, ATAL, ISTE, Madhya Pradesh Government-sponsored, and self-financed workshops across India as well as Misami University, Philipines on Artificial Intelligence in Education: The Future and Futuristic Perspectives both theory and practical sessions. The other titles such as Modern Tools and Software in Teaching Learning Practices, Outcome Based Education, Scientific Educational Practices, Flipped Learning, Blended Learning, Activity Based Learning, Marching towards Quality and Excellence in Higher Educational Institutions, NEP 2022, Emotional Intelligence, Python Essential, Data Analytics, IoT, Machine Learning, Deep Learning, Cyber Security, AR/VR in Medicine, Architecture and Military Applications Instructional Strategies, Assessment techniques, Research Writing, etc. She has 20 international conference presentations, and 32 international journal papers inclusive of SCOPUS & SCI (cumulative impact factor 45). A total of 20 SCOPUS-indexed book chapters. A total of 24 patents are in various states and 18 patents have been granted at both national and international levels. She was appointed as an external examiner for several Ph.D candidates at reputed universities. Under her supervision, one scholar has completed a Ph.D. at Annamalai University. One scholar is pursuing right now at VIT Bhopal University. She has won two Best Paper awards at international conferences, one at the IEEE conference and another one at EAMMIS 2021 (First European, Asian, Middle Eastern North African Conference on Management & Information Systems). She received two awards in the year 2022 on the eve of Teacher's Day 1. Kamal Sharma Award of Academic Excellence - 2022 from Lexicon Group of Institutions, Pune for the Engaged Pedagogies. from the virtual ceremony. 2. Bharat Academic Excellence "UttamaAdyapika" Award from Braino Vision. She published a book on "Theory of Computation" in 2003, "Leading Education in the Age of Disruption" in 2021, and "Smart Cities: Disruptive Technologies Driving the Force", in 2023. She acted as a SPOC to both KAVACH and the Smart India Hackathon in the last three editions. She has created 15 hours of the high-quality online course "Python Essentials" at VITyarthi Online Learning Platform. She has 5 SCOPUS Indexed book edits with three CRS Press, Taylor, and Francis, three IGI Global, and two IEEE Rivers.

Manali Datta is Associate Prof. at Amity University Rajasthan. Having done her Postgraduate studies from Jamia Millia Islamia and Ph.D. from IIT Roorkee, she specializes in structural proteomics and diagnostic development..She has many publications to her credit with citations equal to 256 and H-Index of 9. She has handled projects pertaining to recombinant organisms and diagnostic development. She has 7 patents applied in IPO. Currently, she was involved in development of biosensor capable of detecting kidney malfunction in the preliminary stages. She is actively working on many projects encompassing bioinformatics with wet-lab research in the field of diagnostic development.

Soumya Sankar Ghosh is an Experienced Linguist by profession with almost 10 years of research and job experience in both the field of academics and the IT industry. Skilled in Discourse Analysis, Data Analysis, Semantics, Text-to-Speech, and Pragmatics. In December 2019, I obtained my PhD in Linguistics from Jadavpur University, Kolkata. Currently working as, an Assistant Professor, at VIT Bhopal University Madhya Pradesh, India.

Geeta Khanwani is a PhD Research Scholar and keen to explore more in her field of excellence so that she could contribute more and more relevant information as a budding researcher.

Rita Komalasari is a lecturer at YARSI University. Her current work is focused on Navigating Mental Health Crises: Understanding Pivotal Phases, Health Campaigns, and Community Resilience for Recovery and Reform. Please direct correspondence to rita.komalasari161@gmail.com.

Sunil Kumar, currently an Associate Professor at Faculty of Management Sciences, Shoolini University, possesses extensive academic and research experience. With a background in Business Administration, His research endeavors span multiple domains, including human resource management, e-training, and the application of artificial intelligence in business. His prolific contributions are evidenced by numerous research papers, book chapters, copyrights, and patents. Dr. Kumar has a knack for teaching with expertise in subjects like HR Analytics, Talent Management, Industrial Psychology, and more. He has also successfully guided PhD students and actively contributes to various academic administrative roles.

Monali Mishra is an Associate Professor at Centurion University of Technology and Management, Bhubaneswar-752050, India received MSc degree in Medical Laboratory Technology at CUTM, Odisha, India, in 2019. She is currently pursuing a Ph.D. in Applied and Clinical Microbiology. She had been served as an Assistant Professor, Central Laboratory and OPD in-charge in Department of Medical Laboratory Technology and Center for Medical Diagnostics at CUTM, Odisha, India from 2020-2022 and currently working as an Assistant Professor at DRIEMS School of

Paramedical, Tangi, Cuttack, Odisha Since 2023. She has 4 years of Clinical along with 3.6 years of teaching, training, and skill experience. Her research and skill areas include Clinical Microbiology, Pathology and Hematology and Clinical Biochemistry development. She has 15+ numbers of publications in SCIE, SCOPUS, and UGC-Care indexed Journals, Conferences, and Books. She can be contacted at email: susmitachakrabarty566@gmail.com

Minaxi Parmar, currently working as Assistant Professor at the Central University of Gujarat, Gandhinagar. She holds a PhD degree from Hemchandracharya North Gujarat University, Patan and MLIS degree from Gujarat Vidyapith. Dr. Parmar has teaching experience from the Library and Information Science Department, C U Shah University, Wadhavan, Surendranagar and seven years' experience in librarian positions in various colleges including Ahmedabad Institute of Medical Science, Ahmedabad Institute of Nursing Science Institutions. She teaches Knowledge Organization, Web Technologies, Information Storage and REtrieval, Scientometrics, etc.

Nishi Patel has completed MBA in Healthcare management and worked as intern in various hospitals at national level.

Paturi Jagadeeswar Reddy has completed MBA in Healthcare management and worked as intern in various hospitals at national level.

Shreya Shetye is a Student and Researcher.

Suyesha Singh is an Assistant Professor at the Department of Psychology, School of Humanities and Social Sciences, Manipal University Jaipur, India. She has an experience of over a decade in teaching, research and life skills training. Her research interests include Clinical Psychology, Health Psychology, Psychotherapy and Applied Psychology. She has authored several research papers and articles.

Subir Sinha is an Indian scholar and a Lecture (State Aided College Teacher) in the Department of Journalism and Mass communication of Dum Dum Motijheel College (Affiliated under West Bengal State University). He was formerly attached with the Department of Journalism, Surendranath College (Affiliated under University of Calcutta) and Vijaygarh Jyotish Ray College (Affiliated under University of Calcutta) as a Guest Faculty. He was also remained attached with Indra Gandhi National Open University (IGNOU) under convergence scheme with Dum Dum Motijheel College as an Academic Counsellor of PGJMC for a short period. Among his interest- impact of media, role of new media, social media, communication and development communication are significant. He presented various papers in

National and International seminars and conference and published various articles in various books and journals.

Index

R

S

T

V

W

www.ingramcontent.com/pod-product-compliance
Lightning Source LLC
LaVergne TN
LVHW080637011026
849160LV00014B/1246
* 9 7 8 1 7 9 9 8 9 6 5 3 1 *